Essentials of Ophthalmology

Essentials of Ophthalmology

Editor: Slade Decker

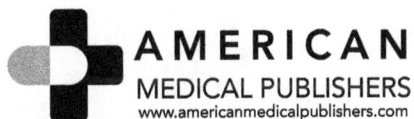

AMERICAN
MEDICAL PUBLISHERS
www.americanmedicalpublishers.com

AMERICAN
MEDICAL PUBLISHERS
www.americanmedicalpublishers.com

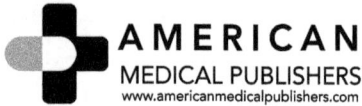

Cataloging-in-Publication Data

Essentials of ophthalmology / edited by Slade Decker.
   p. cm.
Includes bibliographical references and index.
ISBN 978-1-63927-379-9
1. Ophthalmology. 2. Eye--Diseases. 3. Medicine. I. Decker, Slade.
RE48 .E44 2022
617.7--dc23

American Medical Publishers,
41 Flatbush Avenue,
1st Floor, New York,
NY 11217, USA

ISBN 978-1-63927-379-9 (Hardback)

Contents

Preface

This book was inspired by the evolution of our times; to answer the curiosity of inquisitive minds. Many developments have occurred across the globe in the recent past which has transformed the progress in the field.

Ophthalmology is a field that falls under the branch of medicine and surgery. It is concerned with the diagnosis and treatment of eye disorders. Some of the common eye diseases are cataract, glaucoma, macular degeneration, strabismus, proptosis, uveitis, diabetic retinopathy, etc. Some of its common symptoms are blurred and double vision, faded colors, trouble with bright lights, seeing bright floating spots, etc. Eye disorders are diagnosed through specialized eye tests and medical examinations such as ocular tonometry, viscal acuity, ultrasonography, etc. This field makes use of medications, laser therapies and advanced surgeries for the treatment of these eye diseases. Ophthalmology involves certain specialties to deal with certain eye diseases. Some of them are anterior segment surgery, vitreo-retinal surgery, refractive surgery, oculoplastics and orbit surgery. Ophthalmology is an upcoming field of medicine that has undergone rapid developments over the past few decades. This book is compiled in such a manner that it will provide in-depth knowledge about the theory and practice of this field. This book will prove to be immensely beneficial to students and researchers in this field.

This book was developed from a mere concept to drafts to chapters and finally compiled together as a complete text to benefit the readers across all nations. To ensure the quality of the content we instilled two significant steps in our procedure. The first was to appoint an editorial team that would verify the data and statistics provided in the book and also select the most appropriate and valuable contributions from the plentiful contributions we received from authors worldwide. The next step was to appoint an expert of the topic as the Editor-in-Chief, who would head the project and finally make the necessary amendments and modifications to make the text reader-friendly. I was then commissioned to examine all the material to present the topics in the most comprehensible and productive format.

I would like to take this opportunity to thank all the contributing authors who were supportive enough to contribute their time and knowledge to this project. I also wish to convey my regards to my family who have been extremely supportive during the entire project.

Editor

Different patterns of myopia prevalence and progression between internal migrant and local resident school children in Shanghai, China: a 2-year cohort study

Yingyan Ma[1,2†], Senlin Lin[1,2,3†], Jianfeng Zhu[1,2], Xun Xu[1,2], Lina Lu[1,2], Rong Zhao[4], Huijuan Zhao[5], Qiangqiang Li[5], Zhiyuan Hou[3*], Xiangui He[1,2*] and Haidong Zou[1,2*]

Abstract

Background: In 2010, there were ~ 36 million migrant children under 18 y old in China. This study compared patterns of myopia prevalence and progression between migrant and resident children.

Methods: Eight hundred forty-two migrant children from 2 migrant schools and 1081 from 2 local schools in Baoshan District, Shanghai, were randomly chosen. Baseline measurements were taken on children in grades one through four, and children in grades one and two were followed for 2 y. The children underwent comprehensive ophthalmic examinations, including cycloplegic refraction and axial length. The average time per week spent on homework and outdoor activities were investigated.

Results: Migrant children in grades one and two showed a lower myopia prevalence than resident children; however, from grades three to four, the prevalence accelerated and exceeded that of residents. In the follow-up, the myopia incidence did not significantly change from grades one to two in resident children but was significantly higher in grade two in migrant children. Correspondingly, for migrant children, increased progression of refraction and axial length was observed; however, it decreased in resident children. The average time spent on homework increased from grades two to three in parallel with the acceleration of myopia prevalence for migrant children; however, the time spent outdoors did not correspondingly change.

Conclusion: The patterns of myopia prevalence and progression are different between migrant and non-migrant children. The acceleration of myopia in migrant children might be a result of a change in their environment, such as intensive education pressure.

Keywords: Migrant children, Myopia, Progression, Spherical equivalent refraction, Axial length

* Correspondence: zouhaidong@hotmail.com; xianhezi@163.com; zyhou@fudan.edu.cn
†Equal contributors
[1]Department of Preventative Ophthalmology, Shanghai Eye Disease Prevention and Treatment Center, Shanghai Eye Hospital, No. 380 Kangding Road, Shanghai, China
[2]Department of Ophthalmology, Shanghai General Hospital, Shanghai Jiao Tong University, No.100, Haining Road, Shanghai, China
[3]School of Public Health, National Key Laboratory of Health Technology Assessment (National Health and Family Planning Commission), Fudan University, Shanghai, China
Full list of author information is available at the end of the article

Background

With rapid economic development and urbanization during the past few decades in China, a large number of adults and their children have moved from rural to urban areas, constituting 273.95 million internal migrants by 2014 [1, 2]. The 2010 National Population Census revealed ~ 36 million migrant children in China, comprising 12.5% of the population under 18 y old [3]. In addition to the discrepancy in educational opportunities, migrant children are ineligible for other urban social welfare programs, such as public health care and financial assistance [4]. The restrictions on access to urban social welfare, in addition to relatively lower economic and sanitary conditions, make migrant children more vulnerable than urban residents to diseases [1, 5, 6]. Although many studies have focused on the mental health, nutritional problems, vaccination coverage, and communicable diseases of these children [1, 5, 6], very few have been conducted in China on their ocular health [7, 8].

The prevalence of myopia is especially high in children of East-Asian ethnicity [9]. Among 15-y-old children, the prevalence is highest in Singapore (86.2%), followed by Taiwan (80%), Hong Kong (78.2%), and mainland China (59%) [9]. In general, children from urban areas demonstrated an obviously higher prevalence for myopia than those from rural settings [9–11]. In mainland China's Shunyi District, a rural area, myopia prevalence in 15-y-olds was 36.7% for boys and 55% for girls, and was 73.4% for boys and 83.2% for girls in Guanzhou, an urban city [12, 13]. Migrants comprise a special group of children that are usually born in rural areas, but move with their parents to live and study in urban cities, providing a natural condition by which to explore the influence of environmental changes on myopia within the same group of children. Whether their myopia prevalence and progression are as high as that of urban children or are comparatively similar to those of rural children is not clear.

There have been only two cross-sectional studies on myopia prevalence among migrant children in China. One study by He et al. [7] reported that uncorrected refractive error, especially myopia, was the major cause of visual impairment in migrant children. Another study reported that the prevalence of myopia in primary school was 30.3% in migrant children, lower than that in resident children (33.9%), suggesting a protective effect of migration [8]. Nevertheless, the prevalence of myopia changed rapidly as grade level increased, especially during the primary school years; therefore, the cross-sectional research cannot capture the progression of myopia, and cannot identify whether myopia incidence and progression are different between migrants and residents. Longitudinal studies are necessary to understand the patterns of myopia incidence and progression between migrant and resident children.

To determine myopia problems in migrant children in urban China, the present study, through a follow-up of primary school students in both migrant and local schools for 2 y, compared changes in the patterns of refraction and refractive components between the internal migrant children and their local resident counterparts. This study will also provide valuable suggestions for alleviating the disease burden of myopia in this normally fragile population.

Methods

Study settings and participants

Shanghai, one of the most developed regions in China, was the site for our study. According to *Shanghai Statistical Yearbook*, the number of internal migrants had increased dramatically from 3.87 million in 2000 to 11.22 million in 2010, accounting for nearly one-half of the total population of this city [14]. Children of these migrants also accounted for ~ 46.2% of all children in Shanghai in 2010 [15]. Baoshan District, located north of Shanghai, was one of the largest migrant population import areas [16]. In 2010, the average gross domestic product per capita was 54,657 RMB in Baoshan District, lower than that in Shanghai (76,074 RMB) [14, 16].

The increasing migrant population has imposed great pressure on the local urban education system, and as a result, any migrant children without a permanent registered urban residence (Hukou) do not have access to normal public schools. Consequently, most migrant children are enrolled in private schools, which were specifically established for migrants (hereinafter refer to "migrant schools"), to meet the increasing educational demands; however, with much less support from government, those migrant schools were usually without proper equipment and could employ only low-quality teachers [17, 18]. In the present study, two private primary schools, established specifically for internal migrant children and two public primary schools mainly for local resident children (hereinafter refer to "local schools"), were randomly selected in Baoshan District, and children in grades one to four from these schools were included in the study. Grade five students were not included in the study because of the extremely low participation rate most likely from intensive study pressure on the students to enter junior high school. Our study chose the longitudinal research design and followed the students for 2 y, with the first visits from May 2010 to April 2011 and the second visits from May 2012 to April 2013. The order by which each of the four schools was examined was the same during the first and second visits to ensure a 2-y gap between visits to each school. Figure 1 displays the study design. Considering the length of time spent in primary school in Shanghai (five grades), only children from grades one to two were

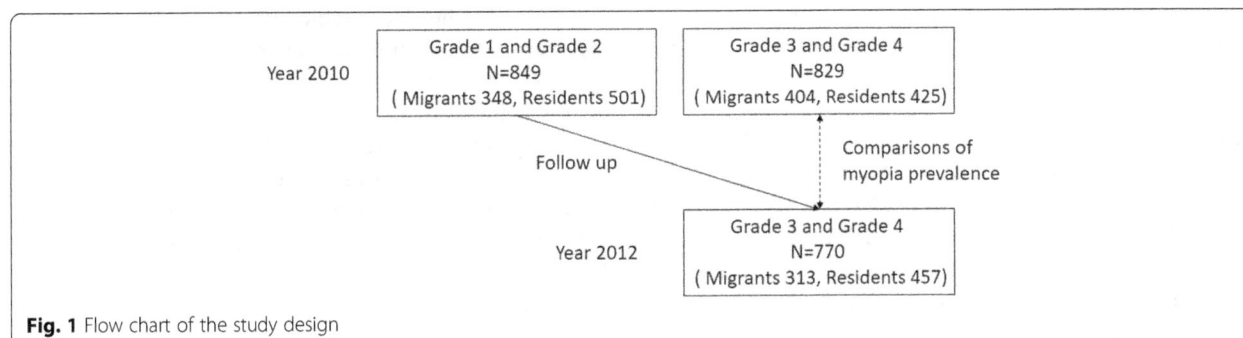

Fig. 1 Flow chart of the study design

chosen and followed for 2 y because those in grades three and four graduated after 2 y. The cluster random sampling technique was used for selecting the students. In the 2010 baseline measurements, 1923 students from grades one through four from four schools were included. Children with severe ocular diseases other than refractive error, such as congenital cataract, and children who would not cooperate with the examinations were excluded from the study.

Examinations

A research group consisting of one ophthalmologist, five optometrists, and two public health doctors was involved in the examinations performed in the schools. Before the formal examinations, members of the research group were trained according to exact protocols and were tested for eligibility of their specific examination item. Children underwent tests for visual acuity (uncorrected) (Standard Logarithmic Visual Acuity E Chart, 5 m), slit lamp examinations, measurements of intraocular pressure by noncontact tonometer, tests for cycloplegia, tests for cycloplegic autorefraction, measurements of corneal curvature radius (CR) using the KR-8800 table-mounted autorefractor (Topcon, Tokyo, Japan), measurements of axial length (AL) using an IOLMaster (v. 5.02, Carl Zeiss Meditec, Oberkochen, Germany), and tests for best corrected visual acuity. Cycloplegia was induced by administering 1 drop 0.5% tropicamide every 5 min and repeating five times. Pupil size and light reflex were examined 20 min after the last drop of tropicamide, and if the pupil dilated ≥6 mm and light reflex was absent, cycloplegia was deemed complete. The average reading of three consecutive measurements of refraction and AL were calculated for data analyses. The ophthalmologist examined children under a slit lamp and determined whether a child was suitable for cycloplegia. The optometrists manipulated the measurement for intraocular pressure, autorefraction, AL, and CR. Any children with uncorrected visual acuity lower than 20/25 in either eye were given subjective optometry to obtain the best corrected visual acuity.

To explore the reason for the changes in the patterns of myopia prevalence with school grade between migrant and resident children, we did a quick assessment in 2010 using questionnaires on the time the children spent on homework and outdoor activities. The questionnaires were distributed to students to record the times for these activities over the previous week with the help of their parents.

Statistical analyses

We used Epidata 3.1 to create a database for recording all measurements. All data were independently entered twice by two research assistants, and all discrepancies were adjudicated. Statistical analyses were conducted using SAS v. 9.3 (SAS Institute, Cary, NC, USA).

Spherical equivalent refraction (SE) was calculated as spherical diopters + 0.5* cylinder diopters. Myopia is defined as SE ≤ – 0.5 diopters (D) in the right eye. Because the right eye is usually largely correlated with the left eye, measurements of the right eye were included in the analyses. The incidence of myopia was defined as not myopic at baseline (2010) and myopic 2 y later in 2012. The progress of SE was calculated as the student's SE in 2010 minus his/her SE in 2012. A positive value reflected progression into a more myopic refraction. Similarly, the progress of AL was calculated as the student's AL in 2012 minus his/her AL in 2010, and the larger the AL value, the higher the myopic refraction.

Chi-squared and t-tests were applied for comparing basic characteristics, myopia prevalence, and refractive status between migrant and resident children at baseline (2010). Multivariate logistic regressions with and without interaction terms were performed to explore the potential risk factors for a 2-y myopia incidence. The first model comprised the main effects of the independent variables, while the second comprised the additional interaction effects between migration and grade. Furthermore, to analyze changes in refractive status, we applied a linear regression to two continuous indicators—2-y SE progression and 2-y AL increase—as dependent variables. Just as in the logistic regression, two models with and without interaction terms were applied for each indicator, respectively. Statistical significance was defined as $p < .05$ (two tailed).

Results

Inclusion of students in the baseline and follow-up

There were 842 students from grades one through four in the two migrant schools, and 1081 students from grades one through four in the two local schools for which baseline data were to be compiled. In the baseline analyses, after excluding those without a written informed consent, those who were uncooperative with the examinations, and those who suffered from severe ocular diseases other than refractive error, 752 (89.3%) children from migrant schools and 926 (85.7%) from local schools were included. Among the 849 (348 for migrants and 501 for residents) students in grades one and two included in the baseline data, 313 (89.9%) migrant students with a mean age of 7.89 y (SD = 0.88) and 457 (91.2%) students of local schools with a mean age of 7.54 y (SD = 0.75) were followed for 2 y, corresponding to the students in grades three and four in 2012. The average followup time for the current population was ~ 24 months.

Prevalence of myopia between 752 children from the migrant schools and 926 children from local schools in the baseline

In the baseline, the myopia prevalence changed from grades one through four between the migrant and resident children. For children in grade one, the prevalence of myopia was similar between the two populations (7.42% for residents and 8.15% for migrants, $P = .78$). For the children from local schools, the myopia prevalence increased steadily from grades one through four; however, the migrant children showed an accelerated prevalence after grade two, resulting in a prevalence of myopia higher than that in resident children by grade four (Fig. 2a).

Comparison of the 2-y myopia incidence, progression, and axial length progression among 313 migrant children and 457 children from local schools who were followed

For those included in the 2-y cohort, in the baseline, the percentage of males was higher in migrant children, and the refractive status was more myopic for parents of children from local schools, while the refractive status and components were not statistically different between the two populations (Table 1). During the 2-y follow-up, the incidence of myopia did not change significantly from grades one (28.2%) to two (26.4%) for the resident children ($P = .6786$); however, the incidence of myopia in grade one migrant children (32.7%) was less than that in grade two migrant children (42.6%) ($P = .0828$, Fig. 3a). Accordingly, increased progression of refraction and axial length toward myopia were observed in migrant children from grades one to two ($p = .0012$ and $p = 0.2211$, respectively), and the progressions decreased in resident children as grades increased ($p = .4471$ and $p = .0026$, respectively) (Figs. 3b, c).

Factors associated with myopia incidence and progression of SE and AL

Logistic regression of myopia incidence is listed in Table 2. For local school children, the incidence of myopia was not significantly associated with grade level (aOR = 0.780, $p = .4048$, model 2); however, for migrant children, students in grade two showed a significantly higher incidence of myopia than those in grade one (aOR$_{interaction}$ = 2.525, $p = .033$) (Table 2, model 2). This pattern change was further confirmed by the changes in SE and AL in the migrants and the children in local schools (Table 3). For the migrant children, the students in grade two showed an increased change of SE compared with those in grade one over 2 y ($p = .0016$). For the children of local schools, the students in grade two showed a decrease in the change in axial length elongation compared with the students in grade one ($p < .001$); however, for the migrant children, the students in grade two showed no significant changes in

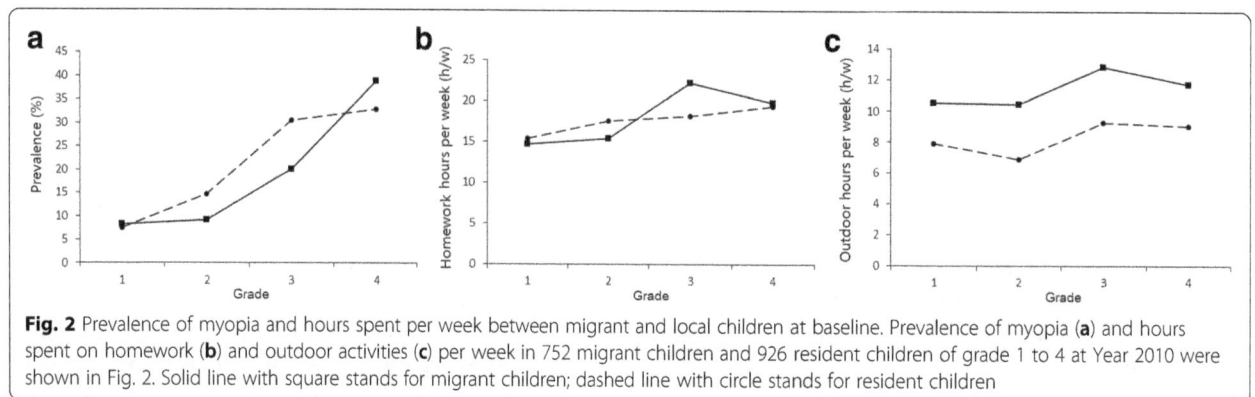

Fig. 2 Prevalence of myopia and hours spent per week between migrant and local children at baseline. Prevalence of myopia (**a**) and hours spent on homework (**b**) and outdoor activities (**c**) per week in 752 migrant children and 926 resident children of grade 1 to 4 at Year 2010 were shown in Fig. 2. Solid line with square stands for migrant children; dashed line with circle stands for resident children

Table 1 Comparison of baseline characteristics between 457 resident and 313 migrant children who completed 2-year follow-up

		Resident $n = 457$	Migrant $n = 313$	Chi-square/t value	P Value
Grade, No (%)	1	227 (49.7)	159 (50.8)	0.0944	0.7587
	2	230 (50.3)	154 (49.2)		
Gender, No (%)	male	233 (51.0)	184 (58.8)	4.5538	0.0328
	female	224 (49.0)	129 (41.2)		
Age, years (SD)		7.54 (0.75)	7.89 (0.88)	5.926	< 0.0001
Parental Myopia, No (%)	0	123 (26.9)	201 (64.2)	107.9569	< 0.0001
	> = 1	87 (19.0)	21 (6.7)		
	unknown	247 (54.1)	91 (29.1)		
Prevalence of Myopia, No (%)		51 (11.2)	25 (8.0)	2.1018	0.1471
SE, Mean (95% CI), D		0.59 (0.50–0.68)	0.46 (0.35–0.57)	1.89	0.0588
AL, Mean (95% CI), mm		22.97 (22.90–23.04)	22.94 (22.85–23.02)	0.62	0.5352

SE spherical equivalent refraction, *AL* axial length

axial length progression compared with those in grade one ($p = .2406$).

Changes in the pattern of myopia prevalence from 2010 to 2012 between migrant children and children in local schools in grades three and four

Additional analyses were conducted of myopia prevalence in students in grades three and four in 2010 (baseline) and those in 2012 (the same cohort of grades one and two in 2010) to explore whether time changes influenced the prevalence of myopia. Figure 4 shows the changes in myopia prevalence in students in grades three and four between 2010 and 2012. For the children in local schools, there were nearly no changes in myopia prevalence (chi-squared test, $p = .4868$ for grade three and $p = .3350$ for grade four); however, for the migrant children in grade four, the prevalence of myopia increased, although not significantly ($p = .0003$ for the grade three and $p = .0972$ for grade four children) (Fig. 4).

Time spent on homework and outdoor activities among 752 children from migrant schools and 926 children from local schools recorded during the baseline visit

As recorded during the baseline visit, the average number of hours spent on homework steadily increased from

grades one to four for the children in local schools; however, that sharply increased from grades two to three for the migrants, which most likely explains the parallel increases in myopia prevalence after grade two (Fig. 2a-c). In contrast, the time spent on outdoor activities showed no corresponding correlation with changes in myopia prevalence in the two populations.

Discussion

The results of the present study showed changes in the pattern of myopia prevalence, incidence, and progression between the internal migrant children and the children in local schools. Unlike the resident children who showed a steady increase in myopia prevalence and a stable myopia incidence and progression, the migrant children presented an accelerated increase in myopia prevalence and refraction progression, resulting in an increased prevalence of myopia with time and revealing an unsatisfied status of myopia, which is worth attention.

In general, in cross-sectional studies, migrant children showed less myopia than resident children, and were even regarded as a protective factor [8]. In the present study, myopia prevalence was low in migrant children in the junior grade, but comparable or a litter higher in the

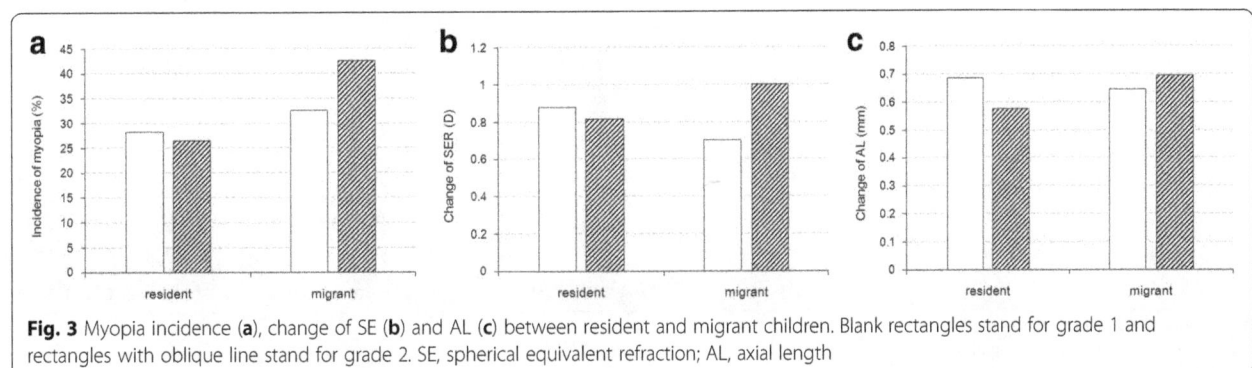

Fig. 3 Myopia incidence (**a**), change of SE (**b**) and AL (**c**) between resident and migrant children. Blank rectangles stand for grade 1 and rectangles with oblique line stand for grade 2. SE, spherical equivalent refraction; AL, axial length

Table 2 Multivariate logistic analysis for myopia incidence (Only including children who were not myopia at baseline)

Variable		MODEL 1	MODEL 2
Migrant		1.162	0.72
		(0.728–1.855)	(0.379–1.368)
Grade 2		1.205	0.780
		(0.788–1.843)	(0.436–1.398)
Grade2*Migrant		–	2.525
			(1.078–5.916)*
Female		1.146	1.198
		(0.724–1.813)	(0.755–1.902)
Parental Myopia	0	REF	REF
	>= 1	1.139	1.131
		(0.575–2.254)	(0.570–2.242)
	Unknown	1.179	1.175
		(0.721–1.928)	(0.718–1.921)
Baseline SE		0.017	0.017
		(0.009–0.033)‡	(0.009–0.032)‡
Baseline AL		0.718	0.721
		(0.503–1.025)	(0.505–1.030)

Odds ratios and 95% confidence intervals were shown
Significance level: *p < 0.05, ‡p < 0.001
SE spherical equivalent refraction, AL axial length

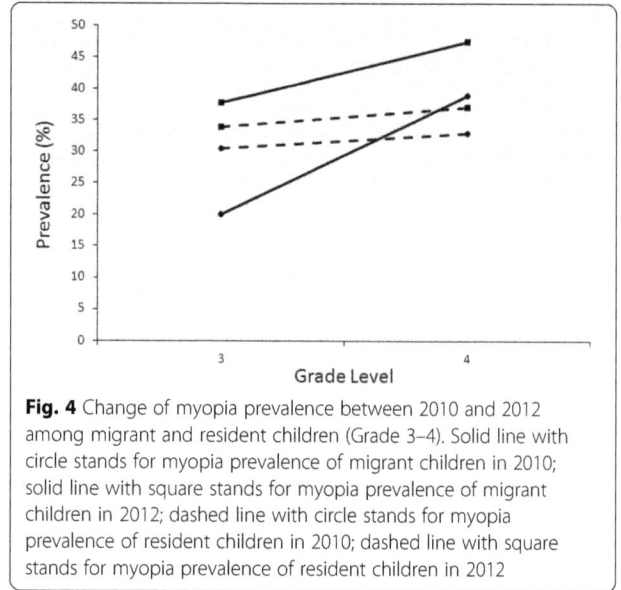

Fig. 4 Change of myopia prevalence between 2010 and 2012 among migrant and resident children (Grade 3–4). Solid line with circle stands for myopia prevalence of migrant children in 2010; solid line with square stands for myopia prevalence of migrant children in 2012; dashed line with circle stands for myopia prevalence of resident children in 2010; dashed line with square stands for myopia prevalence of resident children in 2012

senior grade (grade four) than that of the resident children. Lacking a follow-up study, the incidence and progression of myopia in migrant children remains unknown. Our study found that the crude 2-y incidence of myopia is even higher in migrant children than in resident children, as well as the 2-y progression of refraction

Table 3 Multivariate linear regression analyses for progression of SE and AL in 2 years

		Progression of SE		Progression of AL	
		MODEL 1	MODEL 2	MODEL 1	MODEL 2
Variable					
Migrant		0.0665	−0.1394	0.0637	−0.0276
		(−0.0626 to 0.1957)	(−0.3122 to 0.0333)	(0.0094 to 0.118)*	(−0.1003 to 0.0451)
Grade 2		0.0463	−0.1222	−0.0645	−0.1391
		(−0.0716 to 0.1643)	(−0.2727 to 0.0284)	(−0.1141 to −0.0149)*	(−0.2023 to −0.0758)‡
Grade2*Migrant		–	0.4194	–	0.1855
			(0.1835–0.6553)‡		(0.0864 to 0.2846)†
Female		0.2257	0.2342	0.057	0.0609
		(0.0995 to 0.3520)‡	(0.1089 to 0.3596)‡	(0.0039 to 0.1101)*	(0.0082 to 0.1135)*
Parental Myopia	0	REF	REF	REF	REF
	>= 1	0.3175	0.3261	0.1491	0.1529
		(0.1294 to 0.5055)‡	(0.1395 to 0.5127)‡	(0.0701 to 0.2281)†	(0.0746 to 0.2313)†
	Unknown	0.1644	0.1741	0.0934	0.0975
		(0.0311 to 0.2978)*	(0.0417 to 0.3065)*	(0.0373 to 0.1495)*	(0.0419 to 0.1532)†
Baseline SE		−0.2549	−0.2566	−0.1480	−0.1487
		(−0.3279 to −0.1819)‡	(−0.3290 to −0.1842)‡	(−0.1786 to −0.1173)‡	(−0.1791 to −0.1184)‡
Baseline AL		0.0029	0.003	−0.0233	−0.0233
		(−0.0952 to 0.101)	(−0.0944 to 0.1003)	(−0.0645 to 0.0179)	(−0.0642 to 0.0175)

Coefficients and 95% confidence intervals were shown
Significance level: *p < 0.05, †p < 0.01, ‡p < 0.001
SE spherical equivalent refraction, AL axial length

and axial length. These migrant children, usually from less seriously–affected rural areas, presented a low prevalence of myopia in the junior grade; however, after being affected by the changing environment, showed a myopia prevalence similar to that of the local urban children in the senior grade. Our study captured this catch-up phenomenon, which could be associated with urban environmental factors.

A similar phenomenon was also observed in children of Chinese ethnicity who showed a relatively high prevalence of myopia if living in Singapore, Hong Kong, or Taiwan but a far lower prevalence if living in Australia [9]. In addition, the prevalence of myopia among second-generation (or higher) Indian immigrants in Singapore is higher than that in first-generation immigrants and in Indians living in India and Malaysia [19]. On the contrary, the Yunnan Minority Study [20] reported that people of different ethnicities living under the same environmental conditions shared a similar prevalence of myopia. The results of our study are consistent with those of previous studies and provide sufficient evidence for the importance of environmental factors on myopia incidence and progression.

Long periods of time at near work and short periods of time spent on outdoor activities are the two widely acknowledged environmental risk factors for myopia [21–23]. In the present study, the sudden increase in the time spent on homework might account for accelerated myopia prevalence, especially in migrant children in grades three and four (Fig. 4). Because migrant children come mostly from less-developed areas with a less-rigorous education system, they are usually less educated and have a poor foundation for learning in school. In addition, the migrant schools are usually incapable of recruiting high-level or experienced teachers and have less resources than local public schools; however, as grades increase, the education curriculum becomes more and more difficult; therefore, the migrant children must spend more time studying to catch up with their resident counterparts, resulting in an accelerated increase in the time spent on homework, as observed in our study. The present study did not observe a relationship between outdoor activities and myopia as did other studies conducted on Chinese school children [24, 25], most likely because the number of hours spent outdoors per week was generally low in the present population, which was not enough to have any effect on protection [21].

In addition, migrant children in grades three and four in 2012 presented a higher prevalence of myopia than those in 2010; however, an increase in myopia prevalence in resident children was not observed. The Beijing Myopia Progression Study and the Handan Offspring Myopia Study also reported an increasing prevalence of myopia in the younger generation and suggested a change in environmental factors as the reason [26, 27]. We presumed that in the present population, the study pressure increased with time in migrant children but remained unchanged in resident children. In addition to study pressure, other environmental risk factors existed, which harmed migrant children more than resident children. For example, with electronic devices usually under loose parental control, migrant children might be more involved in watching TV, playing on the computer, and using mobile phones or other electronic devices for entertainment than resident children. Those near work activities could aggravate the incidence or progression of myopia [28]. Hence, it is indicated that there are risk factors for myopia that change with time, making migrant children more vulnerable to myopia than resident children. To determine the reasons behind this, future studies must be conducted that collect detailed data on the risk factors of myopia in those migrant children.

Previous studies have reported that after the onset of myopia, the number of migrant children who wear corrective lenses was ~ 10% lower than that in resident children [29]. In addition, in those children with corrective lenses, 26.1% were inadequately corrected [7]. Not wearing or wearing inappropriate lenses could cause additional visual impairment in myopic children, influencing their study and living habits, reducing their quality of life, and affecting their healthy development [30–32]. Because myopia prevalence especially accelerates from grades three to four in migrant children, a relatively high demand for corrective lenses is anticipated during this period; therefore, reinforcing health education on the importance of wearing corrective lenses, distributing them free, or providing an allowance for prescribing or buying them could be valuable strategies to relieve the burden of reduced visual acuity caused by myopia in those migrant children. Information on myopia prevention methods, such as increasing the amount of time on outdoor activities and making myopia treatment available to slow its progression, such as the use of atropine and orthokeratology lenses, could be presented in the migrant schools to increase everyone's knowledge about the disease.

Study limitations

There were a few limitations to the present study that must be clarified. First, two migrant schools and two local schools were randomly selected. The school-based study design might have resulted in the participants not being representative of the objective population. Although all the children in migrant schools were migrant children who immigrated with their parents, not all children in local schools were resident children. Children with urban Hukou in the local schools could also have moved there from other parts of China; however, they could have lived in Shanghai for a relatively long period to establish local Hukou, thus their environmental risk factors would be similar to those of local resident children. Future studies with a larger sample size and with a design that includes a mixture of both local and migrant children within the same schools are needed to further clarify the phenomenon. Second, we did the followup examinations 2 y from baseline but did not conduct any annually. The followup period might have been too long to determine an accurate myopia incidence or progression in this young population because of their rapidly changing refractive status. Third, detailed information about myopia-related risk factors or information on migration, such as how long they had lived in the city and their original place of residence were not collected in the present study. Only reading and outdoor hours were assessed using a brief investigation; therefore, the reasons for the rapid increase in myopia incidence and progression in migrant children and the discrepancy between the two populations could not be determined. Finally, we used 0.5% tropicamide, which is a relatively weak cycloplegic reagent, in the study. Although evidence has proved that 0.5% tropicamide could be effective in measuring refraction in myopic children with dark pupils [33, 34], it could overestimate a child's refraction toward myopia because of its relatively weak cycloplegic effect [35]; however, becuase the reagent was applied in both migrants and residents using the same standards during the baseline and followup, the differences from the true refraction could be consistent and would not influence the comparisons between migrants and residents.

Conclusions

To the best of our knowledge, this study is the first to document different patterns of myopia incidence and progression among migrant children and resident children in China. Unlike their resident partners, who showed a slow and steady increase in myopia, the migrant children displayed accelerated myopia progression, resulting in rapid elongation of axial length. Although the crude prevalence of myopia could be lower in migrant children than in resident children during the primary school period, the incidence of myopia was higher in the migrants, making this population more at risk for developing myopia. Considering the relatively lower uses of health services in migrants, special attention should be paid to relieve the disease burden of myopia in this population.

Abbreviations
AL: Axial length; CR: Corneal curvature radius; D: Diopters; SE: Spherical equivalent refraction

Acknowledgements
Not applicable.

Funding
The study was funded by Three-year Action Program of Shanghai Municipality for Strengthening the Construction of the Public Health System (2011–2013) (Grant NO.2011–15) and (2015–2017) (Grant NO. GWIV-13.2); National Natural Science Foundation of China for Young Staff (Grant NO. 81402695); Shanghai Natural Science Foundation (Grant no. 15ZR1438400); Shanghai Scientific Research Plan Project (Grant NO. 14411969500); Shanghai Municipal Health Bureau (Grant NO. 12GWZX0301); Key Discipline of Public Health –Eye health in Shanghai (Grant NO. 15GWZK0601) and Shanghai Sailing Program (No. 17YF1416100). The founders didn't participated in the design of the study and collection, analysis, and interpretation of data and in writing the manuscript.

Authors' contributions
MYY, LSL and ZHD designed the experiments; ZR, ZHJ, LQQ, and HXG performed the experiments; ZJF, LLN, HZY, and XX analyzed the data; MYY and LSL wrote the paper. All authors read and approved the final manuscript.

Competing interests
The authors declare that they have no competing interests.

Author details
[1]Department of Preventative Ophthalmology, Shanghai Eye Disease Prevention and Treatment Center, Shanghai Eye Hospital, No. 380 Kangding Road, Shanghai, China. [2]Department of Ophthalmology, Shanghai General Hospital, Shanghai Jiao Tong University, No.100, Haining Road, Shanghai, China. [3]School of Public Health, National Key Laboratory of Health Technology Assessment (National Health and Family Planning Commission), Fudan University, Shanghai, China. [4]Shanghai Shen Kang Hospital Development Center, No.2 Kangding Road, Shanghai, China. [5]Baoshan Center for Disease Prevention and Control, No. 158 Yueming Road, Shanghai, China.

References
1.   Hu X, Cook S, Salazar MA. Internal migration and health in China. Lancet. 2008;372:1717–9.
2.   Statistics Year Book. National Bureau of Statistics of China, 2015. http://www.stats.gov.cn/tjsj/ndsj/. Accessed 28 Nov 2016.
3.   All China Women's Federation. Report on rural left-behind children and urban migrant children. http://www.chinadaily.com.cn/hqpl/zggc/2015-01-17/content_13060717.html. Accessed 21 Feb 2018.
4.   Nielson I, Nyland C, Smyth R, Zhang M, Zhu CJ. Which rural migrants receive social insurance in Chinese cities? Evidence from Jiangsu Survey Data Global Soc Pol. 2005;5:353–81.
5.   Sun X, Chen M, Chan KL. A meta-analysis of the impacts of internal migration on child health outcomes in China. BMC Public Health. 2016;16:66.
6.   Mou J, Griffiths SM, Fong H, Dawes MG. Health of China's rural-urban migrants and their families: a review of literature from 2000 to 2012. Br Med Bull. 2013;106:19–43.
7.   He J, Lu L, Zou H, et al. Prevalence and causes of visual impairment and rate of wearing spectacles in schools for children of migrant workers in shanghai, China. BMC Public Health. 2014;14:1312.
8.   Zhu X, Zhu J, Zou H, et al. Prevalence of ametropia and visual impairment in elementary school students in Baoshan District of shanghai. Chin J Exp Ophthalmol. 2014;32:451–6. (In Chinese)
9.   Rudnicka AR, Kapetanakis VV, Wathern AK, et al. Global variations and time trends in the prevalence of childhood myopia, a systematic review and quantitative meta-analysis: implications for aetiology and early prevention. Br J Ophthalmol. 2016;100:882–90.
10. Wu JF, Bi HS, Wang SM, et al. Refractive error, visual acuity and causes of vision loss in children in Shandong, China. The Shandong children eye study. PLoS One. 2013; https://doi.org/10.1371/journal.pone.0082763.
11. He M, Zheng Y, Xiang F. Prevalence of myopia in urban and rural children in mainland China. Optom Vis Sci. 2009;86:40–4.

12. He M, Zeng J, Liu Y, Xu J, Pokharel GP, Ellwein LB. Refractive error and visual impairment in urban children in southern china. Invest Ophthalmol Vis Sci. 2004;45:793–9.

13. Zhao J, Pan X, Sui R, et al. Refractive error study in children: results from Shunyi District, China. Am J Ophthalmol. 2000;129:427–35.

14. Shanghai Statistical Yearbook 2010. http://www.stats-sh.gov.cn/html/sjfb/201701/1000196.html?pClassID=664&ClassID=665&MatterID=13153. Accessed 21 Feb 2018.

15. Duan C, Lv L, Wang Z, Guo J. The survival and development status of floating children in China: an analysis of the sixth population census data [in Chinese]. S China Popul. 2013;4:44–55. 80

16. Baoshan District Statistical Yearbook 2010. http://bstj.baoshan.sh.cn/fxbg/tjfx2011/201103/t20110303_47412.html. Accessed 21 Feb 2018.

17. Wu X, Zhang Z. Population migration and children's school enrollments in China, 1990–2005. Soc Sci Res. 2015;53:177–90.

18. Lai F, Liu C, Luo R, et al. The education of China's migrant children: the missing link in China's education system. Int J Educ Dev. 2014;37:68–77.

19. Pan CW, Zheng YF, Wong TY, et al. Variation in prevalence of myopia between generations of migrant indians living in Singapore. Am J Ophthalmol. 2012;154:376–81.

20. Pan CW, Chen Q, Sheng X, et al. Ethnic variations in myopia and ocular biometry among adults in a rural community in China: the Yunnan minority eye studies. Invest Ophthalmol Vis Sci. 2015;56:3235–41.

21. French AN, Morgan IG, Mitchell P, Risk RKA. Factors for incident myopia in Australian schoolchildren: the Sydney adolescent vascular and eye study. Ophthalmology. 2013;120:2100–8.

22. He M, Xiang F, Zeng Y, et al. Effect of time spent outdoors at school on the development of myopia among children in China: a randomized clinical trial. JAMA. 2015;314:1142–8.

23. Ramamurthy D, Lin Chua SY, Saw SM. A review of environmental risk factors for myopia during early life, childhood and adolescence. Clin Exp Optom. 2015;98:497–506.

24. Lin Z, Gao TY, B V, et al. Near work, outdoor activity, and myopia in children in rural China: the Handan offspring myopia study. BMC Ophthalmol. 2017;17:203.

25. Lin Z, Vasudevan B, Mao GY, et al. The influence of near work on myopic refractive change in urban students in Beijing: a three-year follow-up report. Graefes Arch Clin Exp Ophthalmol. 2016;254:2247–55.

26. Lin Z, Gao TY, Vasudevan B, et al. Generational difference of refractive error and risk factors in the Handan offspring myopia study. Invest Ophthalmol Vis Sci. 2014;55:5711–7.

27. Liang YB, Lin Z, Vasudevan B, et al. Generational difference of refractive error in the baseline study of the Beijing myopia progression study. Br J Ophthalmol. 2013;97:765–9.

28. Huang HM, Chang DS, Wu PC. The association between near work activities and myopia in children-a systematic review and meta-analysis. PLoS One. 2015; https://doi.org/10.1371/journal.pone.0140419.

29. Wang X, Yi H, Lu L, et al. Population prevalence of need for spectacles and spectacle ownership among urban migrant children in eastern China. JAMA Ophthalmol. 2015;133:1399–406.

30. Chadha RK, Subramanian A. The effect of visual impairment on quality of life of children aged 3-16 years. Br J Ophthalmol. 2011;95(5):642.

31. Kumaran SE, Balasubramaniam SM, Kumar DS, Ramani KK. Refractive error and vision-related quality of life in south Indian children. Optom Vis Sci. 2015;92:272–8.

32. Schneider J, Leeder SR, Gopinath B, et al. Frequency, course, and impact of correctable visual impairment (uncorrected refractive error). Surv Ophthalmol. 2010;55:539–60.

33. Hamasaki I, Hasebe S, Kimura S, et al. Cycloplegic effect of 0.5% tropicamide and 0.5% phenylephrine mixed eye drops: objective assessment in Japanese schoolchildren with myopia. Jpn J Ophthalmol. 2007;51:111–5.

34. Fan DS, Rao SK, Ng JS, et al. Comparative study on the safety and efficacy of different cycloplegic agents in children with darkly pigmented irides. Clin Exp Ophthalmol. 2004;32:462–7.

35. Egashira SM, Kish LL, Twelker JD, et al. Comparison of cyclopentolate versus tropicamide cycloplegia in children. Optom Vis Sci. 1993;70:1019–26.

2

Preoperative preparation of eye with chlorhexidine solution significantly reduces bacterial load prior to 23-gauge vitrectomy in Swedish health care

Nasser J. Gili[1*], Torbjörn Noren[2,3], Eva Törnquist[3], Sven Crafoord[1] and Anders Bäckman[2,4]

Abstract

Background: Bacteria in the conjunctiva present a potential risk of vitreous cavity infection during 23-gauge pars plana vitrectomy (PPV). Current preoperative procedures used in Sweden include irrigation with chlorhexidine solution (CHX) 0.05% only and no iodine solutions. We evaluated the bacterial diversity and load before and after this single antibacterial measure.

Methods: In a prospective, consecutive cohort we investigated bacterial growth in samples from 40 eyes in 39 consecutive individuals subjected to vitrectomy. A conjunctival specimen was collected from each preoperative patient before and after irrigating of eye with CHX, 0.05% solution. Iodine was not used during any part of the surgery. One drop of chloramphenicol was administered prior to surgery. Samples from vitreous cavity were collected at the beginning and end of vitrectomy. All conjunctival specimens were cultured for different species and quantified using colony forming units (CFU).

Results: There was a significant 82% reduction in the total number of CFUs for all bacteria in all eyes ($P < 0.0001$), and 90% reduction for coagulase negative staphylococci (CoNS) alone ($P = 0.0002$). The number of eyes with positive bacterial growth in conjunctival samples decreased from 33 to 18 after irrigation with CHX ($P = 0.0023$). The most common bacteria prior to surgery were CoNS (70%), *Propionibacterium acnes* (55%) and Corynebacterium species (36%). No case of post-vitrectomy endophthalmitis was reported during mean follow-up time, which was 4.6 ± 2.3 (range; 1.5 to 9) months.

Conclusions: Patients undergoing PPV harbored bacteria in conjunctiva capable of causing post-vitrectomy endophthalmitis. Preoperative preparation with CHX significantly reduced the bacterial load in the conjunctival samples subsequently leading to very low inoculation rates in recovered vitreous samples. Thus, CHX used as a single disinfectant agent might be an effective preoperative procedure for eye surgery in Sweden. This is a relatively small study but the results could be a reference for other intraocular surgeries.

Keywords: Conjunctival colonization, chlorhexidine solution, Endophthalmitis, Microorganisms, Small-gauge vitrectomy

* Correspondence: nasser.jadidi-gili@regionorebrolan.se
[1]Department of Ophthalmology, Örebro University Hospital, SE-701 85 Örebro, Sweden
Full list of author information is available at the end of the article

Background

Postoperative endophthalmitis is a serious complication in intraocular surgery. Several different bacterial species are able to cause endophthalmitis after surgical procedures [1, 2], and sometimes with serious consequences and poor final visual outcomes [2, 3]. With the introduction of transconjunctival small-gauge vitrectomy (TSGV) there were reports of increased incidence of acute postoperative endophthalmitis [1, 3]. The commonly used preoperative disinfection of eyes in countries besides Sweden is polyvinylpyrrolidone iodine (povidone iodine (PI)), which has been used for decades, and has been proven effective compared to other prophylactic measures by reducing bacteria (91%) on the ocular surface [4–7] . However, in Swedish health care, chlorhexidine (CHX) is the sole recommended antiseptic agent that is always used for preoperative washing preceding intraocular surgery and CHX was established as antimicrobial agent in 1954 [8]. It has a broad-spectrum bactericidal effect when used at different concentrations from 0.02 to 4% [9–11]. External use on skin and eyelashes includes chlorhexidine alcohol 0.5% and for preoperative irrigation of the ocular surface we use chlorhexidine solution 0.05% [12, 13]. Safety of CHX solutions for ophthalmic use was proved in experimental settings [14], and has been considered equally effective to PI in an outpatient study with 87% versus 91% reduction of bacteria [7]. Recently the safety and adequacy of aqueous chlorhexidine was demonstrated in a multicentre study from Australia where only 3 cases of endophthalmitis were identified in a total of 40,535 intravitreal injection (0.0074%, 1/13512) [15]. The ocular surface is colonized by bacteria and most post-surgical infections are probably originating from these bacteria. It has previously been suggested that an increased risk of intra-vitreous inoculation of pathogenic bacteria is due to transconjunctival approach of TSGV [16]. The trocar-valved cannula system will cut directly through the conjunctiva and into vitreous space and thereby potentially inoculate the vitreous with bacteria. Similar way of microorganisms entering the vitreous cavity was supported by the isolation of bacteria from used intravitreal injection needles [17]. Using molecular analysis of bacterial isolates, other authors demonstrated pathogenic bacteria isolated from vitreous cavity in patients treated from post-surgical endophthalmitis to be closely related to the bacteria isolated from the patients external ocular surface and nose [18]. The preoperative sterilization of the ocular surface should therefore probably be the primary objective to reduce bacteria of the ocular surface, and consequently the risk for endophthalmitis. We designed a prospective outpatient cohort study to assess the bacterial load in the conjunctival sac pre- and post-washing with CHX. We also examined the prevalence of introduced conjunctival flora into the vitreous cavity.

Methods

Patients

A total of 40 eyes of 39 consecutive elective patients who underwent TGSV with 23-gauge trocar (valved cannula) system at University Hospital in Örebro (UHÖ), Sweden, between years 2013 to 2014 were studied. A majority, 82% (32/39), of these outpatients was referred externally from other hospitals, and the follow-up was done at origin, but any post-operative endophthalmitis was treated surgically at the department of ophthalmology, UHÖ. Only patients with macular disease such as epiretinal membrane (ERM), macular hole (MH) and vitreomacular traction syndrome (VMT) were included in study. Exclusion criteria were; a history of vitrectomy or any other form of eye surgery during the last 2 months prior to surgery, any form of eye infection for the last 2 months preoperatively, any current systemic or local antibiotics therapy at the time of surgery, participating in any other study using eye medications, and patients with pathological myopic eye ($\geq$ 6 diopter).

Pre and postoperative procedures

A pre-irrigation sample (Start) was taken using a sterile flocked nylon swab (ESwab Copan liquid-based sampling system; Copan Diagnostics Inc., CA, USA) rolled back and forward once in the inferior conjunctival fornix. The eyelids were then gently retracted and the ocular surface was washed using 30 mL 0.05% chlorhexidine solution (Fresenius Kabi Ab; Uppsala, Sweden). After pausing for 8 $\pm$ 1 min, allowing CHX to drain from the conjunctival sac, the second sample (CHX-treated) was taken using the same procedure as the first sampling.

The eyelids and surrounding skin were cleansed with surgical compresses soaked in 0.5% chlorhexidine alcohol (Fresenius Kabi Ab), followed by sterile draping of lids and eyelashes according to a standard procedure. A single drop of topical antibiotic (chloramphenicol 0.5%; Trimb Healthcare AB, Stockholm, Sweden) was administered on the ocular surface once prior to surgery. All procedures were performed by three experienced surgical consultants.

The first vitreous specimen (V1) was collected at the beginning of vitrectomy, by using a sterile 2.0 mL syringe connected to the aspiration line of a high speed vitreous cutter. A sample of 0.5 to 0.7 mL of vitreous fluid was extracted from the vitreous cavity through controlled manual aspiration. The second sample (V2) (1.0 mL) was manually collected from the sterile infusion fluid (see below) suspension in the eye at the end of vitrectomy through the vitrector aspiration line before removal of the cannulas. No antibiotic was used in the sterile infusion fluid (Balanced Salt Solution (BSS), BSS PLUS; Alcon Laboratories Inc., Forth Worth, USA) during vitrectomy. The vitreous cavity was left with BSS at the end of surgery in 11 cases (27%), whereas gas or air tamponade was used in 29 cases (72%). The integrity of the scleral openings was tested and in 16 procedures (40%) of eyes sclerotomies needed to be sutured at the end of vitrectomy. At the end of the procedure a sub-conjunctival injection of Betapred 0.5 mL (betamethasone 4 mg/mL; Alfasigma S.P.A., Milano, Italy) and Zinacef 0.5 mL (cefuroxime 50 mg/mL; GlaxoSmithKline Ab, Solna, Sweden) were given in the inferior fornix. Postoperative treatment included topical drops of Isopto-Maxidex 1 mg/ml (dexamethasone; Novartis, Switzerland), 3 to 4 times in 4 to 6 weeks, and Cyclogyl 1% (cyclopentolate; Novartis) eye drops, 2 times in 2 weeks. The patients were not routinely treated with any antibiotics postoperatively. All procedures were performed by three experienced surgical consultants.

Bacterial cultures

Conjunctival samples (50 µL) from the ESwab Copan medium (1 mL) were cultured on four differential agar plates (Enriched Chocolate Agar, Colombia Blood Agar, Fastidious Anaerobe Agar and Sabouraud Dextrose Agar). They were incubated aerobically or anaerobically for 7 days. One drop of vitreous aspirate (~30 µL) was inoculated to each of two selective agar plates (Enriched Chocolate Agar and Fastidious Anaerobe Agar) that were incubated as above. The remaining vitreous sample was distributed to supplemented aerobic and anaerobic culture bottles and incubated for 10 days in a Bactec FX-instrument (BD). Terminal subcultures were performed on all negative bottles. Conjunctival isolates were counted quantitatively in colony-forming units (CFU).

Statistics

McNemar's test for case-control comparisons of paired samples (two-tailed) were used for comparing culture result (±), pre- and post CHX-treatment. Wilcoxon Signed-Rank test for paired samples (two-sided) was used to evaluate the significance of the reduction in number of bacterial isolates and bacterial load (CFU). P values less than 0.05 were considered to be statistically significant. Values are expressed as mean ± standard deviation (SD). The calculations were performed using Graphpad Software programs (http://graphpad.com/quickcalcs/) (GraphPad Software, Inc. 2017), and IBM SPSS Statistics 22.0 (Statistical Packages for the Social Science, Chicago, IL, USA).

Results

Demographic data of the eyes and culture results for all pre-irrigation (Start) and CHX-treated samples are summarized in Table 1. The mean patient age was 71.7 ± 5.6 (range; 63 to 85) years. No case of endophthalmitis occurred during the follow up time at the University hospital in Örebro or at referring centres. The mean follow-up time was 4.6 ± 2.3 (range; 1.5 to 9) months.

There was a significant 82% reduction in the total CFU in the eyes in almost all conjunctival samples, post CHX-treatment (Table 1).

Prior to CHX washing 33 of the eyes were culture positive including 61 isolates of 11 different groups of bacteria, and 1 to 3 different isolates/eye (Table 1).

After the preoperative washing with CHX the numbers of culture positive eyes were significantly reduced to 18 ($P = 0.0023$) and the proportion of culture positive eyes for the individual bacterial isolate was reduced. Bacteria were found in the vitreous samples of two patients. A CoNS was isolated after enrichment from vitreous sample (V1) in a healthy patient (eye no. 23, Table 1), and *P. acnes* was isolated after enrichment from second vitreous culture (V2) (eye no. 31, Table 1). Neither of these two patients had the isolated bacteria from the vitreous that matched the bacterial species that were cultured from conjunctiva.

Indications for surgery with different macular diseases are demonstrated in Table 1. One patient had diabetes mellitus (eye no.6) and 2 patients had psoriasis (eye no.17 and 28). The study included 22 phakic and 18 pseudophakic eyes. Intraoperative complications included 2 eyes with retinal tears. In only 16 eyes all 3 sclerotomies were sutured at the end of procedures. In 30 eyes were vitreous cavity left with air or gas at the conclusion of vitrectomy, while 10 eyes were left fluid filled. None of the patients experienced hypotony (defined as IOP ≤ 7 mmHg) on the first postoperative day.

The three most common bacterial isolates were reduced in both CFU, and the number of culture positive eyes (Table 2). The bacterial load for each isolate in the conjunctival sample varied between 20 CFUs to > 1000 CFUs/mL (Table 2).

The less common bacterial isolates were: *Staphylococcus aureus*, Beta- haemolytic Streptococcus grp.G, *Enterococcus faecalis*, Non-fermentative gram negative rod, Alfa- Streptococci, Anaerobic gram positive cocci, *Staphylococcus lugdunesis*, Micrococcus species. These were found in 1 to 3 eyes before and 0 to 2 eyes after CHX.

Discussion

Preoperative preparation of the eye using CHX solution seems to be an efficient strategy for clearing ocular surface of bacteria and preventing intraocular infection. The rate of positive cultures from conjunctival samples decreased significantly in the total bacterial load (CFU), number of isolates and culture positive eyes, after washing with CHX 0.05%. The risk for perioperative inoculation of bacteria in the vitreous cavity was considered low

Table 1 Patient characteristics and bacterial isolates from conjunctival Samples, pre- and post-treatment with chlorhexidine (CHX)

Eye	Gender	Diagnosis	Bacterial isolates		Total CFU/mL	
			Start	CHX	Start	CHX
1	F	ERM	2+	2+	60	380
2	F	MH	3+	–	260	–
3	M	MH	1+	1+	360	240
4	F	MH	3+	–	500	–
5	F	MH	–	–	–	–
6	M[b]	MH	3+	3+	4180	480
7	F	MH	1+	–	40	–
8	M	ERM	1+	–	40	–
9	M	ERM	1+	–	60	–
10	F	ERM	–	–	–	–
11	M	MH	–	–	–	–
12	F	MH	2+	1+	2040	60
13	F	ERM	3+	–	300	–
14	F	MH	–	–	–	–
15	F	ERM	1+	–	20	–
16	F	ERM	2+	3+	60	140
17	F	MH	2+	1+	60	20
18	F	ERM	2+	1+	160	40
19	M	MH	2+	1+	660	280
20	F	ERM	1+	–	60	–
21	M	ERM	3+	1+	620	40
22	M	ERM	2+	–	40	–
23	F	MH	–	1+	–	40
24	F	MH	1+	1+	140	20
25	F	ERM	1+	–	40	–
26	M	VMT	3+	–	540	–
27	M	ERM	3+	–	340	–
28	F	MH	–	2+	–	40
29	F	MH	2+	2+	2400	240
30	M	ERM	2+	–	1040	–
31	M	ERM	2+	1+	420	140
32	M	ERM	–	1+	–	120
33	F	ERM	2+	–	100	–
34	M	ERM	2+	1+	220	40
35	M	ERM	1+	–	60	–
36	M	ERM	3+	–	940	–
37	F	MH	1+	2+	1000	880
38	F	ERM	1+	–	1000	–
39	F	MH	1+	1+	200	40
40	F	ERM	1+	–	20	–

Table 1 Patient characteristics and bacterial isolates from conjunctival Samples, pre- and post-treatment with chlorhexidine (CHX) *(Continued)*

Eye	Gender	Diagnosis	Bacterial isolates		Total CFU/mL	
			Start	CHX	Start	CHX
All culture positive eyes			33	18		
Reduction				45%		
P value				0.0023[a]		
All isolates/All CFU			61	26	17,980 CFU	3240 CFU
Reduction				57%		82%
P value				0.0004[b]		<0.0001[b]

Culture positive (+) isolates/sample: 1, 2 or 3. Culture negative (–).
[a] McNemar's test for case-control of paired samples (culture ±) two-tailed.
[b] Wilcoxon Signed-Rank test for paired samples, two tailed

during 23-gauge PPV as no case of endophthalmitis was observed in this study using this Swedish standard preoperative procedure. The number of positive conjunctival culture prior to CHX was comparable to previous reports (range; 67 to 80.2%) [12, 19], and as well as that CoNS as the most common culture positive result from an eye. The same bacterial flora was isolated from samples from vitreous cavity in patients treated for endophthalmitis [18]. Culture positivity in conjunctival samples from treated eyes was reduced by 45% after CHX irrigation. Also, the number of different bacterial isolates in the conjunctiva was reduced from 61 isolates to 26 isolates. Furthermore, the total number of detectable bacteria decreased by 82%, after rinsing of eye with CHX and even greater efficacy was observed for CoNS (90%). These major reductions in bacterial load, number of different bacterial genus/species and culture positive eyes were most likely the result of effective action of CHX solution and support its use as an antiseptic agent in Swedish eye surgery procedures. However, the complete surgical procedure used may also have influenced the outcome of results. Our findings are also comparable to results from other studies on disinfection methods in eye surgery used in other parts of the world. The use of povidone-iodine (5%), which reported a 91% decrease of number of colonies and 50 to 61% reduction of number of species after sterilization of ocular surface [4, 5] showed similar results as well as one CHX/PI comparative outpatient study [7]. Apart from commonly isolated bacteria like CoNS, Corynebacterium species and *P. acnes* other kind of bacteria were sparsely found only in the conjunctiva of a few eyes (Table 2). Among these, *S. aureus* and *E. faecalis* are important microorganisms causing post-surgical endophthalmitis with very poor visual outcomes despite emergency treatment [20].

In this study CoNS and *P. acnes* were isolated from vitreous samples (V1) respective (V2) (Table 1), both only positive after enrichment broth incubation. The

Table 2 The bacterial load in eyes carrying the most commonly found isolates, pre- and post-chlorhexidine (CHX)

Bacteria	CoNS		Propionibacterium acnes		Corynebacterium species	
CFU/ mL	Start	CHX	Start	CHX	Start	CHX
20–40	11	8	6	3	2	0
41–200	10	1	5	2	4	1
201–1000	1	0	4	5	5	0
> 1000	1	0	2	0	1	0
All eyes	23	9	17	10	12	1
Reduction		61%		41%		92%
P value		0.0037[a]		0.0961[a]		0.0026[a]
Total CFU/mL	2900	300	9180	2440	4100	60
Reduction		90%		73%		99%
P value		0.0002[b]		0.0143[b]		0.0022[b]

[a]McNemar's test for a case control of paired samples, two-tailed. [b]Wilcoxon Signed-Rank test for paired samples, two tailed

source is therefore minute and of unclear significance. The risk for inoculation of bacteria into vitreous cavity in our series of 23-gauge TSGV (post–irrigation with CHX) seems low in comparison to 18% (18/98) using intravitreal injection [17]. Our bacterial isolation rate (2.5%) from the vitreous (V1) at initiation of 23-gauge vitrectomy was significantly lower than the rate of 22.5% (9/40 eyes) reported by Tominaga et al. during 25-gauge PPV [16]. However, at the completion of vitrectomy both studies reported comparable culture positivity (0 to 2.5%) from vitreous cavity (V2). Any vitreous contamination by low number bacteria of for example CoNS and *P. acnes* is probably removed during the vitrectomy extraction or secondary by the immune defense system of the patient preventing an intraocular infection. A positive bacterial culture from vitreous space at the end of vitrectomy does not necessarily lead to postoperative endophthalmitis [21]. At the Department of Ophthalmology, Örebro University Hospital, Örebro, Sweden, we experienced an unexpected increase of incidence of endophthalmitis during 2007 to 2012, using small 23-gauge vitrectomy (0.381%; 11/2885; 1 case per 262 patients, unpublished data N. J. Gili et al.). This was nearly 13 times higher compared to similar publications of Oshima et al. (0.030%; 2/6600) and Wu et al. (0.028%; 1/3615) [22, 23]. The endophthalmitis was caused by similar bacteria isolated in this current study. The present study demonstrates the clearance of colonizing bacteria in the conjunctiva, especially of CoNS, after washing with CHX. However, the individual patient samples were not always reduced after CHX. This could in at least one case (eye no. 1, Table 1) be the result of differences in sampling efficiency. The used culture methods and a limited detection level of 20 CFU could also influence the results (Table 1). No case of endophthalmitis was recorded during this study and follow-up. We might need to look at other causes and risk factors

not presented in this study to find out the reasons for upsurge of endophthalmitis in 2007 to 2012. This study has some weaknesses. A relatively small number of patients were included. The surgical procedures and samplings were performed by three different surgeons in our department. There was also a risk for false negative result when analysing vitreous culture, due to difficulty in culturing low number of bacteria from small volume of vitreous sample.

Conclusions

Current preoperative procedures used in Sweden include irrigation with chlorhexidine solution (CHX) 0.05% only and no iodine solutions. One drop of chloramphenicol was administered prior to surgery. We found that patients undergoing PPV harbored bacteria in conjunctiva capable of causing post-vitrectomy endophthalmitis. Preoperative preparation with CHX significantly reduced the bacterial load in the conjunctival samples subsequently leading to very low inoculation rates in recovered vitreous samples. Thus, CHX used as a single disinfectant agent may be an effective preoperative procedure for eye surgery in Sweden. This is a relatively small study but the results could be a reference for other intraocular surgeries. Further studies could give more information on the risks for endophthalmitis when using CHX only.

Abbreviations
CFU: Colony-forming units; CHX: chlorhexidine; CHX-treated: Post-irrigation sample; CoNS: Coagulase-Negative Staphylococci; ERM: Epiretinal membrane; F: Female; M: Male; MH: Macular hole; PI: povidone iodine; PPV: Pars plana vitrectomy; SD: Standard deviation; Start: Pre-irrigation sample; TSGV: Transconjunctival small-gauge vitrectomy; UHÖ: University Hospital in Örebro; V1/V2: Vitreous specimens; VMT: Vitreomacular traction syndrome

Funding
This research was funded by Örebro University Hospital (Sweden) and Örebro county Council-Research funds upheld weeks of working hours.

Authors' contributions
NJG, TN and ET conceived the study design. NJG collected the data. AB, NJG, TN, SC and ET analyzed and interpreted the data. AB and NJG drafted the manuscript. All authors edited the manuscript. All authors read and approved the final manuscript.

Competing interests
The authors declare that they have no competing interests.

Author details
[1]Department of Ophthalmology, Örebro University Hospital, SE-701 85 Örebro, Sweden. [2]Faculty of Medicine and Health, Örebro University, Örebro, Sweden. [3]Department of Laboratory Medicine, Örebro University Hospital, Örebro, Sweden. [4]Department of Clinical Research Laboratory, Örebro University Hospital, Örebro, Sweden.

References
1. Scott IU, Flynn HW Jr, Dev S, Shaikh S, Mittra RA, Arevalo JF, et al. Endophthalmitis after 25-gauge and 20-gauge pars plana vitrectomy: incidence and outcomes. Retina. 2008;28(1):138–42.
2. Park JC, Ramasamy B, Shaw S, Ling RH, Prasad S. A prospective and nationwide study investigating endophthalmitis following pars plana vitrectomy: clinical presentation, microbiology, management and outcome. Br J Ophthalmol. 2014;98(8):1080–6.
3. Kunimoto DY, Kaiser RS. Incidence of endophthalmitis after 20- and 25-gauge vitrectomy. Ophthalmology. 2007;114(12):2133–7.
4. Apt L, Isenberg S, Yoshimori R, Paez JH. Chemical preparation of the eye in ophthalmic surgery. III. Effect of povidone-iodine on the conjunctiva. Arch Ophthalmol. 1984;102(5):728–9.
5. Isenberg SJ, Apt L, Yoshimori R, Khwarg S. Chemical preparation of the eye in ophthalmic surgery. IV. Comparison of povidone-iodine on the conjunctiva with a prophylactic antibiotic. Arch Ophthalmol. 1985;103(9): 1340–2.
6. Ciulla TA, Starr MB, Masket S. Bacterial endophthalmitis prophylaxis for cataract surgery: an evidence-based update. Ophthalmology. 2002;109(1): 13–24.
7. Barkana Y, Almer Z, Segal O, Lazarovitch Z, Avni I, Zadok D. Reduction of conjunctival bacterial flora by povidone-iodine, ofloxacin and chlorhexidine in an outpatient setting. Acta Ophthalmol Scand. 2005;83(3):360–3.
8. Davies GE, Francis J, Martin AR, Rose FL, Swain G. 1:6-Di-4'-chlorophenyldiguanidohexane (hibitane); laboratory investigation of a new antibacterial agent of high potency. Br J Pharmacol Chemother. 1954;9(2): 192–6.
9. Emilson CG. Susceptibility of various microorganisms to chlorhexidine. Scand J Dent Res. 1977;85(4):255–65.
10. Anderson MJ, Horn ME, Lin YC, Parks PJ, Peterson ML. Efficacy of concurrent application of chlorhexidine gluconate and povidone iodine against six nosocomial pathogens. Am J Infect Control. 2010;38(10):826–31.
11. Oakley CL, Vote BJ. Aqueous chlorhexidine (0.1%) is an effective alternative to povidone-iodine for intravitreal injection prophylaxis. Acta Ophthalmol. 2016;94(8):e808–e9.
12. Montan PG, Setterquist H, Marcusson E, Rylander M, Ransjo U. Preoperative gentamicin eye drops and chlorhexidine solution in cataract surgery. Experimental and clinical results Eur J Ophthalmol. 2000;10(4):286–92.
13. Czajka MP, Byhr E, Olivestedt G, Olofsson EM. Endophthalmitis after small-gauge vitrectomy: a retrospective case series from Sweden. Acta Ophthalmol. 2016;94(8):829–35.
14. Hamill MB, Osato MS, Wilhelmus KR. Experimental evaluation of chlorhexidine gluconate for ocular antisepsis. Antimicrob Agents Chemother. 1984;26(6):793–6.
15. Merani R, McPherson ZE, Luckie AP, Gilhotra JS, Runciman J, Durkin S, et al. Aqueous chlorhexidine for intravitreal injection antisepsis: a case series and review of the literature. Ophthalmology. 2016;123(12):2588–94.
16. Tominaga A, Oshima Y, Wakabayashi T, Sakaguchi H, Hori Y, Maeda N. Bacterial contamination of the vitreous cavity associated with transconjunctival 25-gauge microincision vitrectomy surgery. Ophthalmology 2010;117(4):811–817.e1.
17. Stewart JM, Srivastava SK, Fung AE, Mahmoud TH, Telander DG, Hariprasad SM, et al. Bacterial contamination of needles used for intravitreal injections: a prospective, multicenter study. Ocul Immunol Inflamm. 2011;19(1):32–8.
18. Speaker MG, Milch FA, Shah MK, Eisner W, Kreiswirth BN. Role of external bacterial flora in the pathogenesis of acute postoperative endophthalmitis. Ophthalmology. 1991;98(5):639–49. discussion 50
19. Tervo T, Ljungberg P, Kautiainen T, Puska P, Lehto I, Raivio I, et al. Prospective evaluation of external ocular microbial growth and aqueous humor contamination during cataract surgery. J Cataract Refract Surg. 1999; 25(1):65–71.
20. Major JC Jr, Engelbert M, Flynn HW Jr, Miller D, Smiddy WE, Davis JL. Staphylococcus aureus endophthalmitis: antibiotic susceptibilities, methicillin resistance, and clinical outcomes. Am J Ophthalmol. 2010;149(2):278–83.e1.
21. Shimada H, Nakashizuka H, Hattori T, Mori R, Mizutani Y, Yuzawa M. Effect of operative field irrigation on intraoperative bacterial contamination and postoperative endophthalmitis rates in 25-gauge vitrectomy. Retina. 2010; 30(8):1242–9.
22. Oshima Y, Kadonosono K, Yamaji H, Inoue M, Yoshida M, Kimura H, et al. Multicenter survey with a systematic overview of acute-onset endophthalmitis after transconjunctival microincision vitrectomy surgery. Am J Ophthalmol 2010;150(5):716–725.e1.
23. Wu L, Berrocal MH, Arevalo JF, Carpentier C, Rodriguez FJ, Alezzandrini A, et al. Endophthalmitis after pars plana vitrectomy: results of the Pan American collaborative retina study group. Retina. 2011;31(4):673–8.

3

A cost-effectiveness study of ICT training among the visually impaired in the Netherlands

Nathalie J. S. Patty*⬤, Marc Koopmanschap and Kim Holtzer-Goor

Abstract

Background: Due to the ageing population, the number of visually impaired people in the Netherlands will increase. To ensure the future availability of services in rehabilitative eye care, we aim to assess the cost-effectiveness of information and communication technology (ICT) training among visually impaired adults from a societal perspective, using primary data from two large rehabilitative eye care providers in the Netherlands.

Methods: Participants were asked to fill in a questionnaire, which used six different instruments at three different time points: pre training, post training and three months post training. We investigated whether the participants' quality of life and well-being improved after the training and whether this improvement persisted three months post training. Economic evaluation was conducted by comparing costs and outcomes before and after training. Quality of life and well-being were derived from the EQ-5D and ICECAP-O, respectively. Costs for productivity losses and medical consumption were obtained from the questionnaires. Information regarding the costs of training sessions was provided by the providers.

Results: Thirty-eight participants filled in all three questionnaires. The mean age at baseline was 63 years (SD = 16). The effect of ICT training on ICT skills and participants' well-being was positive and persisted three months after the last training session. Assuming these effects remain constant for 10 years, this would result in an incremental cost-effectiveness ratio (ICER) of € 11,000 per quality-adjusted life-year (QALY) and € 8000 per year of well-being gained, when only the costs of ICT training are considered. When the total costs of medical consumption are included, the ICER increases to € 17,000 per QALY gained and € 12,000 per year of well-being gained. Furthermore, when the willingness-to-pay threshold is € 20,000 per year of well-being, the probability that ICT training will be cost-effective is 75% (91% when including only the costs of ICT training).

Conclusion: Our study suggests that ICT training among the visually impaired is cost-effective when the effects of ICT training on well-being persist for several years. However, further research involving a larger sample and incorporating long-term effects should be conducted.

Keywords: Cost-effectiveness, ICECAP-O, Visually impaired, Eye care, Rehabilitation, ICT training

* Correspondence: patty@eshpm.eur.nl
Erasmus School of Health Policy & Management, Erasmus University, P.O. Box 1738, 3000, DR, Rotterdam, The Netherlands

Background

In the Netherlands, approximately 320,000 people live with a visual impairment of both eyes (visual acuity of < 0.3 and logMAR approximately < 0.5 with applicable corrections); of these, approximately 45,000 are considered blind (visual acuity of < 0.05 and logMAR < 1.3). The probability of becoming visually impaired increases with age, and 85% of all visually impaired people in the Netherlands are 50 years or older. It has been estimated that due to the ageing population, the number of visually impaired people in the Netherlands will increase to approximately 400,000 in 2020 if eye care remains at its current standard [1, 2].

Social health insurance in the Netherlands financially covers assistance and rehabilitative care for people with visual impairments as a part of standard care. These rehabilitative services include support and counseling, with the objective of enabling people to live as independently as possible. As people with visual impairments face distinct barriers in relation to information and communication technology (ICT) tools [2], one of the rehabilitative services covered is ICT training. ICT skills are essential for social interactions and information searching and hence necessary for full participation in society [2]. To maintain financial coverage for such rehabilitative care services, it is important to understand what the health and/or well-being gains are in relation to the financial investments for these services. Cost-effectiveness analysis (CEA) aims to assess the costs and gains of healthcare policies, services or interventions and hence inform decision-makers about the benefits and costs of specific services [3].

To our knowledge, only three studies have assessed the cost-effectiveness of interventions within rehabilitative eye care, and none of these investigated ICT training. Eklund et al. [4] investigated whether a health education program provided by community-based occupational therapists to small groups of people with age-related macular degeneration would be cost-effective compared to individually tailored programs (the usual type of care). The primary outcome measure was perceived security in performing daily activities. The results indicated that the small-group health education program was cost-effective compared to individually tailored programs. In the US, Stropue et al. [5] compared an outpatient program with a residential patient program for visually impaired veterans and found that the costs and effects (in terms of functional visual ability) had increased for both groups four months after the end of the rehabilitative care period. However, the residential patient program was more costly, and after adjusting for the baseline characteristics, the residential program was also more effective. To our knowledge, the most recent study investigating the cost-effectiveness of interventions within rehabilitative eye care was conducted by Bray et al. [6]. Compared to the previously mentioned two studies, this study compared electronic vision enhancement systems with optical low vision aids. Bray et al. [6] concluded that the electronic vision enhancement systems may be a cost-effective mean of improving near vision visual function. However, their results could not be proven cost-effective when using generic utility instruments (EQ-5D) and capability measurements (ICECAP-A).

For people with visual impairments, rehabilitative eye care services such as ICT training, can be seen as a means to increase independence and enable participation in society [2]. However, in the context of continuously rising healthcare expenditures, it is essential to optimally allocate healthcare resources. To date, there has been a limited amount of studies, which estimate the cost-effectiveness of interventions for visually impaired and no evidence of the cost-effectiveness of ICT training among visually impaired. Therefore, the aim of the present study was to assess the cost-effectiveness of ICT training for the visually impaired, as offered by two large rehabilitative eye care providers in the Netherlands, by comparing the situation before and after receiving ICT training.

Methods

The study was carried out among visually impaired clients of two large rehabilitative eye care providers in the Netherlands who were enrolled in ICT training between July 2014 and January 2015. Annually, about 180 people received ICT training, not simultaneously with other training. Enrollees were eligible and invited by the trainers to participate if they were not receiving any other training that could bias the outcome. The ICT training included computer training (e.g., use of Word, the Internet and email) and training sessions on the use of iPhones, iPads and digital assistant devices. Because the training was tailored to each individual's needs (differing in the length of training), no other equivalent training was available and the waiting time for being enrolled in the training was short, the study compared each enrollee's outcomes before and after receiving ICT training. Furthermore, as the ICT training was a part of standard rehabilitative care, the use of a control group without such training was considered impossible and unethical. The outcomes were also re-measured three months after the end of the training to investigate whether the effect of the training persisted.

Recruitment took place as follows. Those who were interested in the ICT training were assigned to an assessor who performed the intake and judged whether the ICT training would be feasible and appropriate. During the intake, enrollees were asked if they were willing to participate in the study. Those willing to participate then gave their informed consent. After recruitment, participants completed the first questionnaire (questionnaire pre training). Based on the intake, a revalidation plan consisting of an estimation of the scope, content and length of the training was set up by the assessor. Immediately after the last training session, enrollees were asked to fill in the second questionnaire (questionnaire post training). The last questionnaire was completed three months after the end of the training (questionnaire three months post training). The questionnaires were sent to participants by mail or digitally. In some cases when enrollees struggled filling in the questionnaire, and did not have anyone who could help them with filling in the questionnaire, researchers filled out the questionnaire together with the enrollees via telephone. See Fig. 1 for the enrollment process, dropout rates and the time points for questionnaires.

At each time point (pre training, post training and three months post training), participants were asked to fill in the same questionnaire, the pre training questionnaire additionally asked participants about their highest completed level of education and their main daily activity. The questionnaire used six different instruments, each presented in the exact same order at each time point. The respondents received the questionnaire in Dutch.

The first instruments of the questionnaire included standardized questions for measuring health-related quality of life and well-being, the EQ-5D (5-level version) and the ICECAP-O. The EQ-5D (a generic health related quality of life instrument) that comprises of five health dimensions (mobility, self-care, activity, pain/discomfort and anxiety/depression) and produces 'utilities' that can be used to calculate quality-adjusted life-years (QALYs) [7]. Similarly, the ICECAP-O consists of five attributes (attachment, security, role, enjoyment and control), one question per dimension and four answering categories per question. The ICECAP-O measures 'years of full capability', based on attributes of well-being that have been found to be important for the elderly [8]. The ICECAP-O produces a weighted index for capability, with a score of one representing full capability and a score of zero no capability. As this capability index is defined by an individual's well-being [8], we will in the following sections present the ICECAP-O outcomes in terms of 'years of well-being', where a score of one represents the best possible well-being and a score of zero the worst possible well-being. During discussions with the ICT trainers about the practical concerns of the process of gathering the data, we were informed that the majority of the participants receiving ICT training were elderly (above the age of 60). Therefore, the explicit decision was made to use the ICECAP-O, as it is specifically aimed at measuring the well-being among elderly.

The third and fourth instruments used in the questionnaire comprised the Medical Consumption Questionnaire (iMCQ) [9] and the Productivity Cost Questionnaire (iPCQ). The iMCQ was used to determine respondents'

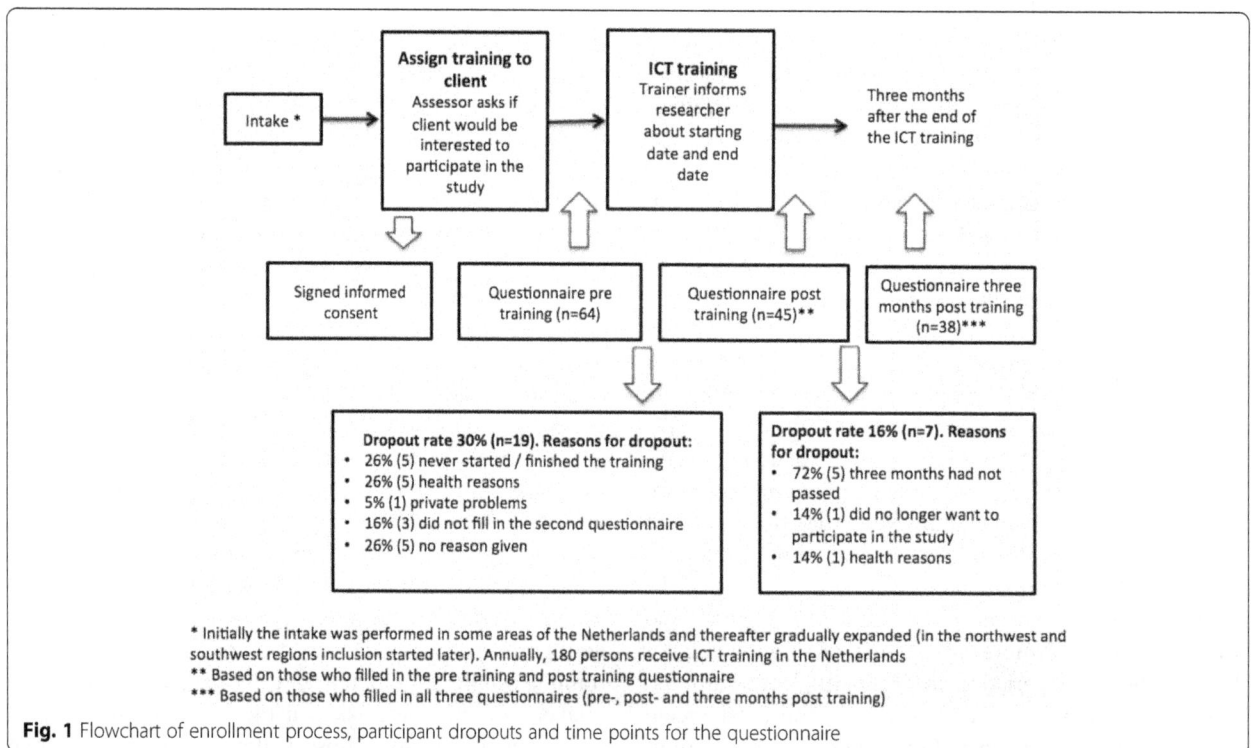

Fig. 1 Flowchart of enrollment process, participant dropouts and time points for the questionnaire

healthcare consumption during the previous two or three months, depending on the length of their training. Those who had received training for three months or longer were asked about their healthcare consumption during the preceding three months, while those who had received training for less than three months were asked about their healthcare consumption during the past two months, which was then extrapolated to three months. The iPCQ [10], which encompasses questions related to presenteeism at or absenteeism from paid work and productivity losses due to unpaid work, was used to determine productivity losses.

The final two instruments of the questionnaire were the Care-related Quality of Life (CarerQol-7D, hereafter referred to as CarerQol) and an adapted version of the Dutch Activity Inventory (D-AI) [11, 12]. The D-AI measures rehabilitation needs of visually impaired persons and rehabilitation outcomes, hence addressing the ICT needs as measured by the D-AI, is the vehicle towards possible improvement in well-being (ICECAP-O) and health-related quality of life (EQ-5D). The adapted version of the D-AI that was used included only those items relevant for evaluating the effect of the training on enrollees' ICT skills. This resulted in 14 questions with six answering categories for each question (easy, fairly easy, difficult, very difficult, impossible, not applicable). To obtain an overall picture of ICT skills, a sum score was calculated for all 14 items (possible range 0–56). The CarerQol was used to assess the potential effect of ICT training on informal caregivers, as it is a standardized instrument for measuring and valuing the impact of providing informal care. Hence, informal caregivers were asked to complete the last part of the questionnaire.

Reference prices from the Dutch costing manual [13] were used to calculate the costs for productivity losses and medical consumption. Information regarding the total costs of the training sessions (including overheads) was provided by the rehabilitation centers.

To examine whether the outcomes before and immediately after the training differed, a t-test was conducted, as health outcomes are generally distributed normally. However, we also performed a Wilcoxon signed-rank test to validate the results. In addition, we conducted a multiple regression to investigate whether the number of training sessions, the participants' gender or their age influenced the D-AI sum score. The cost-effectiveness analysis was performed comparing the outcomes and costs pre training and post training ($n = 45$). Four different approaches were used to calculate the incremental cost-effectiveness ratios (ICERs). The first and second were the incremental costs per QALY gained and the incremental costs per well-being year gained. The 'utilities' derived from the EQ-5D were used to calculate the QALYs, and the 'utilities' derived from ICECAP-O were

used to calculate costs per 'years of well-being'. Furthermore, we used two types of costs: the costs for ICT training alone and the combined total medical costs and costs for ICT training. Applying bootstrapping, 5000 replications were generated for the outcomes and costs before and after the training. For each replication, an ICER was calculated.

Results

We limit the results to those respondents who filled in the pre training questionnaire and post training questionnaire ($n = 45$). This number is limited as some ICT trainers, although informed about the study, had to be reminded repeatedly to include clients. Respondents who had not completed the ICT training within the study period or who dropped out because of other reasons were excluded from the analysis (the dropout rates and reason for drop out can be found in Fig. 1). Among the respondents who filled in all three questionnaires ($n = 38$), an additional analysis was conducted to determine whether the effects of ICT training were persistent.

ICT training costs

The mean cost of the ICT training per participant who had filled in the pre- and post-questionnaire was € 3011, and the average number of sessions per participant was 20 (range 2–63). Respondents with a higher level of education (university- or applied sciences degree) had on average slightly fewer ICT training sessions (on average 17 sessions) compared to those with a lower education level. The average cost (including overheads) per hour was € 129. In an additional scenario-analysis, we also included the costs generated by those who dropped out. The 14 respondents, who started training but dropped out, had on average 9.42 sessions. The average cost per session was € 150. In total, these sessions cost € 19,800. Distributing these costs among the 45 respondents who completed the training, gives an additional cost of (€ 19,800 / 45=) € 440 per participant. As a result, in the scenario analysis, the mean costs of the ICT training per participant became (€ 3011 + € 440 =) € 3451. Unfortunately, we do not know whether these 14 persons had benefits of their (shorter) ICT-training.

Baseline characteristics

Of the 45 participants who completed the questionnaire pre training and post training, 58% (26) were women; see Table 1. The mean age was 63 years (range 27–90 years), and the mean quality of life score (EQ-5D) was 0.70 (range 0.1–1.0). Participants experienced trouble mainly with respect to daily activities, pain/discomfort and mobility; the percentages of participants with at least moderate problems in terms of daily activities, pain and mobility were 29%, 36% and 42%, respectively. Turning to well-being,

Table 1 Participant characteristics and results pre- and post-training

n = 45	Pre training	Post training
Gender (women)[a]	57.8	
Mean age (SD) range[a]	63 (17) 27–90	
Main daily activity (%)[a]		
Employed (paid work)	11.4	
Homemaker	15.9	
Incapable of working due to sickness or disability	34.1	
Early retirement	38.6	
Highest completed education (%)[a]		
No education	6.7	
Primary school	8.9	
Secondary education	57.8	
Higher education	24.5	
Other	2.2	
EQ-5D		
Mean utility score (SD) range	0.70 (0.24) 0.1–1	0.73 (0.22) 0.1–1
Mean VAS (SD) range	71 (16) 20–100	71 (16) 30–100
At least moderate problems (%)		
Mobility	28.8	37.8
Self-care	4.4	4.4
Daily activities	35.5	31.1
Pain/discomfort	42.2	31.1
Anxiety/depression	15.5	11.1
ICECAP-O		
Mean (SD) range	0.77 (0.13) 0.4–1	0.81 (0.13) 0.5–1
Outcome per item (%)		
Little/no friendship and love	24.4	22.2
Some concern/a lot of concern about the future	33.3	22.2
Able to do a few things to feel valued/unable to do any of the things to feel valued	26.6	20
Little/no enjoyment and pleasure	24.4	17.8
Able to be independent in a few things/unable to be independent	57.8	40
D-AI		
Mean sum score (SD) range	22.98 (11.9) 6–56	13.13 (8.7) 1–36
Difficult, very difficult or impossible (%)		
Computer skills	64.4	21.0
Screen	81.9	62.3
Keyboard	37.8	15.5
Mouse	63.3	38.0
Hotkeys	70.2	31.4
Word processor	55.3	25.8
Photographs	82.2	52.4

Table 1 Participant characteristics and results pre- and post-training *(Continued)*

n = 45	Pre training	Post training
Internet	70.4	29.6
E-mail	42.9	11.9
Computer games	76.2	57.1
Using ICT without pain/complaints	58.1	33.3
Braille	74.9	40.0
Speech programs	39.3	10.8
Magnification software	46.9	14.4
iMCQ/iPCQ		
Mean productivity costs per 3 months	€ 1094	€ 1086
Mean medical costs per 3 months	€ 1681	€ 1825
CarerQol	n = 27	n = 26
Mean (SD) range	84 (12.0) 44–97	82 (16.8) 29–100
Mean VAS (SD) range	7.4 (1.0) 5–9	7.6 (0.9) 5–9

[a]Respondents were only asked to report this in the pre training questionnaire

the mean score for the ICECAP-O was 0.77 (range 0.4–1.0), and participants experienced the most restrictedness with respect to the 'control' domain (a low level of perceived independence): 58% felt that they were independent in only a few things or were completely dependent on others. Twenty-seven participants reported having an informal caregiver, and their mean CarerQol-score was 84 (range 14–97). The mean D-AI sum score was 23 (out of 56), indicating that participants largely struggled with various items presented in the D-AI questionnaire. For example, 82% of the participants had difficulty viewing photographs and 82% had difficulty reading the screen. In addition, 70% experienced difficulty with using the Internet and 43% with email. Regarding medical consumption, 38% of the participants received some form of home care, mainly practical household help. Furthermore, 77% had seen their general practitioner at least once during the preceding three months. The mean medical cost per participant was € 1681 for three months, the main cost driver being home care. Out of the total sample, only 11% (5) were employed. The mean productivity losses at the baseline were € 1094 per respondent for three months, solely due to their decreased ability to undertake unpaid work.

Impact of the ICT training

The health-related quality of life measured with the EQ-5D improved slightly after the ICT training, from 0.70 to 0.73. Participants experienced less pain/discomfort and anxiety/depression and fewer problems with daily activities than before the training. However, the percentage of participants who had at least moderate problems with their mobility increased from 29% at the start of the training to 38% after the last training session. Furthermore, an increase in well-being (ICECAP-O) was observed immediately after the training, with a mean score of 0.81 compared to 0.77 before the training. The most notable improvements were seen within the domains 'security' (an 11% decrease in reporting some or a lot of concern about the future) and 'control' (an 18% decrease in reporting independence in only a few things or none at all); see Table 1. The mean D-AI score (ICT skills) decreased from the initial outcome by 9.9 points, to 13.1, indicating a positive effect on ICT skills. The most noteworthy changes were observed in the areas of computer skills, the Internet and use of hotkeys.

Twenty-six participants had an informal caregiver at the end of the training, and their mean CarerQol score was 82, largely similar to the score before the training. The iMCQ revealed that 30% of the participants received home care and 60% had visited their general practitioner at least once during the preceding two or three months. The mean medical costs per respondent were € 1825 during the last three months, with the main cost drivers being hospital admissions and home care. Productivity costs per respondent were € 1086 for three months, mainly due to the productivity losses of unpaid work. Table 1 provides a more detailed description of the outcomes before and after the training.

To investigate the differences in outcomes before (pre training) and after the training (post training), a paired t-test was conducted. The utility and VAS score of the EQ-5D and the CarerQol VAS did not differ statistically ($p > 0.05$). The improvement in well-being (measured by ICECAP-O) was, however, statistically significant ($p < 0.03$). Examining each domain of the ICECAP-O, the most substantial, although non-significant, improvements were found in 'enjoyment' ($p = 0.38$), 'security' ($p = 0.23$) and 'control' ($p = 0.06$). Before the training, 24% of the respondents stated that they felt 'only little enjoyment or pleasure' or 'none', and this decreased to 18% after the training. In addition, while 42% of the respondents felt they were 'completely independent' or 'independent in many things'

before the training, this increased to 60% after the training.

We observed improvements in ICT skills: The mean D-AI score decreased (improved) by 10 points ($p < 0.01$), and all ICT skills except computer games and braille improved; see Table 1. To further validate these results, a Wilcoxon signed-rank test was conducted, and it yielded the same results as the t-test.

Notably, the medical costs were slightly higher post training compared to pre training, due to the hospital admissions of five participants during the ICT training period, but not at a statistically significant level ($p = 0.69$). Productivity costs remained constant and were predominantly related to unpaid work ($p = 0.98$). In addition, a regression analysis was conducted to investigate whether the number of training sessions, participants' gender or age influenced the D-AI sum score. The analysis showed that an extra training session leads to a 0.15 decrease in the sum score (positive effect). However, this was not statistically significant, and the model had limited explanatory power. The mean CarerQol score after the training was slightly lower than before the training, but this difference was not statistically significant ($p = 0.28$). Table 2 shows the outcomes before and after the training.

Does the effect of ICT training persist?

Three months after the last training session, respondents were asked to fill in the last questionnaire. The sample consisted of 38 participants, among whom 17 had an informal caregiver. A t-test comparing the scores immediately following the training (post training) and the scores three months later (three months post training) was conducted to analyze whether the effects of the ICT training were persistent. The mean D-AI score remained 13 after three months, indicating a persistent improvement in ICT skills. The mean utility score for EQ-5D appeared to be slightly higher after three months, but this was not statistically significant. The mean score for measuring well-being remained constant. The t-test revealed a

Table 2 Outcomes pre-, post-, and three months post- training

Outcomes pre-, post-, and three months post-training

	Pre training (mean)	Post training (mean)	Three months post training (mean)	p-value (pre- and post-training)	95% CI differences (pre-and post-training)	p-value (pre- and post-training)	95% CI differences (pre- and post-training)
ICECAP-O	0.77	0.81	0.81	0.03*	0.00 - 0.08	0.91	−0.03 - 0.04
EQ-5D	0.70	0.73	0.75	0.36	− 0.03 - 0.08	0.45	−0.04 - 0.08
EQ-5D VAS	71.02	71.26	70.68	0.92	−4.84 - 5.33	0.80	− 04.94 - 3.84
D-AI sum score	22.98	13.13	12.97	0.01*	−6.51 - -13.17	0.81	−3.48 - 2.74
CarerQol[a]	83.07	81.81	77.02	0.69	−7.65 - 5.13	0.01*	− 10.96 - -1.58
CarerQol VAS	7.40	7.61	6.97	0.28	−0.16 - 0.54	0.03*	− 1.13 - -0.49

*p < 0.05
[a]The t-test for CarerQol is based on caregivers who filled in the questionnaire pre- and post-training, n = 24

significant increase in the mean CarerQol ($p = 0.01$) and CarerQol VAS ($p = 0.03$). Table 2 shows the outcomes.

Cost-effectiveness

Because medical costs were slightly (but not significantly) higher post training (€ 1825) compared to pre training (€ 1682), we could not rule out that higher medical costs after the training may have had an impact on participants' health-related quality of life and/or well-being. Therefore, we decided to include medical costs in the calculations.

As ICT training was shown to have persistent positive effects on health and well-being after the last training session, and the mean age among the participants was 63 years, which meant that their remaining life expectancy was 18 years [14], we assumed that the health and well-being effects would remain constant for 10 years. Because this assumption of 10 years is uncertain, we also calculated the ICERs for five and 15 years.

The results show that when only the costs for ICT training are included, the incremental costs were € 11,362 per QALY and € 7821 per well-being year gained. In contrast, when both the costs for ICT training and medical costs are considered, the costs were € 16,785 per QALY gained and € 11,553 per well-being year gained. If we assume that the effect persists for five years, the cost-effectiveness (including only the costs for ICT training) changes to € 22,725 per QALY and € 15,642 per well-being year gained. If we assume that the effect lasts for 15 years, the result is € 7575 per QALY gained and € 5214 per well-being year gained. As scenario-analysis, we also included the estimates for costs and cost-effectiveness including training costs of dropouts, assuming that the training produced no beneficial effect for the dropouts. This results in a limited increase in cost per QALY (and per year of well-being) gained. Table 3 provides an overview of the cost-effectiveness outcomes.

Uncertainty analysis

Figure 2 illustrates the cost-effectiveness plane for the replicated ICERs, based on total medical costs and costs for the ICT training per gained year of well-being. The plane shows that 89% of the replicates were plotted in

the northeast quadrant, indicating an increase in costs and effects. However, 1% of the replicates were plotted in the southwest quadrant, indicating a 1% chance of negative effects and increased costs. Lower costs as well as favorable effects were observed in 10% of the replicates. This is depicted in the southeast quadrant.

In addition, Fig. 3 presents an acceptability curve with different thresholds. When the willingness to pay is € 20,000 per year of well-being, then the probability that ICT training will be cost-effective is 75% (73% when including the training costs of the dropouts). With a threshold of € 50,000 per year of well-being, the probability that the ICT training is cost-effective is 95%.

When only the costs of ICT training were included (excluding the change in medical costs), the results of the bootstrapping analysis indicated that in 99% of the cases, well-being was gained with limited additional costs.

Discussion

In the context of increasing healthcare expenditures, optimal allocation of healthcare resources is essential. To ensure future availability of services in rehabilitative eye care, it is important to investigate the costs and effects of such services. However, recent cost-effectiveness studies for rehabilitative eye care are lacking. Therefore, the aim of this study was to assess the cost-effectiveness of rehabilitative eye care with respect to ICT training for the visually impaired offered by two large rehabilitative eye care providers in the Netherlands.

The results of our cost-effectiveness study indicate that ICT training among the visually impaired has positive effects on the participants' ICT skills and well-being. These effects also seem to persist at least three months after the last training session. Given the quality of life score of 0.7 for the respondents, their disease severity is 0.15 in terms of proportional shortfall (i.e. equity weighting, combining QALY loss with the remaining QALY expectations in the absence of the disease [15]), which implies that the willingness to pay for a year of well-being or QALY will be at most € 20,000 in the Netherlands [16]. This indicates that ICT training for the visually impaired is cost-effective as per Dutch

Table 3 Costs, effects and cost-effectiveness of ICT training per respondent who completed training

	QALYs gained	Well-being years gained	Differences in costs	Costs per extra QALY	Costs per extra year of well-being gained
Costs of training	0.265	0.385	€ 3011	€ 11,362	€ 7821
Cost of training (incl. costs of dropouts)	0.265	0.385	€ 3451	€ 13,023	€ 8964
Training and medical costs	0.265	0.385	€ 4448	€ 16,785	€ 11,553
Costs for training and 5-year persistent effects	0.133	0.193	€ 3011	€ 22,725	€ 15,642
Costs for training and 15-year persistent effects	0.398	0.578	€ 3011	€ 7575	€ 5214

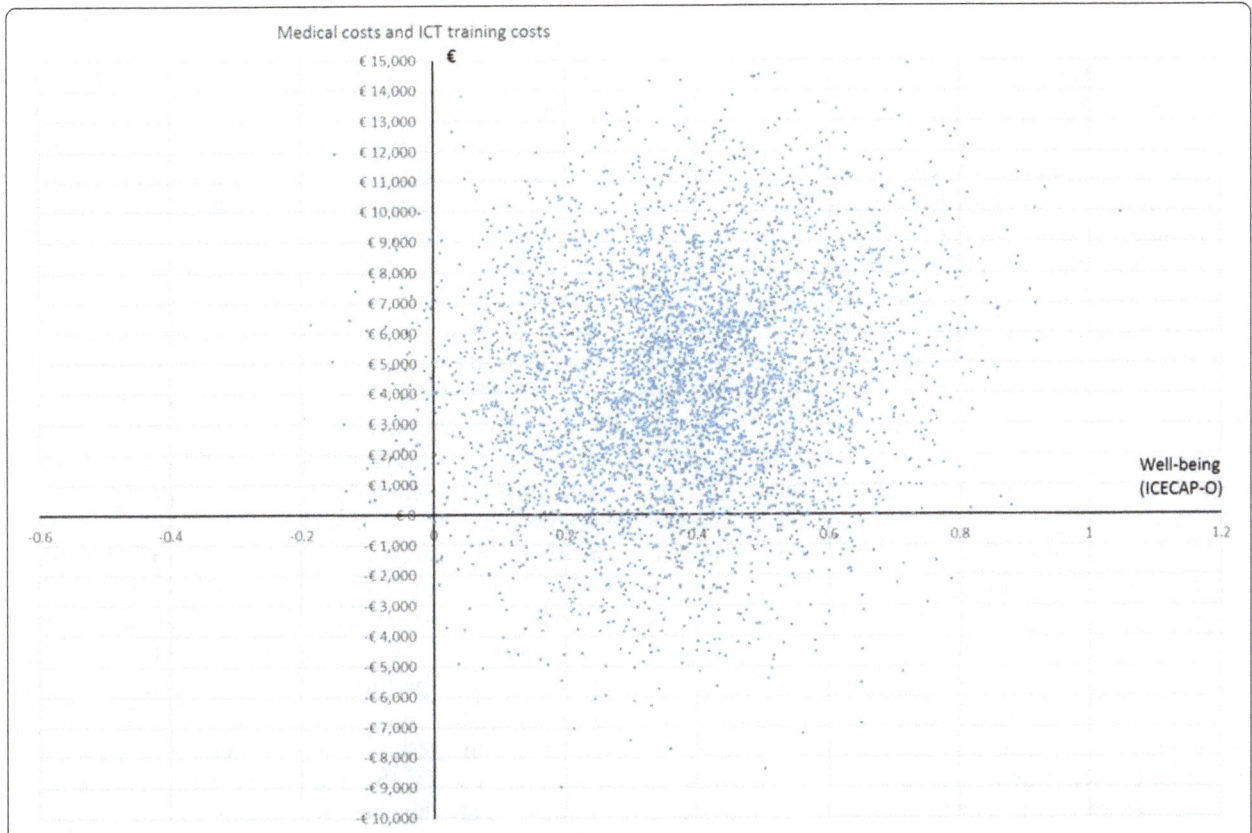

Fig. 2 Cost-effectiveness plane (well-being, total medical costs and costs of ICT training)

standards, under the assumption that the effects of ICT training are persistent for 10 years.

As previously mentioned, three cost-effectiveness studies have been conducted in the area of rehabilitative eye care. Two of these studies are rather outdated, and do not use generic health technology assessment (HTA) instruments nor do they present ICERs, which makes direct comparisons with other rehabilitative (eye) care programs impossible. The third study by Bray et al. [6] is more recent and up to HTA quality standards. It showed a quite small increase in QALYS and well-being (capability) years of electronic vision enhancement systems in comparison with optical magnifiers, for people with a visual impairment. The nature of vision enhancement

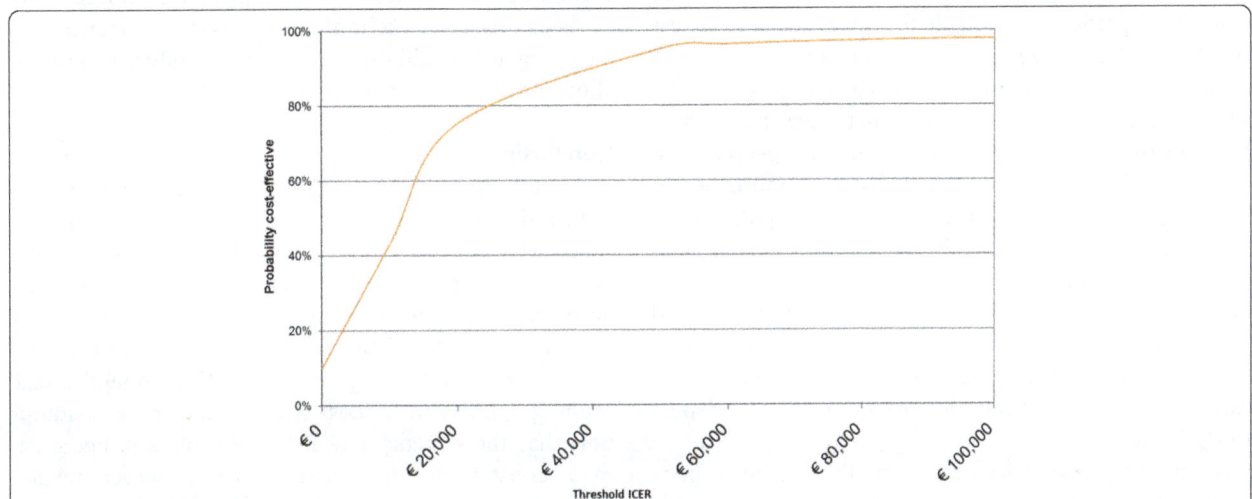

Fig. 3 Acceptability curve for well-being and medical and ICT training costs

systems is quite different from the rehabilitative intervention evaluated in this study.

We used several generic HTA instruments (ICECAP-O, EQ-5D, CarerQol) along with a program-targeted outcome (D-AI). Our study suggests that ICECAP-O and EQ-5D have different levels of sensitivity. The overall EQ-5D score did not statistically change from before the training to after (although the underlying domains 'mobility' and 'pain/discomfort' showed some changes), while the respondents' ICT skills increased. However, the 0.04 increase in the ICECAP-O score was relevant and statistically significant. The relevance of the 0.04 gain in well-being (capability) can be illustrated by Flynn et al. [17], analyzing 622 older people in Britain. The difference in well-being between 'good' and 'fairly good' general health was estimated as 0.029, between 'fairly good sleep quality' and 'very good sleep quality' was 0.028. Both differences appear relevant in terms of health, but are still smaller than the well-being increase as found in our study. However, further investigations should be conducted to determine the sensitivity of generic HTA instruments in the area of rehabilitative eye care. We therefore recommend that generic HTA instruments along with program-targeted instruments should be applied when determining the cost-effectiveness of rehabilitative eye care. In addition, we also experienced a very limited amount of missing values among the generic HTA instruments, which indicates that these instruments are practically applicable in the area of rehabilitative eye care.

This is the first study to use the ICECAP-O in connection with rehabilitative care for the visually impaired; Bray et al. [6] used the ICECAP-A that measures capabilities for non-elderly. We suggest that the ICECAP-O should be used more often within this type of care and that its validity and applicability should be established. Deriving well-being scores from the ICECAP-O can be considered particularly suitable for this cost-effectiveness study, as ICT training can be perceived to have a broader impact on well-being [8]. Furthermore, our results, like those of other studies that have investigated the effectiveness of rehabilitative care for people with visual impairments, show little evidence of improvement in the generic health-related quality of life [18]. In today's society, where ICT skills are essential for full societal participation, ICT skills can be seen as a crucial determinant that can hinder societal exclusion [2] and hence affect a person's well-being. Therefore, measuring only the health-related quality of life would likely underestimate the effects of rehabilitative eye care with respect to ICT training.

Regarding productivity costs, only five of the respondents held a paid job (11%), and only one of these reported absenteeism. This respondent was on sick leave for the entire training period but did not show any deterioration in EQ-5D, ICECAP-O or D-AI scores pre training and post training. Therefore, we excluded these productivity costs, as we did not expect in this case that productivity costs would have an impact on quality of life and well-being.

However, this study has some limitations. First, the sample size was rather small, and the results should therefore be interpreted with caution. It is advisable that economic evaluations of rehabilitative eye care should be conducted on a larger sample. Second, no control group was available, nor was randomization possible. ICT training is not a new intervention but rather a part of standard care; hence, a control group without ICT training would have been unethical. As such, this study should be seen as a 'pragmatic trial' (opposed to a 'strict clinical trial'), with the aim of estimating the cost-effectiveness of the current practice with all its flaws, providing more external validity. Therefore, for example, strict registration of those who rejected to participate in the study during the intake was not performed. Third, this study did not investigate the long-term effects of ICT training, although our results show persistent effects after three months. In the cost-effectiveness analysis, we assumed that the positive effects of ICT training would persist for 10 years. However, it remains unclear exactly how long the positive effects of rehabilitative eye care interventions will persist [18]. To address the uncertainty regarding persistence, we included a more conservative assumption of five years in our cost-effectiveness analysis, which still showed to be cost-effective. However, as mentioned above, we strongly recommend further empirical research to investigate the long-term effects of ICT training in a larger group of people with visual impairments. As technology is constantly evolving, ICT requires users to keep up with technological advances. Hence, we also suggest evaluating the (cost-) effectiveness of short refresher courses in ICT training.

Conclusion

This study suggests that ICT training among the visually impaired has positive effects on well-being and ICT skills, which also seem to persist five months after the last training session. As the respondents in our study have limited disease severity, the willingness to pay for the training in the Netherlands will be at most € 20,000 for a year of well-being or QALY. Consequently, ICT training appears to be cost-effective under the assumption that the effects of ICT training on well-being remain constant for five or 10 years. However, further research involving a larger sample and incorporating long-term effects should be conducted. As this is, to our knowledge, one of the first cost-effectiveness studies in the area of rehabilitative eye care, we hope that this study sets the scene for future economic evaluation of rehabilitative eye care.

Abbreviations

CEA: Cost-effectiveness analysis; D-AI: Dutch Activity Inventory; HTA: Health technology assessments; ICER: Incremental cost-effectiveness ratio; ICT: Information and communication technology; iMCQ: iMTA Medical Consumption Questionnaire; iPCQ: iMTA Productivity Cost Questionnaire; QALY: Quality adjusted life-years

Acknowledgements

We would like to thank Mathilde Berghout for helping coordinate the study and gathering the data.

Funding

This study was funded by Bartiméus and Koninklijke Visio in the Netherlands. The funders commented on the study design and a late draft of the manuscript. The funders had no role in the collection, analysis or interpretation of data, and no role in the decision to submit the article for publication.

Authors' contributions

KH-G and MK set up the study. NP and KH-G gathered the data and, when necessary, filled in the questionnaire together with the respondents via telephone. NP conducted the statistical analysis and cost-effectiveness analysis. MK and NP interpreted the results. NP drafted the manuscript and MK helped draft and revise the manuscript. KH-G provided critical input for the final version of the manuscript. All authors have read and approved the final version of the manuscript.

Competing interests

The authors declare that they have no competing interests.

References

1. VISION 2020 Netherlands. Vision 2020: the right to sight: the Netherlands. 2005. http://www.vision2020.nl/contents/V2020NLrapport.pdf. Accessed 15 Dec 2016.
2. Puffelen C, van der Geest T, van der Meij H. The use of digital skills by visually disabled people to participate in society. 2008. In: IADIS International Conference on ICT, Society and Human Beings. p. 85–90.
3. Drummond MF, Sculpher MJ, Claxton K, Stoddart GL, Torrance GW. Introduction to economic evaluation. In: Methods for economic evaluation of health care programmes. 4th ed. Oxford: Oxford University Press; 2015. p. 1–13.
4. Eklund K, Sonn U, Nystedt P, Dahlin-Ivanoff S. A cost-effectiveness analysis of a health education programme for elderly persons with age-related macular degeneration: a longitudinal study. Disabil Rehabil. 2005;27(20):1203–12.
5. Stroupe KT, Stelmack JA, Tang XC, Reda TJ, Moran D, Rinne S, et al. Economic evaluation of blind rehabilitation for veterans with macular diseases in the Department of Veterans Affairs. Ophthalmic Epidemiol. 2008;15(2):84–91.
6. Bray N, Brand A, Taylor J, Hoare Z, Dickinson C, Edwards R. Portable electronic vision enhancement systems in comparison with optical magnifiers for near vision activities: an economic evaluation alongside a randomized crossover trial. Acta Ophtalmol. 2016; https://doi.org/10.1111/aos.13255.
7. Versteeg MM, Vermeulen KM, Evers SM, de Wit GA, Prenger R, Stolk EA. Dutch tariff for the five-level version of EQ-5D. Value Health. 2016; https://doi.org/10.1016/j.jval.2016.01.003.
8. Coast J, Flynn TN, Natarajan L, Sproston K, Lewis J, Louviere JJ, et al. Valuing the ICECAP capability index for older people. Soc Sci Med. 2008; https://doi.org/10.1016/j.socscimed.2008.05.015.
9. Bouwmans C, Hakkaart-van Roijen L, Koopmanschap M, Krol M, Severens H, Brouwer W. Handleiding iMTA medical cost questionnaire (iMCQ). Rotterdam: iMTA. In: Erasmus Universiteit Rotterdam; 2013. https://www.imta.nl/questionnaires/. Accessed 10 Oct 2017.
10. Bouwmans C, Krol M, Severens H, Koopmanschap M, Brouwer W, Hakkaart-van Roijen L. The iMTA productivity cost questionnaire: a standardized instrument for measuring and valuing health-related productivity losses. Value Health. 2015; https://doi.org/10.1016/j.jval.2015.05.009.
11. Bruijning J, van Nispen R, van Rens G. Feasibility of the Dutch ICF activity inventory: a pilot study. BMC Health Serv Res. 2010; https://doi.org/10.1186/1472-6963-10-318.
12. Bruijning J, van Nispen R, Verstraten P, van Rens G. A Dutch ICF version of the activity inventory: results from focus groups with visually impaired persons and experts. Opthalmic Epidemol. 2010; https://doi.org/10.3109/09286586.2010.528133.
13. Hakkaart-van Roijen L, van der Linden N, Bouwmans C, Kanters T, Swan Tan S. Kostenhandleiding: Methodologie van kostenonderzoek en referentieprijzen voor economische evaluaties in de gezondheidszorg. 2015. https://www.zorginstituutnederland.nl/over-ons/publicaties/publicatie/2016/02/29/richtlijn-voor-het-uitvoeren-van-economische-evaluaties-in-de-gezondheidszorg. Accessed 13 Apr 2018.
14. Statistics Netherlands. Statline Levensverwachting: geslacht, geboortegeneratie. 2017. https://opendata.cbs.nl/statline/#/CBS/nl/dataset/80333ned/table?ts=1523620703808. Accessed 13 Apr 2018.
15. Stolk EA, Pickee SJ, Ament AH, Busschbach JJ. Equity in health care prioritisation: an empirical inquiry into social value. Health Policy. 2005; https://doi.org/10.1016/j.healthpol.2005.01.018.
16. Zorg Instituut Nederland. Rapport kosteneffectiviteit in de praktijk. 2015. https://www.zorginstituutnederland.nl/publicaties/rapport/2015/06/26/kosteneffectiviteit-in-de-praktijk. Accessed 9 Jan 2016.
17. Flynn TN, Chan P, Coast J, Peters TJ. Assessing quality of life among British older people using the ICEPOP CAPability (ICECAP-O) measure. Appl Health Econ and Health Policy. 2011; https://doi.org/10.2165/11594150-000000000-00000.
18. Binns AM, Bunce C, Dickinson C, Harper R, Tudor-Edwards R, Woodhouse M, et al. How effective is low vision service provision? A systematic review. Surv Ophthalmol. 2012; https://doi.org/10.1016/j.survopthal.2011.06.06.006.

4

Association between blood pressure and retinal arteriolar and venular diameters in Chinese early adolescent children, and whether the association has gender difference

Yuan He[1], Shi-Ming Li[1], Meng-Tian Kang[1], Luo-Ru Liu[2], He Li[2], Shi-Fei Wei[1], An-Ran Ran[1], Ningli Wang[1]* and the Anyang Childhood Eye Study Group

Abstract

Background: To establish the independent association between blood pressure (BP) and retinal vascular caliber, especially the retinal venular caliber, in a population of 12-year-old Chinese children.

Methods: We have examined 1501 students in the 7th grade with mean age of 12.7 years. A non-mydriatic fundus camera (Canon CR-2, Tokyo, Japan) was used to capture 45^0 fundus images of the right eyes. Retinal vascular caliber was measured using a computer-based program (IVAN). BP was measured using an automated sphygmomanometer (HEM-907, Omron, Kyoto, Japan).

Results: The mean retinal arteriolar caliber was 145.3 μm (95% confidence interval [CI], 110.6–189.6 μm) and the mean venular caliber was 212.7 μm (95% CI, 170.6–271.3 μm). After controlling for age, sex, axial length, BMI, waist, spherical equivalent, birth weight, gestational age and fellow retinal vessel caliber, children in the highest quartile of BP had significantly narrower retinal arteriolar caliber than those with lower quartiles (P for trend< 0.05). Each 10-mmHg increase in BP was associated with narrowing of the retinal arterioles by 3.00 μm (multivariable-adjusted $P < 0.001$), and the results were consist in three BP measurements. The association between BP measures and retinal venular caliber did not persist after adjusting for fellow arteriolar caliber. And there was no significant interaction between BP and sex, age, BMI, and birth status.

Conclusions: In a large population of adolescent Chinese children, higher BP was found to be associated with narrower retinal arterioles, but not with retinal venules. Sex and other confounding factors had no effect on the relationship of BP and retinal vessel diameter.

Keywords: Hypertension, Adolescents, Retinal arteriolar diameter, Retinal venular diameter, Blood pressure

* Correspondence: xiaowwnnll@163.com
[1]Beijing Tongren Eye Center, Beijing Tongren Hospital, Beijing
Ophthalmology & Visual Science Key Lab, Beijing Institute of Ophthalmology,
Capital Medical University, Beijing, China
Full list of author information is available at the end of the article

Background

Major component of the circulatory system is composed of the microcirculation, which plays an important role in maintaining cardiovascular health. There is a widespread influence of blood pressure (BP) on the structure and function of microcirculation system. Early in the late nineteenth century, Marcus Gunn had put forward the statement that there were associations between microvascular abnormalities and cardiovascular diseases [1].

The retina is a unique structure of the eyes, where the in vivo microcirculation can be directly visualized and monitored non-invasively. Retinal microcirculation shares the same anatomic architecture and physiological feature with other terminal organs elsewhere in the body [2]. These characteristics increase its utility as a tool to study the clinical performance of microvascular diseases. Recently, with the improvement of retinal imaging particularly the computer-assistant analysis techniques from digital retinal images [3], plenty of epidemiological studies in adult populations have displayed that abnormal changes in retinal vascular caliber (predominantly retinal arteriolar and venular caliber) are closely associated with some systemic vascular abnormalities such as cardiovascular risk factors [4], hypertension [5], coronary heart disease [6], risk of diabetes and stroke [7], cerebral infarcts and white matter lesions [8], and renal disease [9], independent of other risk factors.

Despite increasing data on the risk prediction of retinal vascular caliber measurement in different population-based studies, there had been still some controversial opinions on association between retinal vascular changes and BP, especially for the retinal venular changes. Understanding the impacts of BP and changes to the retinal microvasculature in persons with different background is an important aspect of the study on microcirculation disease. Children are generally free of many systemic conditions and eye diseases (such as glaucoma or diabetic retinopathy, etc.) that could bring about confounding effects on observed associations. High BP in children and adolescents is more and more common in western countries [10], and BP levels and prevalence of hypertension has increased dramatically among children and adolescents in China [11]. It is encouraging that there are some studies on the association of BP and retinal vessel caliber in children recently, but substantial data on children group are still needed to provide the reference data.

In this study, we investigated the independent association between blood pressure measures and changes to the retinal microvasculature in a relatively large population of 12-year-old Chinese children. This study also assessed the potential modifying influences of age, BMI, birth parameters, especially sex, on the associations between BP and retinal vessel caliber.

Methods

Study population

The Anyang Childhood Eye Study (ACES) is a school-based cohort study designed to observe the occurrence and development of myopia as well as other diseases in school children living in Anyang urban area, Henan Province, Central China. Detailed methodology of the study has been previously described [12]. In briefly, 1501 students in 7th grade average aged 12.7 years have been examined from October 2011 to December 2011. The flowchart of participants included in the present study was shown in Fig. 1. Ethics approval was obtained from the institutional review board of Beijing Tongren Hospital, Capital Medical University, and followed the tenets of the declaration of Helsinki. Informed written consent was obtained from at least one parent. Verbal assent was obtained from each child.

Retinal photography and measurement of retinal vascular caliber

The children were examined at health examination station of the Anyang Eye Hosptial. A non-mydriatic fundus camera (Canon CR-2, Tokyo, Japan) was used to capture 45^0 fundus images centering on optic disc and macular area of children's right eyes by a well-trained operator [12]. Children with abnormal fundus images would also undergo left eye measurements, and we analyzed one picture for each child.

According to a standardized protocol described previously [3], the computer-imaging program (IVAN, University of Wisconsin, Madison, WI) was used to measure calibers of all retinal arterioles and venules located in zone 0.5 to 1 disc diameter from the optic disc margin (zone B). The program automatically combined vessel diameters from the six largest arterioles and six largest venules into a pair of indices. The central retinal arteriolar and venular equivalents (CRAE and CRVE) represent the average arteriolar and venular caliber for each eye, respectively. One grader masked to children's identity and characteristics performed all measurements. Before starting the measurement, 50 randomly selected retinal images were repeatedly measured by the grader with an interval of 2 weeks. The reliability was high with intraclass correlation coefficients of 0.85 for arteriolar caliber and 0.97 for venular caliber.

Blood pressure measurement

Blood pressure of children was measured in a seated position after 5 min of rest using an automated sphygmomanometer (HEM-907, Omron, Kyoto, Japan) with appropriate cuff size (bladder length ≈80% and width at least 40% of the arm circumference, covering the upper arm but not obscuring the antecubital fossa). Systolic and diastolic blood pressure (SBP and DBP, respectively)

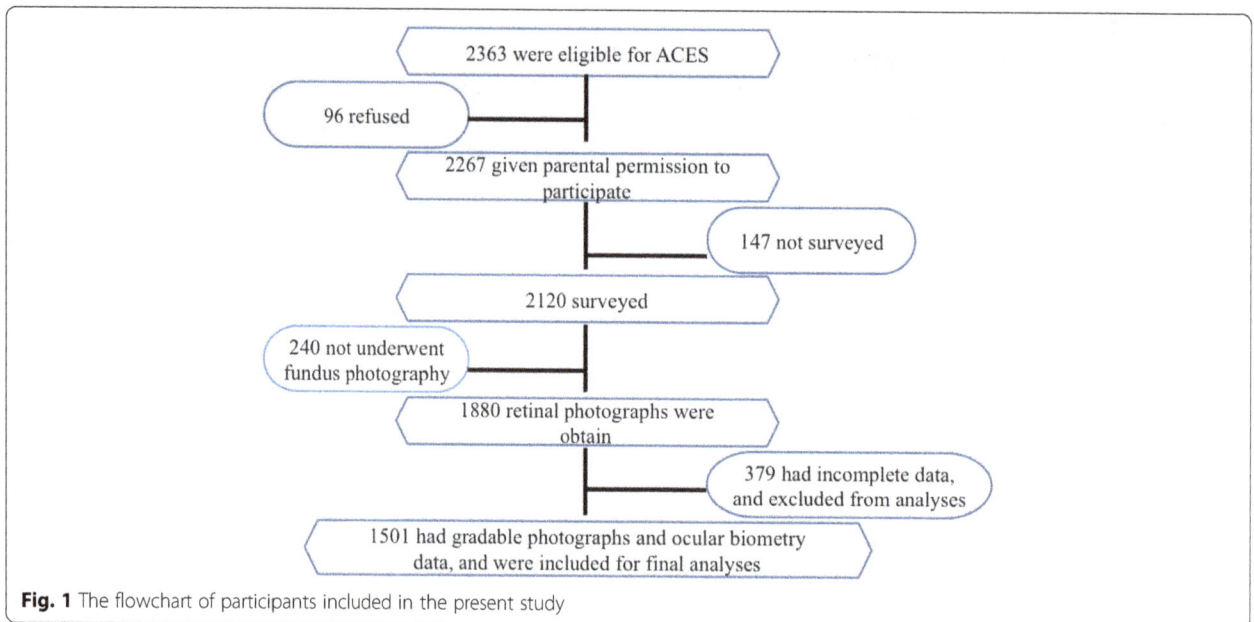

Fig. 1 The flowchart of participants included in the present study

readings were taken. Two readings were taken 5 min apart and averaged for analysis. Mean arterial blood pressure (MABP) was computed as 2/3 of the diastolic plus 1/3 of the systolic value.

Other measurements

Any abnormality of anterior segment (any abnormalities of the anterior segment of the eye, such as corneal leukoplakia, cataract, pupil abnormalities, iris anterior adhesion, etc.) was observed and recorded using a slit-lamp (YZ5J, 66 Vision Tech Co, Suzhou, China). Cycloplegic spherical equivalent refraction was measured using an autorefractor (HRK7000 A, Huvitz, Gunpo, South Korea) with three readings taken and averaged. An optical coherence biometry (IOL-master 1322–734, Carl Zeiss Meditec AG, Jena, Germany) was applied to evaluate the optical axial length (AL) value along the visual axis (line connecting the fixation point to the fovea, specifically from the anterior surface of the cornea to the retinal pigment epithelium layer of the fovea), with five repeated measurements taken and averaged. Height and weight were measured using an automatic and professional integrated set. Body mass index (BMI) was calculated as weight/height^2 (kg/m^2). Waist circumference was measured with a tape measure and was defined as the narrowest part of the student's trunk. Birth information including gestational weeks, birth weight and birth length were collected by administrating questionnaires to the participating students' parents.

Statistical analysis

SAS (v9.3, SAS Institute Inc., Cary, NC, USA) was used to perform statistical analysis. BP was categorized into quartiles as well as being analyzed as a continuous variable (i.e. each 10 mmHg increase). The retinal arteriolar, venular calibers, and arteriolar to venular ratio (AVR) were compared across blood pressure quartiles based on three models, Model 1 was analyzed without any adjustment, Model 2 adjusted for multivariate variables (age, sex, axial length, BMI, waist, spherical equivalent, birth weight, and gestational age) and then Model 3 adjusted additionally for fellow retinal vessel diameter. The test of trend was determined by regarding quartiles of BP as continuous ordinal variables. Multiple linear regressions were used to estimate the absolute changes in retinal arteriolar and venular caliber for a 10-mmHg increase in SBP, DBP, and MABP. Potential modifiers were examined in stratified analyses of age, sex, BMI, and birth parameters. All probabilities quoted are two-sided, and a significant P value was defined as < 0.05.

Results

Table 1 shows the study characteristics of the children included for crosss-sectional analyses. Compared with boys, girls had higher systolic and mean arterial blood pressure, higher waist and BMI, and had less myopia and longer axial length.

Table 2 shows the mean retinal vascular caliber and AVR by quartiles of systolic, diastolic and mean arterial blood pressure in three different models. Children with highest quartile of BP were more likely to have narrower retinal arteriolar caliber than those in the lowest quartile after multivariable-adjustment (all $P < 0.01$), with a mean difference of 6–7 μm between the highest and lowest quartiles, and the results were consistent for three BP measurements. As for retinal venular diameter, in Model

Table 1 Basic characteristics of the children included in the study

Characteristics	Male	Female	p
	(n = 792)	(n = 709)	
Age (year)	12.66 (0.50)	12.73 (0.49)	**0.004**
Spherical equivalent refraction (diopters)	−1.78 (2.08)	− 1.32 (2.02)	**< 0.001**
Axial length (mm)	23.93 (1.01)	24.35 (1.09)	**< 0.001**
Systolic blood pressure (mm Hg)	104.55 (10.87)	107.36 (10.35)	**< 0.001**
Diastolic blood pressure (mm Hg)	65.35 (7.57)	65.45 (7.21)	0.758
Mean arterial blood pressure (mm Hg)	78.42 (8.23)	79.41 (7.63)	**0.005**
BMI (kg/m^2)	19.32 (3.22)	20.28 (3.91)	**< 0.001**
Waist (cm)	69.04 (7.84)	71.92 (10.14)	**< 0.001**

Data are mean (SD). *BMI* body mass index; Significant p values are bolded. Significant p values are bolded

1, children with higher BP had significantly narrower CRVE ($P < 0.001$ for trend for three BP measurements), and in Model 2, only children with higher SBP were found to have narrower CRVE than those with lower SBP ($P = 0.038$ for trend), however, this association did not persist after adjusting for fellow vessel caliber. In Model 1 and Model 2, children with higher BP quartiles had consistently and significantly narrower AVR ($P < 0.001$ for trend), and the results were consistent for three BP measurements.

Table 3 shows the multivariable linear regression between retinal vascular caliber and BP. In model 1 and model 2, for each 10-mmHg increase in SBP, DBP and MABP, CRAE decreased by 3.07–4.40 μm ($P < 0.001$) and CRVE decreased by 1.47–2.69 μm ($P < 0.001$). In model 3 adjusted for fellow vessel caliber additionally, each 10-mmHg increase in BP was associated with 2.34–3.47 μm decrease in retinal arteriolar caliber ($P < 0.001$), but no significant change in CRVE ($p > 0.42$) was observed. AVR decreased by 0.010 to 0.014 for every 10-mmHg increase in BP in Model 1, Further adjustment for age, gender, axial length, BMI, waist, spherical equivalent, birth weight and gestational age had no impact on the magnitude of this effect (AVR reduction 0.007 to 0.012).

Subgroup analysis stratified by potential effect modifiers was presented in Tables 4, 5 and 6. Associations were consistent across subgroups stratified by age, sex, BMI, and birth parameters.

It is worth noting that, there were no significant interactions between sex, and BP on retinal vessel diameters. The impact of BP on the diameters of retinal vessels showed no gender differences between boys and girls. In model 2, each 10-mmHg increase in BP was associated with 3.41–4.91 μm ($P < 0.001$) and 2.73–3.89 μm ($P < 0.001$) decrease in CRAE for boys and girls respectively, and in model 3, the decrease of CRAE reduced to 2.57–3.81 μm ($P < 0.001$) and 2.12–3.12 μm ($P < 0.001$) for boys and girls respectively (Table 4). And for CRVE,

each 10-mmHg increase in BP resulted in 2.03–2.68 μm ($P < 0.05$) decrease for boys and 2.15–2.76 μm ($P < 0.05$) decrease for girls in model 2, but when CRAE was additionally adjusted in model 2, there is no significant association between BP and CRVE in either boys nor girls, which was consistent in three BP measurements (Table 5).

Discussion

In this population of 12-year-old Chinese children, we found that increasing blood pressure was significantly associated with narrowing retinal arteriolar caliber and smaller AVR, but not with retinal venular caliber. After controlling for age, gender, axial length, BMI, waist, spherical equivalent, birth parameters and fellow retinal vessel, each 10-mmHg increase in BP was associated with an approximate 3~ 4 μm reduction in CRAE, and the changes were consistent of three BP measurements. The similar pattern and magnitude of change were also found in the relationship of BP with CRVE prior of taking confounding fellow arteriolar diameter into account, but after the fellow vessel were further adjusted, the change no longer had significant difference. And there was no significant interaction between BP and age, sex, BMI and birth status.

Both cross-sectional and longitudinal studies had provided substantial evidence that there is significant association between elevated blood pressure or hypertension and narrower central retinal arteriole caliber in adult populations [13–19]. However, there is conflicting evidence on retinal venular diameter as marker related to hypertension. Some studies [16, 18–22] suggested that retinal venular widening may be independently associated with risk of hypertension, others [15, 19, 23–25] had found no association, whereas some other researchers announced that both retinal venular and arteriolar caliber were inversely related to blood pressure, independent of age, gender, and smoking [26].

Table 2 Mean retinal arteriolar diameter, retinal venular diameter, and AVR (mean and standard error) stratified by SBP, DBP and MABP

		n	Range (mm Hg)	Rentinal Arteriolar Diameter (μm)			Rentinal Venular Diameter (μm)			AVR	
				Model 1	Model 2	Model 3	Model 1	Model 2	Model 3	Model 1	Model 2
SBP	First quartile	375	79 to 100	149.02 ± 1.31	148.70 ± 0.62	147.91 ± 0.56	214.54 ± 0.63	214.91 ± 0.79	212.96 ± 0.71	0.696 ± 0.004	0.688 ± 0.007
	Second quartile	365	101 to 107	146.17 ± 0.62	146.19 ± 0.61	146.20 ± 0.54	213.16 ± 0.30	212.65 ± 0.69	212.12 ± 0.69	0.687 ± 0.002	0.685 ± 0.008
	Third quartile	373	107 to 113	144.24 ± 0.54	144.22 ± 0.60	144.36 ± 0.54	212.23 ± 0.20	212.30 ± 0.76	212.89 ± 0.68	0.681 ± 0.002	0.683 ± 0.008
	Fourth quartile	388	113 to 142	141.63 ± 1.36	141.99 ± 0.61	142.62 ± 0.55	210.97 ± 0.65	210.91 ± 0.78	212.76 ± 0.70	0.672 ± 0.004	0.680 ± 0.009
	P for trend			**< 0.001**	**0.001**	**< 0.001**	**< 0.001**	**0.038**	0.941	**< 0.001**	**< 0.0001**
DBP	First quartile	323	49 to 61	147.96 ± 2.50	149.14 ± 0.65	148.15 ± 0.58	214.04 ± 1.21	215.49 ± 0.82	213.29 ± 0.75	0.692 ± 0.007	0.687 ± 0.007
	Second quartile	407	61 to 65	145.95 ± 2.18	146.21 ± 0.57	146.19 ± 0.51	213.06 ± 1.05	212.73 ± 0.73	212.19 ± 0.65	0.686 ± 0.007	0.685 ± 0.008
	Third quartile	360	66 to 70	144.49 ± 2.20	144.53 ± 0.61	144.92 ± 0.55	212.35 ± 1.06	211.60 ± 0.77	212.01 ± 0.69	0.682 ± 0.007	0.683 ± 0.008
	Fourth quartile	411	70 to 90	142.99 ± 2.28	141.84 ± 0.58	142.31 ± 0.52	211.62 ± 1.10	211.36 ± 0.73	213.29 ± 0.66	0.677 ± 0.007	0.682 ± 0.010
	P for trend			**< 0.001**	**0.005**	**0.009**	**< 0.001**	0.078	0.970	**< 0.001**	**< 0.0001**
MABP	First quartile	370	60 to 75	148.62 ± 1.80	149.31 ± 0.61	148.24 ± 0.55	214.36 ± 0.87	215.75 ± 0.78	213.47 ± 0.71	0.695 ± 0.005	0.687 ± 0.007
	Second quartile	366	75 to 79	145.96 ± 1.55	145.81 ± 0.60	145.98 ± 0.54	213.07 ± 0.75	212.18 ± 0.77	211.87 ± 0.69	0.686 ± 0.005	0.685 ± 0.008
	Third quartile	400	79 to 84	144.28 ± 1.59	144.36 ± 0.58	144.56 ± 0.52	212.25 ± 0.77	212.12 ± 0.73	212.62 ± 0.66	0.681 ± 0.005	0.683 ± 0.008
	Fourth quartile	365	84 to 102	142.14 ± 1.84	141.50 ± 0.62	142.21 ± 0.56	211.22 ± 0.89	210.67 ± 0.79	212.78 ± 0.72	0.674 ± 0.005	0.680 ± 0.010
	P for trend			**< 0.001**	**0.011**	**0.004**	**< 0.001**	0.086	0.738	**< 0.001**	**< 0.0001**

Model 1:unadjusted model; Model 2: adjusted for age, gender, axial length, BMI, waist, spherical equivalent, birth weight and gestational age; Model 3: adjusted for fellow vessel diameter additionally. *SBP* systolic blood pressure, *DBP* diastolic blood pressure, *MABP* mean arterial blood pressure, *AVR* arteriolar to venular ratio. Significant *p* values are bolded

Table 3 Multivariate Linear Regression Models of Retinal Vascular Caliber and Blood Pressure

	Retinal arteriolar diameter (μm)		Retinal venular diameter (μm)		AVR	
	Mean (95%CI)	P	Mean (95%CI)	P	Mean (95%CI)	P
SBP						
Model 1	−3.23(− 3.96 to −2.52)	**< 0.001**	−1.57(− 2.50 to − 0.63)	**< 0.001**	−0.01 (− 0.013 to − 0.007)	**< 0.001**
Model 2	− 3.07 (− 3.79 to − 2.34)	**< 0.001**	− 2.06 (− 2.97 to − 1.15)	**< 0.001**	− 0.007(− 0.010 to − 0.004)	**< 0.001**
Model 3	−2.34 (− 3.00 to − 1.69)	**< 0.001**	− 0.34 (− 1.18 to 0.50)	0.428	–	–
DBP						
Model 1	−3.85(− 4.88 to −2.82)	**< 0.001**	− 1.47 (− 2.78 to − 0.15)	**< 0.001**	−0.013 (− 0.017 to − 0.009)	**< 0.001**
Model 2	− 4.02 (− 4.96 to − 3.08)	**< 0.001**	− 2.34 (− 3.53 to − 1.15)	**< 0.001**	− 0.011(− 0.015 to − 0.007)	**< 0.001**
Model 3	−3.20 (− 4.05 to − 2.35)	**< 0.001**	− 0.06 (− 1.16 to 1.03)	0.909	–	–
MABP						
Model 1	− 4.37(−5.35 to −3.39)	**< 0.001**	− 1.84 (− 3.11 to − 0.56)	**< 0.001**	−0.014 (− 0.019 to − 0.010)	**< 0.001**
Model 2	− 4.40 (− 5.34 to − 3.47)	**< 0.001**	−2.69 (− 3.88 to − 1.50)	**< 0.001**	− 0.012(− 0.016 to − 0.007)	**< 0.001**
Model 3	−3.47 (− 4.31 to − 2.62)	**< 0.001**	−0.21 (− 1.31 to 0.89)	0.712	–	–

Model 1:unadjusted model; Model 2: adjusted for age, gender, axial length, BMI, waist, spherical equivalent, birth weight and gestational age; Model 3: adjusted for fellow vessel diameter additionally. *SBP* systolic blood pressure, *DBP* diastolic blood pressure, *MABP* mean arterial blood pressure, *AVR* arteriolar to venular ratio. Significant *p* values are bolded

In addition, smaller retinal arteriolar caliber was also found to be associated with current alcohol consumption, greater body mass index and higher levels of total homocysteine [20], incident clinical stroke, carotid atherosclerosis, incident heart disease and cardiovascular mortality, as well as metabolic syndrome [13]. Larger venular calibers had been shown to be associated with atherosclerosis [27], inflammation [20–22, 27–30], stroke, cardiovascular mortality [13, 31], cigarette smoking [20, 27, 32, 33], and the metabolic syndrome (hyperglycemia, central obesity, and dyslipidemia) [16, 34]. These findings suggested that retinal venular widening may has pleiotropic associations with cardiovascular risk factors and diseases, and was not a specific biomarker for hypertension [35].

There have been some studies on relationship of blood pressure with retinal vessel calibers in children. Mitchell [36] reported that higher childhood blood pressure was associated with retinal arteriolar narrowing but not with retinal venular caliber in children aged 6–8 years. They found that each 10-mmHg increase in systolic blood pressure was associated with narrowing of retinal arterioles by 2.08 μm in Sydney children and 1.43 μm in Singapore children. In high school students aged 12.7 years, they found that elevated blood pressure was associated with narrower retinal arterioles, and also with wider retinal venules in boys, with each 10-mmHg increase in MABP associated with 2.02-mm decrease in retinal arteriolar caliber, and 2.19 μm increase in CRVE in boys (the Sydney Childhood Eye Study. SCES) [37]. In a later study on Singapore children aged 4~ 5 years, Li et al. [38] found that higher systolic blood pressure was associated with narrower retinal arterioles and wider retinal venules, with each 10-mmHg increase associated with 2.00 μm of retinal arteriolar narrowing and 2.51 μm of retina venular widening. In 2012, Hanssen examined 578 school children aged 11.1 ± 0.6 years from secondary schools in Germany and found that diastolic blood pressure was not only independently associated with arteriolar narrowing, but also with venular narrowing [39]. Imhof found that systolic and diastolic BP were associated with arteriolar narrowing in 391 Switzerland children with an average age of 7.3 years, but they failed to find the association between BP and venular diameter [40].

According to the results of the above studies, we found that just like the roles of retinal venular diameter play on the BP in adults, the relationship between retinal venular diameter and BP in the childhood population is still in controversy.

Unlike the SCES [37] (The subjects of this study were comparable in age to our research), we didn't catch the finding that higher BP was associated with wider retinal venules in preadolescent boys. We speculated here that there are some possible reasons contributing to the discrepancy between the two results.

First, at present, there were some epidemiological studies on adolescent BP, but these studies had not reached the uniform conclusion related to the gender difference. Some studies showed a higher frequency of elevated BP in males than in females in children population based research [41], but these results differed from those obtained by Rosner B, whose study found that the prevalence of elevated BP significantly increased among girls (8.2% versus 12.6%; *P* = 0.007), but was only of borderline significance among boys (15.8% versus 19.2%; *P*

Table 4 Subgroup analysis stratified by potential effect modifiers of retinal Arteriolar Diameter with BP, stratified by potential modifiers

Potential Effect Modifiers			n	Retinal Arteriolar Diameter (µm)					
				Model 1	p	Model 2	P	Model 3	P
SBP	Age	10 + 11	70	−1.97 ± 1.66	0.238	−0.60 ± 1.79	0.736	−1.28 ± 1.54	0.411
		12	1122	−3.63 ± 0.43	**< 0.01**	− 3.31 ± 0.42	**<.001**	− 2.46 ± 0.39	**<.001**
		13 + 14 + 15	309	−2.6 ± 0.82	**< 0.01**	− 2.60 ± 0.84	**0.002**	−1.98 ± 0.73	**0.007**
	Sex	Male	792	−3.1 ± 0.52	**< 0.01**	− 3.41 ± 0.52	**<.001**	−2.57 ± 0.45	**<.001**
		Female	709	−3.05 ± 0.52	**< 0.01**	− 2.73 ± 0.52	**<.001**	−2.12 ± 0.49	**<.001**
	BMI	Upper 50%	750	−2.37 ± 0.57	**< 0.01**	−2.39 ± 0.5	**<.001**	−1.72 ± 0.49	**<.001**
		Lower 50%	751	−4.03 ± 0.55	**< 0.01**	−3.71 ± 0.52	**<.001**	−2.89 ± 0.46	**<.001**
	Birth weight	Upper 50%	778	−3.69 ± 0.53	**< 0.01**	−3.09 ± 0.53	**<.001**	−2.35 ± 0.48	**<.001**
		Lower 50%	723	−2.87 ± 0.51	**< 0.01**	−2.97 ± 0.52	**<.001**	−2.28 ± 0.47	**<.001**
	Gestational age	Term	1372	−3.27 ± 0.39	**< 0.01**	− 3.10 ± 0.39	**<.001**	−2.33 ± 0.35	**<.001**
		Preterm	129	−3.06 ± 1.09	**< 0.01**	−2.46 ± 1.12	**0.03**	−2.21 ± 1.02	**0.033**
DBP	Age	10 + 11	70	−1.84 ± 2.04	0.370	−0.78 ± 2.18	0.722	− 1.81 ± 1.88	0.342
		12	1122	−4.85 ± 0.62	**< 0.01**	−4.74 ± 0.56	**<.001**	−3.76 ± 0.51	**<.001**
		13 + 14 + 15	309	−1.35 ± 1.11	**< 0.01**	−2.27 ± 1.08	**0.037**	−1.36 ± 0.95	0.154
	Sex	Male	792	−4.2 ± 0.74	**< 0.01**	− 4.65 ± 0.69	**<.001**	−3.67 ± 0.60	**<.001**
		Female	709	−3.68 ± 0.72	**< 0.01**	−3.46 ± 0.67	**<.001**	−2.79 ± 0.62	**<.001**
	BMI	Upper 50%	750	−3.33 ± 0.75	**< 0.01**	−3.73 ± 0.68	**<.001**	−3.06 ± 0.62	**<.001**
		Lower 50%	751	−4 ± 0.75	**< 0.01**	−4.30 ± 0.68	**<.001**	−3.34 ± 0.60	**<.001**
	Birth weight	Upper 50%	778	−3.83 ± 0.73	**< 0.01**	−3.73 ± 0.66	**<.001**	−3.01 ± 0.59	**<.001**
		Lower 50%	723	−3.92 ± 0.75	**< 0.01**	−4.31 ± 0.70	**<.001**	−3.42 ± 0.64	**<.001**
	Gestational age	Term	1372	−3.89 ± 0.55	**< 0.01**	−3.95 ± 0.51	**<.001**	−3.10 ± 0.46	**<.001**
		Preterm	129	−3.32 ± 1.57	**< 0.01**	−4.35 ± 1.50	**0.005**	−3.69 ± 1.39	**0.009**
MABP	Age	10 + 11	70	−2.21 ± 2.03	0.280	−0.81 ± 2.17	0.709	−1.83 ± 1.88	0.334
		12	1122	−5.22 ± 0.58	**< 0.01**	−5.01 ± 0.56	**<.001**	−3.91 ± 0.51	**<.001**
		13 + 14 + 15	309	−2.41 ± 1.09	**< 0.01**	−3.00 ± 1.09	**0.006**	−2.04 ± 0.95	**0.034**
	Sex	Male	792	−4.40 ± 0.70	**< 0.01**	−4.91 ± 0.68	**<.001**	−3.81 ± 0.59	**<.001**
		Female	709	−4.21 ± 0.70	**< 0.01**	−3.89 ± 0.68	**<.001**	−3.12 ± 0.64	**<.001**
	BMI	Upper 50%	750	−3.58 ± 0.75	**< 0.01**	−3.88 ± 0.68	**<.001**	−3.06 ± 0.63	**<.001**
		Lower 50%	751	−4.90 ± 0.73	**< 0.01**	− 4.87 ± 0.68	**<.001**	−3.81 ± 0.60	**<.001**
	Birth weight	Upper 50%	778	−4.68 ± 0.71	**< 0.01**	−4.31 ± 0.68	**<.001**	−3.40 ± 0.61	**<.001**
		Lower 50%	723	−4.11 ± 0.70	**< 0.01**	−4.42 ± 0.68	**<.001**	−3.49 ± 0.62	**<.001**
	Gestational age	Term	1372	−4.40 ± 0.53	**< 0.01**	−4.38 ± 0.51	**<.001**	−3.39 ± 0.46	**<.001**
		Preterm	129	−3.98 ± 1.49	**< 0.01**	−4.23 ± 1.47	**0.005**	−3.66 ± 1.35	**0.008**

Model 1:unadjusted model; Model 2: adjusted for age, gender, axial length, BMI, waist, spherical equivalent, birth weight and gestational age; Model 3: adjusted for fellow vessel diameter additionally. *SBP* systolic blood pressure, *DBP* diastolic blood pressure, *MABP* mean arterial blood pressure. Term means pregnancy lasts longer than 37 weeks, and preterm represents that the duration of pregnancy is less than 37 weeks. Significant p values are bolded

= 0.057), after analyzing a population-based sample of 3248 children in National Health and Nutrition Examination Survey (NHANES) III (1988–1994) and 8388 children in continuous NHANES (1999–2008), aged 8 to 17 years [42]. The female subjects in our study were more frequently shown to have elevated BP compared to males. The SCES did not present whether there was a significant difference between girl and boy blood pressure. If the BP of two genders were basically similar, the difference of the retinal venular caliber maybe associated with other reasons.

Second, in the SCES, with regard to the mechanism underlying the conclusion that higher blood pressure was associated with wider retinal venules in boys, the author deduced that maybe it was because sex hormones had an protective effect on the retinal circulation, as a

Table 5 Subgroup analysis stratified by potential effect modifiers of retinal Venular Diameter with BP, stratified by potential modifiers

Potential Effect Modifiers			n	Retinal Venular Diameter (µm)					
				Model 1	p	Model 2	P	Model 3	P
SBP	Age	10 + 11	70	0.40 ± 2.16	0.855	1.43 ± 1.99	0.476	1.78 ± 1.71	0.302
		12	1122	−2.1 ± 0.55	**< 0.001**	−2.52 ± 0.54	<.001	−0.73 ± 0.50	0.148
		13 + 14 + 15	309	− 0.53 ± 1.08	0.622	−1.61 ± 1.06	0.129	0.02 ± 0.94	0.986
	Sex	Male	792	−1.12 ± 0.66	0.092	−2.03 ± 0.65	**0.002**	0.14 ± 0.57	0.809
		Female	709	−1.72 ± 0.69	**0.013**	−2.15 ± 0.68	**0.002**	−0.85 ± 0.64	0.186
	BMI	Upper 50%	750	−1.66 ± 0.75	**0.028**	−2.11 ± 0.69	**0.002**	−0.84 ± 0.64	0.186
		Lower 50%	751	−2.67 ± 0.69	**< 0.001**	−2.13 ± 0.64	**0.001**	0.06 ± 0.58	0.923
	Birth weight	Upper 50%	778	−1.97 ± 0.68	**0.004**	−2.05 ± 0.67	**0.002**	−0.27 ± 0.61	0.654
		Lower 50%	723	−1.19 ± 0.67	0.074	−2.06 ± 0.66	**0.002**	−0.43 ± 0.61	0.478
	Gestational age	Term	1372	−1.61 ± 0.5	**0.001**	−2.19 ± 0.49	<.001	−0.46 ± 0.45	0.309
		Preterm	129	−1.13 ± 1.55	0.467	−0.88 ± 1.64	0.594	0.62 ± 1.53	0.688
DBP	Age	10 + 11	70	2.59 ± 2.64	0.330	2.16 ± 2.42	0.376	2.62 ± 2.08	0.213
		12	1122	−2.42 ± 0.79	**0.002**	−2.91 ± 0.72	<.001	−0.31 ± 0.67	0.648
		13 + 14 + 15	309	0.3 ± 1.45	0.838	−2.33 ± 1.36	0.089	−0.92 ± 1.20	0.442
	Sex	Male	792	−1.11 ± 0.94	0.239	−2.38 ± 0.86	**0.006**	0.60 ± 0.76	0.433
		Female	709	−1.96 ± 0.96	**0.042**	−2.35 ± 0.86	**0.007**	−0.69 ± 0.82	0.4
	BMI	Upper 50%	750	−1.42 ± 0.99	0.151	−2.12 ± 0.89	**0.017**	−0.10 ± 0.82	0.907
		Lower 50%	751	−2.11 ± 0.95	**0.026**	−2.46 ± 0.84	**0.004**	0.07 ± 0.76	0.93
	Birth weight	Upper 50%	778	−1.47 ± 0.93	0.112	−1.98 ± 0.84	**0.018**	0.18 ± 0.76	0.811
		Lower 50%	723	−1.48 ± 0.98	0.132	−2.65 ± 0.90	**0.003**	−0.28 ± 0.83	0.733
	Gestational age	Term	1372	−1.59 ± 0.71	**0.024**	−2.37 ± 0.64	<.001	−0.15 ± 0.58	0.798
		Preterm	129	−0.02 ± 2.2	0.994	−2.43 ± 2.23	0.278	0.18 ± 2.12	0.931
MABP	Age	10 + 11	70	1.92 ± 2.65	0.469	2.13 ± 2.41	0.38	2.61 ± 2.07	0.213
		12	1122	−2.75 ± 0.76	**< 0.001**	−3.32 ± 0.71	<.001	− 0.59 ± 0.67	0.38
		13 + 14 + 15	309	− 0.12 ± 1.43	0.933	−2.48 ± 1.37	0.072	−0.62 ± 1.21	0.609
	Sex	Male	792	−1.34 ± 0.89	0.133	−2.68 ± 0.85	**0.002**	0.47 ± 0.75	0.535
		Female	709	−2.25 ± 0.94	**0.017**	−2.76 ± 0.88	**0.002**	−0.90 ± 0.84	0.284
	BMI	Upper 50%	750	−1.89 ± 0.99	0.056	−2.63 ± 0.89	**0.003**	−0.55 ± 0.83	0.513
		Lower 50%	751	−2.85 ± 0.93	**0.002**	−2.74 ± 0.83	**0.001**	0.13 ± 0.76	0.868
	Birth weight	Upper 50%	778	−2.13 ± 0.91	**0.020**	−2.52 ± 0.86	**0.003**	−0.02 ± 0.78	0.978
		Lower 50%	723	−1.55 ± 0.92	0.093	−2.80 ± 0.87	**0.001**	−0.38 ± 0.81	0.643
	Gestational age	Term	1372	−1.94 ± 0.68	**0.004**	−2.78 ± 0.64	<.001	−0.33 ± 0.59	0.577
		Preterm	129	−0.72 ± 2.13	0.736	−2.07 ± 2.18	0.345	0.49 ± 2.07	0.812

Model 1: unadjusted model; Model 2: adjusted for age, gender, axial length, BMI, waist, spherical equivalent, birth weight and gestational age; Model 3: adjusted for fellow vessel diameter additionally. SBP systolic blood pressure, DBP diastolic blood pressure, MABP mean arterial blood pressure. Term means pregnancy lasts longer than 37 weeks, and preterm represents that the duration of pregnancy is less than 37 weeks. Significant p values are bolded

proportion of girls would have commenced puberty. But it was interesting that Zou found that in 76,869 Chinese girls, the rate of high blood pressure in menstruation group from 11 to 13 years was significant higher than that in the same age group of non-menstruation [43]. Similarly, there was conflicting evidence that hormone treatment could effectively reduce the risk of coronary heart disease, data from two large randomized clinical trials, the women's health initiative (WHI) [44] and the heart estrogen and progestin replacement study (HERS) [45], found an increase in cardiovascular incidences in women taking hormone replacement therapy. In some adult population based studies, estrogen replacement therapy was found to be associated with narrower retinal arteriolar and venular calibers [46], independent of blood pressure and other vascular factors, but other

Table 6 Subgroup analysis stratified by potential effect modifiers of AVR with BP, stratified by potential modifiers

Potential Effect Modifiers			n	AVR			
				Model 1	p	Model 2	P
SBP	Age	10 + 11	70	−0.010 ± 0.006	**0.118**	−0.007 ± 0.007	0.37
		12	1122	−0.010 ± 0.002	**<.001**	−0.007 ± 0.002	**<.001**
		13 + 14 + 15	309	−0.010 ± 0.003	**0.002**	−0.007 ± 0.004	0.05
	Sex	Male	792	−0.010 ± 0.002	**<.001**	−0.009 ± 0.002	**<.001**
		Female	709	−0.009 ± 0.006	**<.001**	−0.006 ± 0.002	**0.02**
	BMI	Upper 50%	750	−0.006 ± 0.002	**0.020**	−0.005 ± 0.002	0.06
		Lower 50%	751	−0.010 ± 0.002	**<.001**	−0.010 ± 0.002	**<.001**
	Birth weight	Upper 50%	778	−0.010 ± 0.002	**<.001**	−0.007 ± 0.002	**0.001**
		Lower 50%	723	−0.010 ± 0.002	**<.001**	−0.007 ± 0.002	**0.002**
	Gestational age	Term	1372	−0.010 ± 0.002	**<.001**	−0.007 ± 0.001	**<.001**
		Preterm	129	−0.010 ± 0.004	**0.035**	−0.008 ± 0.007	**0.015**
DBP	Age	10 + 11	70	−0.016 ± 0.008	**0.046**	−0.009 ± 0.009	0.314
		12	1122	−0.015 ± 0.002	**<.001**	−0.013 ± 0.002	**<.001**
		13 + 14 + 15	309	−0.007 ± 0.005	0.136	−0.003 ± 0.004	0.493
	Sex	Male	792	−0.016 ± 0.003	**<.001**	−0.014 ± 0.003	**<.001**
		Female	709	−0.011 ± 0.006	**0.003**	−0.009 ± 0.003	**0.009**
	BMI	Upper 50%	750	−0.011 ± 0.003	**<.001**	−0.011 ± 0.003	**<.001**
		Lower 50%	751	−0.012 ± 0.003	**<.001**	−0.012 ± 0.003	**<.001**
	Birth weight	Upper 50%	778	−0.013 ± 0.019	**<.001**	−0.011 ± 0.003	**<.001**
		Lower 50%	723	−0.013 ± 0.003	**<.001**	−0.012 ± 0.003	**<.001**
	Gestational age	Term	1372	−0.013 ± 0.002	**<.001**	−0.011 ± 0.002	**<.001**
		Preterm	129	−0.015 ± 0.007	**0.03**	−0.012 ± 0.007	0.137
MABP	Age	10 + 11	70	−0.016 ± 0.008	**0.048**	−0.009 ± 0.009	0.302
		12	1122	−0.015 ± 0.002	**<.001**	−0.013 ± 0.002	**<.001**
		13 + 14 + 15	309	−0.010 ± 0.005	**0.02**	−0.006 ± 0.005	0.192
	Sex	Male	792	−0.016 ± 0.002	**<.001**	−0.014 ± 0.002	**<.001**
		Female	709	−0.013 ± 0.003	**<.001**	−0.009 ± 0.003	**0.005**
	BMI	Upper 50%	750	−0.010 ± 0.003	**<.001**	−0.010 ± 0.003	**0.002**
		Lower 50%	751	−0.014 ± 0.003	**<.001**	−0.012 ± 0.003	**<.001**
	Birth weight	Upper 50%	778	−0.015 ± 0.003	**<.001**	−0.012 ± 0.003	**<.001**
		Lower 50%	723	−0.014 ± 0.003	**<.001**	−0.007 ± 0.007	**<.001**
	Gestational age	Term	1372	−0.014 ± 0.002	**<.001**	−0.012 ± 0.002	**<.001**
		Preterm	129	−0.016 ± 0.006	**0.018**	−0.012 ± 0.007	0.108

Model 1:unadjusted model; Model 2: adjusted for age, gender, axial length, BMI, waist, spherical equivalent, birth weight and gestational age. *SBP* systolic blood pressure, *DBP* diastolic blood pressure, *MABP* mean arterial blood pressure, *AVR* arteriolar to venular ratio. Term means pregnancy lasts longer than 37 weeks, and preterm represents that the duration of pregnancy is less than 37 weeks.Significant *p* values are bolded

researchers failed to found relationship between hormonal status in women and retinal vessel caliber [22]. Therefore, more and further researches were needed to acquire a greater depth of understanding on whether the hormone would have an effect on vessel diameter and would produce what kind of impact.

Third, the prevalence of child obesity is increasing rapidly worldwide, and the BMI may play an active role in the result of association of blood pressure and CRVE. Although a lot of literatures showed that the BMI was higher among boys than that of girls [47], Cole TJ reported that in population of 2–17 years of age, the prevalence of overweight is 25% in girls and 27% in boys, and obesity is 7 and 9% in males and females respectively [48]. In our studies, girls had a significantly higher BMI than boys ($P < 0.0001$). Obesity might influence the change of blood pressure by some mechanisms such as glomerular and tubular effects, and some of these mechanisms are sex dependent [49]. In the SCES research, they did not present the particular values of BMI for boys and girls. If the boys were more likely overweight just like that in other studies, they had a better chance to get wider venule than the same-aged girls. Although the BMI had been adjusted, high BMI might accompany by some possible physical abnormalities such as dyslipidemia, hyperglycemia and inflammation, which could result in wider retinal venules simultaneously.

Forth, lack of regular moderate-to-vigorous intensity physical activity is a well-known risk factor for cardiovascular disease, increasingly amount of studies have been focusing on the relationship between physical activity and retinal microcirculation and cardiovascular diseases [50]. Physical activity has been shown to be able to improve coronary endothelial function, reduce systemic blood pressure and improve early markers of atherosclerosis in pre-pubertal obese children. The association of higher levels of physical activity with better retinal vessel health have been demonstrated in adults as well as in children population [39, 51–53]. Before and during adolescence, girls usually undergo a lower level of physical exercise and greater decline in active physical activity than boys [54], which might explain the difference to some extent. Correspondingly, in our study, girls had higher waist circumference and BMI, which might result from insufficiency of physical activity compared with boys.

In addition to the reasons analyzed above, the association between blood pressure and retinal venular caliber might be affected by other factors such as smoking status [55], genetic and sex determinants, as well as ethnic differences. In summary, the association between BP and retinal venular caliber is a result of the interplay of many complicated reasons, maybe elevated blood pressure was associated with wider retinal venules in preadolescent boys, but due to the influence by comprehensive factors, the change was not significantly manifest in our study.

In the past, researchers had generally attributed a lower arteriolar-to-venular ratio (AVR) to generalized arteriolar narrowing and suggested that this ratio may provide information that would predict incident cardiovascular diseases. But with the advent of semi-automatic examination, it makes it possible to measure arteries and veins in retinal fundus separately. Since 2004, Ikram [27] and other researchers confirmed that elevated blood pressures were associated with smaller arteriolar diameters, but larger venular diameters were related to atherosclerosis, inflammation, and cholesterol levels. Hence, the idea that the AVR overall reflects generalized arteriolar narrowing should be reevaluated by taking into account the separate arteriolar and venular diameters. Therefore, many scholars suggested that arteriolar and venular diameters should be examined separately, especially in etiologic research [23]. In our study, we found that increasing blood pressure was significantly associated with narrowing retinal arteriolar caliber and smaller AVR, but not with retinal venular caliber.

Our results once again stressed the necessity of additional adjustment of concomitant vessels. We found a relationship between higher SBP and smaller CRVE, however, when CRAE was added to the final multivariate-adjusted model (model 3), the relationship between SBP and CRVE became nonsignificant, and further adjustment of the caliber of the CRVE diminished the reduction magnitude of CRAE when BP increased, suggesting the possibility of a confounding effect of fellow vessel caliber on this association. A significant association between narrower venular caliber and hypertension was initially reported in the Rotterdam Eye Study [23], but this result was diminished after additional adjustment with retinal arteriolar caliber, and the same conclusion was obtained by Myers [22]. The difference of the results illustrated the importance of correcting concomitant vessels.

Strengths of this study include its random cluster sample of a large number of representative healthy schoolchildren. The samples were free of influences from systemic disease processes or eye diseases on retinal vessel measurements. We also used a previously validated standardized protocol of quantitative retinal imaging program for retinal vessel measurement. However, some potential limitations of our study demand consideration. First, the study design is cross-sectional and does not provide temporal information on the associations. Second, the possible selection bias giving rise from the exclusion of students by ineligibility and ungradable retinal photographs may play a part on the real association between BP and retinal vessel diameters. Finally, we failed to acquire further information from our samples such as smoking status, family history, blood lipid levels, blood glucose, which may have an impact on the results.

In conclusion, this study shows that in population of 12-year-old Chinese children, increasing blood pressure was significantly associated with narrower retinal arteriolar caliber but not with retinal venular caliber, and possible confounding factors such as sex et al. had no effect on the relationship between BP and retinal vessel diameters. This finding provided further insight into the relationship of elevated BP on the microcirculation that occurs in early life. The association of wider retinal venular caliber and hypertension has not yet been consistently found, which should remain one of our highest research priorities.

Abbreviations

BMI: Body mass index; BP: Blood pressure; CRAE: Central retinal arteriolar equivalents; CRVE: Central retinal venular equivalents; DBP: Diastolic blood pressure; MABP: Mean arterial blood pressure; SBP: Systolic blood pressure

Acknowledgements

The authors thank the support from the Anyang city government for helping to organize the survey. We acknowledge the University of Wisconsin Fundus Photograph Reading Center and Nicola Ferrier of the School of Engineering at University of Wisconsin for providing the software of measuring retinal vessels calibers.

Authors' contributions

YH performed all of the retinal vessel pictures and wrote the whole manuscript. S-ML designed the study and supervised the progress of the entire study. M-TK, L-RL and HL participated in the design of the experiment, data collection and analysis. S-FW and A-RR undertook the statistical analysis of sample data. NW designed the study, supervised the progress of the entire study, revised the manuscript and finally agreed to submission. All authors read and approved the final manuscript.

Competing interests

All of the authors declare that they have no competing interests.

Author details

[1]Beijing Tongren Eye Center, Beijing Tongren Hospital, Beijing Ophthalmology & Visual Science Key Lab, Beijing Institute of Ophthalmology, Capital Medical University, Beijing, China. [2]Anyang Eye Hospital, Anyang, Henan, China.

References

1. Gunn R. Opthalmocsopic evidence of (1) arterial changes associated with chronic renal diseases and (2) of increased arterial tension. Trans Ophthalmol Soc UK. 1892;12:124–5.
2. Schneider R, Rademacher M, Wolf S. Lacunar infarcts and white matter attenuation. Ophthalmologic and microcirculatory aspects of the pathophysiology. Stroke. 1993;24(12):1874–9.
3. Hubbard LD, Brothers RJ, King WN, Clegg LX, Klein R, Cooper LS, Sharrett AR, Davis MD, Cai J. Methods for evaluation of retinal microvascular abnormalities associated with hypertension/sclerosis in the atherosclerosis risk in communities study. Ophthalmology. 1999;106(12):2269–80.
4. Seidelmann SB, Claggett B, Bravo PE, Gupta A, Farhad H, Klein BE, Klein R, Di Carli M, Solomon SD. Retinal vessel calibers in predicting long-term cardiovascular outcomes: the atherosclerosis risk in communities study. Circulation. 2016;134(18):1328–38.
5. Rizzoni D, Muiesan ML. Retinal vascular caliber and the development of hypertension: a meta-analysis of individual participant data. J Hypertens. 2014;32(2):225–7.
6. Gopinath B, Chiha J, Plant AJ, Thiagalingam A, Burlutsky G, Kovoor P, Liew G, Mitchell P. Associations between retinal microvascular structure and the severity and extent of coronary artery disease. Atherosclerosis. 2014;236(1):25–30.
7. Kawasaki R, Xie J, Cheung N, Lamoureux E, Klein R, Klein BE, Cotch MF, Sharrett AR, Shea S, Wong TY. Retinal microvascular signs and risk of stroke: the multi-ethnic study of atherosclerosis (MESA). Stroke. 2012; 43(12):3245–51.
8. Hughes AD, Falaschetti E, Witt N, Wijetunge S, Thom SA, Tillin T, Aldington SJ, Chaturvedi N. Association of Retinopathy and Retinal Microvascular Abnormalities with Stroke and cerebrovascular disease. Stroke. 2016;47(11): 2862–4.
9. Lim LS, Cheung CY, Sabanayagam C, Lim SC, Tai ES, Huang L, Wong TY. Structural changes in the retinal microvasculature and renal function. Invest Ophthalmol Vis Sci. 2013;54(4):2970–6.
10. Karatzi K, Protogerou AD, Moschonis G, Tsirimiagou C, Androutsos O, Chrousos GP, Lionis C, Manios Y. Prevalence of hypertension and hypertension phenotypes by age and gender among schoolchildren in Greece: the healthy growth study. Atherosclerosis. 2017;259:128–33.
11. Liang YJ, Xi B, Hu YH, Wang C, Liu JT, Yan YK, Xu T, Wang RQ. Trends in blood pressure and hypertension among Chinese children and adolescents: China health and nutrition surveys 1991-2004. Blood Press. 2011;20(1):45–53.
12. Li SM, Liu LR, Li SY, Ji YZ, Fu J, Wang Y, Li H, Zhu BD, Yang Z, Li L, et al. Design, methodology and baseline data of a school-based cohort study in Central China: the Anyang childhood eye study. Ophthalmic Epidemiol. 2013;20(6):348–59.
13. Henderson AD, Bruce BB, Newman NJ, Biousse V. Hypertension-related eye abnormalities and the risk of stroke. Rev Neurol Dis. 2011;8(1–2):1–9.
14. Wong TY, Hubbard LD, Klein R, Marino EK, Kronmal R, Sharrett AR, Siscovick DS, Burke G, Tielsch JM. Retinal microvascular abnormalities and blood pressure in older people: the cardiovascular health study. Br J Ophthalmol. 2002;86(9):1007–13.
15. Sharrett AR, Hubbard LD, Cooper LS, Sorlie PD, Brothers RJ, Nieto FJ, Pinsky JL, Klein R. Retinal arteriolar diameters and elevated blood pressure: the atherosclerosis risk in communities study. Am J Epidemiol. 1999;150(3):263–70.
16. Jeganathan VS, Sabanayagam C, Tai ES, Lee J, Sun C, Kawasaki R, Nagarajan S, Huey-Shi MH, Sandar M, Wong TY. Effect of blood pressure on the retinal vasculature in a multi-ethnic Asian population. Hypertension research : official journal of the Japanese Society of Hypertension. 2009;32(11):975–82.
17. Sun C, Liew G, Wang JJ, Mitchell P, Saw SM, Aung T, Tai ES, Wong TY. Retinal vascular caliber, blood pressure, and cardiovascular risk factors in an Asian population: the Singapore Malay eye study. Invest Ophthalmol Vis Sci. 2008;49(5):1784–90.
18. Kawasaki R, Cheung N, Wang JJ, Klein R, Klein BE, Cotch MF, Sharrett AR, Shea S, Islam FA, Wong TY. Retinal vessel diameters and risk of hypertension: the multiethnic study of atherosclerosis. J Hypertens. 2009;27(12):2386–93.
19. Wong TY, Klein R, Klein BE, Meuer SM, Hubbard LD. Retinal vessel diameters and their associations with age and blood pressure. Invest Ophthalmol Vis Sci. 2003;44(11):4644–50.
20. Wong TY, Islam FM, Klein R, Klein BE, Cotch MF, Castro C, Sharrett AR, Shahar E. Retinal vascular caliber, cardiovascular risk factors, and inflammation: the multi-ethnic study of atherosclerosis (MESA). Invest Ophthalmol Vis Sci. 2006;47(6):2341–50.
21. Liew G, Sharrett AR, Wang JJ, Klein R, Klein BE, Mitchell P, Wong TY. Relative importance of systemic determinants of retinal arteriolar and venular caliber: the atherosclerosis risk in communities study. Archives of ophthalmology (Chicago, Ill : 1960). 2008;126(10):1404–10.
22. Myers CE, Klein R, Knudtson MD, Lee KE, Gangnon R, Wong TY, Klein BE. Determinants of retinal venular diameter: the beaver dam eye study. Ophthalmology. 2012;119(12):2563–71.
23. Ikram MK, Witteman JC, Vingerling JR, Breteler MM, Hofman A, de Jong PT. Retinal vessel diameters and risk of hypertension: the Rotterdam study. Hypertension. 2006;47(2):189–94.
24. Tanabe Y, Kawasaki R, Wang JJ, Wong TY, Mitchell P, Daimon M, Oizumi T, Kato T, Kawata S, Kayama T, et al. Retinal arteriolar narrowing predicts 5-year risk of hypertension in Japanese people: the Funagata study. Microcirculation (New York, NY : 1994). 2010;17(2):94–102.
25. Wang JJ, Rochtchina E, Liew G, Tan AG, Wong TY, Leeder SR, Smith W, Shankar A, Mitchell P. The long-term relation among retinal arteriolar narrowing, blood pressure, and incident severe hypertension. Am J Epidemiol. 2008;168(1):80–8.
26. Leung H, Wang JJ, Rochtchina E, Tan AG, Wong TY, Klein R, Hubbard LD, Mitchell P. Relationships between age, blood pressure, and retinal vessel diameters in an older population. Invest Ophthalmol Vis Sci. 2003;44(7):2900–4.
27. Ikram MK, de Jong FJ, Vingerling JR, Witteman JC, Hofman A, Breteler MM, de Jong PT. Are retinal arteriolar or venular diameters associated with markers for cardiovascular disorders? The Rotterdam study. Invest Ophthalmol Vis Sci. 2004;45(7):2129–34.
28. Wong TY, Duncan BB, Golden SH, Klein R, Couper DJ, Klein BE, Hubbard LD, Sharrett AR, Schmidt MI. Associations between the metabolic syndrome and retinal microvascular signs: the atherosclerosis risk in communities study. Invest Ophthalmol Vis Sci. 2004;45(9):2949–54.
29. de Jong FJ, Ikram MK, Witteman JC, Hofman A, de Jong PT, Breteler MM. Retinal vessel diameters and the role of inflammation in cerebrovascular disease. Ann Neurol. 2007;61(5):491–5.

30. Yim-Lui Cheung C, Wong TY, Lamoureux EL, Sabanayagam C, Li J, Lee J, Tai ES. C-reactive protein and retinal microvascular caliber in a multiethnic asian population. Am J Epidemiol. 2010;171(2):206–13.

31. McGeechan K, Liew G, Macaskill P, Irwig L, Klein R, Klein BE, Wang JJ, Mitchell P, Vingerling JR, de Jong PT, et al. Prediction of incident stroke events based on retinal vessel caliber: a systematic review and individual-participant meta-analysis. Am J Epidemiol. 2009;170(11):1323–32.

32. Klein R, Klein BE, Knudtson MD, Wong TY, Tsai MY. Are inflammatory factors related to retinal vessel caliber? The beaver dam eye study. Archives of ophthalmology (Chicago, Ill : 1960). 2006;124(1):87–94.

33. Kifley A, Liew G, Wang JJ, Kaushik S, Smith W, Wong TY, Mitchell P. Long-term effects of smoking on retinal microvascular caliber. Am J Epidemiol. 2007;166(11):1288–97.

34. Nguyen TT, Wang JJ, Sharrett AR, Islam FM, Klein R, Klein BE, Cotch MF, Wong TY. Relationship of retinal vascular caliber with diabetes and retinopathy: the multi-ethnic study of atherosclerosis (MESA). Diabetes Care. 2008;31(3):544–9.

35. Ding J, Wai KL, McGeechan K, Ikram MK, Kawasaki R, Xie J, Klein R, Klein BB, Cotch MF, Wang JJ, et al. Retinal vascular caliber and the development of hypertension: a meta-analysis of individual participant data. J Hypertens. 2014;32(2):207–15.

36. Mitchell P, Cheung N, de Haseth K, Taylor B, Rochtchina E, Islam FM, Wang JJ, Saw SM, Wong TY. Blood pressure and retinal arteriolar narrowing in children. Hypertension. 2007;49(5):1156–62.

37. Gopinath B, Baur LA, Wang JJ, Teber E, Liew G, Cheung N, Wong TY, Mitchell P. Blood pressure is associated with retinal vessel signs in preadolescent children. J Hypertens. 2010;28(7):1406–12.

38. Li LJ, Cheung CY, Liu Y, Chia A, Selvaraj P, Lin XY, Chan YM, Varma R, Mitchell P, Wong TY, et al. Influence of blood pressure on retinal vascular caliber in young children. Ophthalmology. 2011;118(7):1459–65.

39. Hanssen H, Siegrist M, Neidig M, Renner A, Birzele P, Siclovan A, Blume K, Lammel C, Haller B, Schmidt-Trucksass A, et al. Retinal vessel diameter, obesity and metabolic risk factors in school children (JuvenTUM 3). Atherosclerosis. 2012;221(1):242–8.

40. Imhof K, Zahner L, Schmidt-Trucksass A, Hanssen H. Association of body composition and blood pressure categories with retinal vessel diameters in primary school children. Hypertension research : official journal of the Japanese Society of Hypertension. 2016;39(6):423–9.

41. Reed KE, Warburton DE, McKay HA. Determining cardiovascular disease risk in elementary school children: developing a healthy heart score. Journal of sports science & medicine. 2007;6(1):142–8.

42. Rosner B, Cook NR, Daniels S, Falkner B. Childhood blood pressure trends and risk factors for high blood pressure: the NHANES experience 1988-2008. Hypertension. 2013;62(2):247–54.

43. Zou ZY, Ma J, Wang HJ, Fu LG, Dong B, Yang YD. Association between early age at menarche and blood pressure in Chinese girls aged 7 to 17 years. Zhonghua yu fang yi xue za zhi [Chinese journal of preventive medicine]. 2013;47(8):726–30.

44. Rossouw JE, Anderson GL, Prentice RL, LaCroix AZ, Kooperberg C, Stefanick ML, Jackson RD, Beresford SA, Howard BV, Johnson KC, et al. Risks and benefits of estrogen plus progestin in healthy postmenopausal women: principal results from the Women's Health Initiative randomized controlled trial. Jama. 2002;288(3):321–33.

45. Hulley S, Grady D, Bush T, Furberg C, Herrington D, Riggs B, Vittinghoff E. Randomized trial of estrogen plus progestin for secondary prevention of coronary heart disease in postmenopausal women. Heart and estrogen/progestin replacement study (HERS) research group. Jama. 1998;280(7):605–13.

46. Wong TY, Knudtson MD, Klein BE, Klein R, Hubbard LD. Estrogen replacement therapy and retinal vascular caliber. Ophthalmology. 2005; 112(4):553–8.

47. Kelishadi R, Heshmat R, Motlagh ME, Majdzadeh R, Keramatian K, Qorbani M, Taslimi M, Aminaee T, Ardalan G, Poursafa P, et al. Methodology and early findings of the third survey of CASPIAN study: a National School-based Surveillance of Students' high risk behaviors. International journal of preventive medicine. 2012;3(6):394–401.

48. Cole TJ, Bellizzi MC, Flegal KM, Dietz WH. Establishing a standard definition for child overweight and obesity worldwide: international survey. BMJ (Clinical research ed). 2000;320(7244):1240–3.

49. Regitz-Zagrosek V, Lehmkuhl E, Weickert MO. Gender differences in the metabolic syndrome and their role for cardiovascular disease. Clin. Res. Cardiol.: official journal of the German Cardiac Society. 2006;95(3):136–47.

50. Gerber M, Endes K, Herrmann C, Colledge F, Brand S, Donath L, Faude O, Puhse U, Hanssen H, Zahner L. Does physical fitness buffer the relationship between psychosocial stress, retinal vessel diameters, and blood pressure among primary schoolchildren? Biomed Res Int. 2016;2016:6340431.

51. Tikellis G, Anuradha S, Klein R, Wong TY. Association between physical activity and retinal microvascular signs: the atherosclerosis risk in communities (ARIC) study. Microcirculation (New York, NY : 1994). 2010; 17(5):381–93.

52. Anuradha S, Healy GN, Dunstan DW, Klein R, Klein BE, Cotch MF, Wong TY, Owen N. Physical activity, television viewing time, and retinal microvascular caliber: the multi-ethnic study of atherosclerosis. Am J Epidemiol. 2011; 173(5):518–25.

53. Imhof K, Zahner L, Schmidt-Trucksass A, Faude O, Hanssen H. Influence of physical fitness and activity behavior on retinal vessel diameters in primary schoolchildren. Scand J Med Sci Sports. 2016;26(7):731–8.

54. Nader PR. National Institute of child H, human development study of early child C, youth development N: frequency and intensity of activity of third-grade children in physical education. Arch Pediatr Adolesc Med. 2003;157(2):185–90.

55. Karp I, O'Loughlin J, Paradis G, Hanley J, Difranza J. Smoking trajectories of adolescent novice smokers in a longitudinal study of tobacco use. Ann Epidemiol. 2005;15(6):445–52.

5

Evaluation of the effectiveness of combined femtosecond laser-assisted cataract surgery and femtosecond laser astigmatic keratotomy in improving post-operative visual outcomes

Jing Wang, Jiangyue Zhao, Jun Xu and Jinsong Zhang[*] ⓘ

Abstract

Background: To determine postoperative refractive and visual outcomes and astigmatic changes after femtosecond laser astigmatic keratotomy in femtosecond laser-assisted cataract surgery (FLACS).

Methods: This was a prospective interventional case series. Patients with age-related cataract and corneal astigmatism (1.0–3.0D) were treated with FLACS and femtosecond laser astigmatic keratotomy (FSAK). All patients underwent examinations before and 3 months after surgery; visual acuity, subjective and objective refraction, and corneal astigmatism were evaluated and recorded for all patients by using an OPD-Scan III topographer. Vector analysis of astigmatic changes was performed by using the Alpins vector method.

Results: Twenty-five patients were included in the study. Postoperatively, refractive and corneal astigmatism were both reduced significantly ($P < 0.05$), concurrent with improved uncorrected distance visual acuity and corrected distance visual acuity. The rate of spectacle use was significantly reduced at 3 months postoperatively ($P = 0.001$). The mean magnitude of the target-induced astigmatism vector (1.40 ± 0.37D) was slightly higher than the mean magnitude of the surgically induced astigmatism vector (1.22 ± 0.46D). The magnitude of error (-0.18 ± 0.36D), as well as the correction index (0.88 ± 0.29), demonstrated slight undercorrection. The angle of error was $0.85 \pm 13.69°$, which was close to zero.

Conclusions: Combined femtosecond laser-assisted cataract surgery and astigmatic keratotomy may be an effective approach to manage preoperative astigmatism in cataract surgery, although slight undercorrection may exist during short-term follow-up.

Trial registration: ChiCTR-TRC-14004977

Keywords: Femtosecond laser-assisted cataract surgery, Femtosecond laser astigmatic keratotomy, Astigmatism, Effectiveness

* Correspondence: cmu_zhangjinsong1@163.com
Department of Ophthalmology, the Fourth Affiliated Hospital of China Medical University, Eye Hospital of China Medical University,The Key Lenticular Laboratory of Liaoning Province, Shenyang 110005, China

Background

Modern cataract surgery has gradually evolved into a precise science, both for restoring visual acuity and for achieving emmetropia. Between 18 and 25% of patients undergoing cataract surgery exhibit > 1.5 diopters (D) of corneal astigmatism; 34–48% have > 1.0D [1, 2]. Naturally occurring and residual corneal astigmatism after cataract surgery both cause reduced uncorrected visual acuity and can contribute to glare, monocular diplopia, asthenopia, and other symptoms, leading to patient dissatisfaction. Treating preexisting corneal astigmatism to help meet patients' demands for complete, spectacle-free visual rehabilitation is a challenge for the modern ophthalmic surgeon.

Two major techniques for the correction of preexisting corneal astigmatism during cataract surgery are corneal incision and toric intraocular lens (IOL) implantation [3–5]. Primary corneal incisions (PIs) at the steeper corneal meridian, opposite clear corneal incisions (OCCIs), limbal relaxing incisions (LRIs), and astigmatic keratotomy (AK) are available options for astigmatism management by modifying the corneal incision. AK is an acceptable and effective procedure for correcting astigmatism, especially in patients with pre-existing corneal astigmatism. This technique uses paired or unpaired, partial-thickness incisions of a predetermined length at the steeper corneal meridian, in order to induce flattening of the steeper meridian while steepening the flatter meridian, known as the coupling effect. Good clinical outcomes of manual AK have been reported [6, 7]. However, manual AK is often associated with unpredictable results, and its accuracy and reproducibility are limited by the depth, length, and location of the incisions. Advances in femtosecond laser-assisted cataract surgery (FLACS) technology have provided a new alternative for performing AK. Femtosecond laser astigmatic keratotomy (FSAK) is a technique that uses a femtosecond laser to make paired or unpaired, partial-thickness, arcuate incisions of a pre-specified length at the steeper corneal meridian [8, 9]. Programmed and standardized FSAK can create incisions with a precise angle, depth, and location, which can significantly improve the predictability of corneal astigmatism correction. The purpose of this study was to determine postoperative refractive and visual outcomes and astigmatic changes after FSAK in FLACS.

Methods

Study design and patients

This prospective interventional case series included patients at the Department of Ophthalmology, the Fourth Affiliated Hospital of China Medical University, between July 2014 and July 2015. The clinical study focused on the safety and effectiveness of FSAK; it was performed in accordance with the tenets of the Declaration of Helsinki and approved by the institutional ethics committee. Each patient was informed of the risks and benefits of the procedure and provided written informed consent. All patients underwent a detailed preoperative ophthalmologic evaluation, including slit-lamp biomicroscopy, fundus evaluation, measurement of axial length and biometry, corneal topography, and noncontact specular microscopy. Patients who presented with the following were excluded from the study: corneal astigmatism >3D, poorly dilated (< 6.0 mm) pupil, small palpebral fissure, nystagmus or obvious eyelid spasm, clear corneal leukoma, hypermature cataract, glaucoma, inflammatory or infectious pathology of the eye, or other pre-existing eye diseases, such as iris neovascularization, exfoliation syndrome, diabetic retinopathy, history of uveitis, optic atrophy, or ocular tumors.

Surgical technique

Procedure for FLACS combined with FSAK

All surgeries were performed by the same experienced surgeon with the contact system LenSx (Alcon, Fort Worth, TX, USA) for laser pretreatment and Infiniti (Alcon) machine for phacoemulsification. Before surgery, all patients were treated with levofloxacin eye drops (Cravit Santen) four times daily for 3 days and pranoprofen eye drops (Pranopulin, Senju) four times daily for 1 day. On the day of surgery, patients received tropicamide and phenylephrine eye drops (Mydrin-P, Santen) for pupillary dilation (> 6.0 mm) and proparacaine hydrochloride (Alcaine, Alcon) for topical anesthesia. The patients were placed in a supine position and a speculum was placed to open the eye. Docking and suction procedures were completed by adjusting the position of the patient interface (PI) (SoftFit™) to ensure that the curved contact lens applanated the cornea. A spectral-domain optical coherence tomography (OCT) imaging device was utilized to scan the patient's eye and locate specific target areas. After manual verification of each procedural step (corneal incisions, capsulotomy, and lens fragmentation parameters), laser treatment was performed. The patient was then transferred for the subsequent operation. After the corneal incisions and arcuate incisions were separated by blades, the anterior chamber was filled with a viscoelastic solution (Provisc; Alcon). Next, the cut anterior capsule was removed by using capsulorhexis forceps, and hydrodissection was performed. After hydrodissection, phacoemulsification of the nucleus and aspiration of the residual cortex were performed with the Infiniti phacoemulsification system. Finally, a monofocal aspheric foldable IOL (Acrysof IQ; Alcon) was implanted in the capsular bag and the corneal incisions were hydrated.

FSAK design

Combined phacoemulsification and arcuate keratotomy was performed by using the LenSx (version 2.23) femtosecond laser platform, which was guided by a real-time intraoperative spectral-domain OCT. On the basis of measurements of the corneal astigmatic axis made by preoperative corneal topography, a single arcuate keratotomy incision was paired with the 3.0-mm primary corneal incision for phacoemulsification, which was located at the corneal steep meridian. The width of FSAK was calculated online by using the Donnenfield Nomogram (http://www.lricalculator.com); a conversion arc, 9.0 mm in diameter, was needed by using LRI-incision size multiplied by 9/11. Before surgery began, the patient was seated at a slit-lamp with head aligned vertically and the corneal limbus was marked at the 0° and 180° positions with a sterile marker. The femtosecond laser energy was set at 3.0 μJ, and spot and layer separation were set at 4 μm. Keratotomy incision was placed at 85% depth of corneal thickness; the side-cut angle was set at 90 degrees at a 9.0-mm arc diameter. The primary corneal incision had a tri-planar configuration with a width of 3.0 mm, and was located at the steeper corneal meridian. One secondary incision with a width of 1.0 mm was located 90 degrees from the primary corneal incision. An example of the programmed FSAK in FLACS is shown in Fig. 1.

Preoperative and postoperative examinations

All patients underwent examinations before surgery and 3 months after surgery, performed by the same ophthalmic technician. Preoperatively, all patients underwent an extensive ophthalmic evaluation that included slit-lamp examination, tonometry, uncorrected distance visual acuity (UDVA), corrected distance visual acuity (CDVA), manifest refraction, dilated fundoscopy, non-contact specular microscopy (SP2000P, Topcon), and corneal topography (OPD-Scan III, Nidek). At the 3-month follow up, slit-lamp examination, tonometry, UDVA, CDVA, manifest refraction, and corneal topography were repeated. Preoperative and postoperative UDVA and CDVA, manifest refraction spherical equivalent (MRSE), and the refractive and corneal astigmatisms were recorded; vector analysis of the astigmatic changes was performed by using the Alpins vector method.

Vector analysis of astigmatic changes

Keratometric astigmatic changes were evaluated 3 months postoperatively by vector analysis with the Alpins method [10–12]. The Alpins method allows evaluation by three fundamental vectors: (1) target-induced astigmatism (TIA) vector, defined as the astigmatic change that the surgery was intended to induce, (2) surgically induced astigmatism (SIA) vector, defined as the astigmatic change that the surgery actually induced, and (3) difference vector (DV), defined as the induced astigmatic change that would enable the initial surgery to achieve its intended target.

Furthermore, relationships among these three fundamental vectors were calculated at follow-up: (1) magnitude of error (ME), defined as the arithmetic difference between the magnitudes of SIA and TIA (ME > 0 indicates overcorrection and ME < 0 indicates undercorrection),

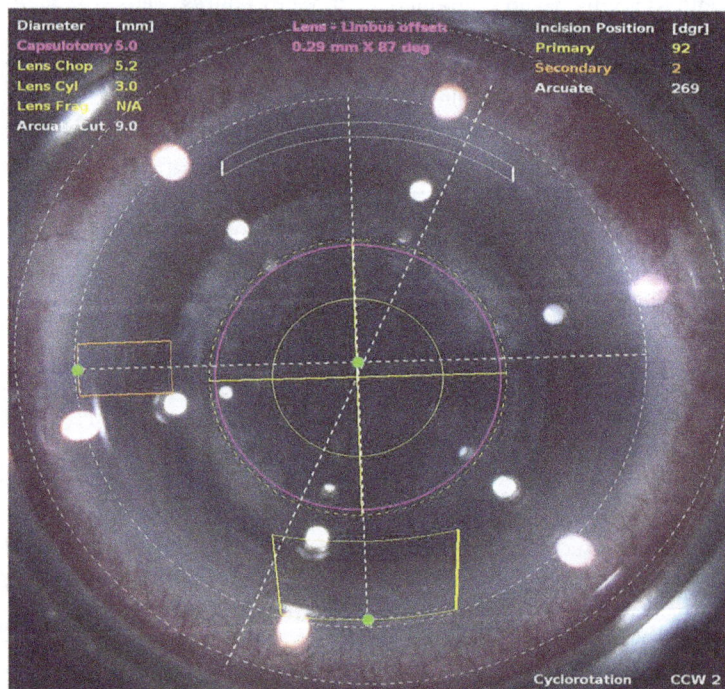

Fig. 1 An example of the programmed femtosecond laser-assisted astigmatic keratotomy in femtosecond laser assisted cataract surgery

(2) angle of error (AE), which is the angle described by the vectors of SIA versus TIA (AE close to zero indicates no significant systematic error of misaligned treatment), (3) correction index (CI), the ratio of SIA to TIA (CI > 1 indicates overcorrection; CI < 1 indicates undercorrection), (4) index of success (IOS), which is the ratio of DV to TIA (indicates the success rate in correction of astigmatism), (5) flattening index (FI), the proportion of SIA that is effective in reducing astigmatism at the intended meridian.

Statistical analysis

All descriptive statistical analyses were performed with SPSS software (version 17.0, SPSS, Inc.). The numerical data were expressed as $\chi \pm s$ and the percentage data were expressed in %. A P-value < 0.05 was considered statistically significant. Student's t-test was applied to compare refractive astigmatism, corneal astigmatism, MRSE, UDVA, and CDVA preoperatively and 3 months postoperatively. The χ^2 test was used to analyze the rate of wearing spectacles.

Results

This study analyzed 25 eyes of 25 patients. Of the 25 eyes, 11 (44%) belonged to men and 14 (56%) to women. The mean age of the patients was 68.56 ± 8.41 years at the time of surgery (range: 55–89 years). FLACS combined with FSAK was successfully performed on all 25 patients without incision-related complications.

Visual acuity and astigmatic change

The mean preoperative refractive astigmatism was 1.57 ± 1.27D, which was significantly reduced to 0.70 ± 0.36D at 3 months postoperatively ($P = 0.001$). There was a statistically significant reduction in corneal astigmatism from preoperative levels (1.41 ± 0.39D) to levels (0.69 ± 0.31D) at 3 months postoperatively ($P = 0.000$). The MRSE showed no significant difference ($P = 0.087$) between preoperative and postoperative values. Statistically significant improvements in UDVA and CDVA were noted at 3 months postoperatively ($P = 0.005$ and $P = 0.009$, respectively). Table 1 shows astigmatic change and visual acuity outcomes in detail.

Rate of wearing spectacles

Three months after the surgery, only three patients (12%) needed spectacles for distant vision, which was significantly lower than the rate of 60% preoperatively ($P = 0.001$). All patients reported improvement in quality of vision and were satisfied with the treatment.

Vector analysis of astigmatism

Table 2 shows vector analysis outcomes with the Alpins method. The mean magnitude of TIA was 1.40 ± 0.37D, whereas the mean magnitude of SIA was slightly lower: 1.22 ± 0.46D (Fig. 2). The DV was 0.70 ± 0.29D and ME was − 0.18 ± 0.36D. These numbers demonstrate a slight undercorrection 3 months postoperatively. This analysis was confirmed by the CI (0.88 ± 0.29), IOS (0.51 ± 0.19), and FI (0.78 ± 0.25) values. A scatter plot of TIA vs. SIA at 3 months after FLACS combined with FSAK is shown in Fig. 2; this plot shows undercorrection, as well as TIA that is almost >1D. The AE (Fig. 3) was 0.85 ± 13.69°, which shows that the SIA was counter-clockwise to the TIA. A wide spread of AE was noted among all eyes (horizontal axis), signifying variable alignment of flattening. The AE is positive if SIA is on an axis counterclockwise to TIA, whereas AE is negative if SIA is clockwise to TIA. Figures 2 and 3 show a combination error related to the magnitude of the treatment and the axis of the treatment. Figures 4 and 5 show the distributions of preoperative and postoperative corneal astigmatism, respectively. The postoperative centroid is closer to zero and the ellipse around the centroid is smaller than that in the preoperative figure; this represents a significant reduction in corneal astigmatism after surgery.

Discussion

With progress in refractive cataract surgery, demands for precision have increased among both doctors and patients. Cataract surgery can simultaneously correct refractive problems, such as myopia, astigmatism, and presbyopia, along with restoring vision and improving quality of life. However, astigmatism remains a significant obstacle in achieving emmetropia; astigmatism can produce glare, monocular diplopia, asthenopia, and visual distortions, even at relatively low levels of astigmatism. Therefore, correction of preexisting corneal astigmatism is particularly

Table 1 Preoperative and 3 months postoperative astigmatic change and visual acuity outcomes

	Refractive astigmatism (D)	Corneal astigmatism (D)	MRSE (D)	UDVA (logMAR)	CDVA (logMAR)
Preoperative	1.57 ± 1.27	1.41 ± 0.39	− 1.93 ± 4.98	0.72 ± 0.23	0.40 ± 0.10
3 m-Postoperative	0.70 ± 0.36	0.69 ± 0.31	− 0.15 ± 0.91	0.13 ± 0.11	0.09 ± 0.10
t	3.674	10.115	−1.782	3.091	2.855
P	0.001*	0.000*	0.087	0.005*	0.009*

MRSE manifest refraction spherical equivalent, UDVA uncorrected distance visual acuity, CDVA corrected distance visual acuity
*$P \leq 0.05$

Table 2 Vector analysis outcome using Alpins method

	Mean	Range [a]
TIA(D)	1.40 ± 0.37	1.25, 1.55
SIA(D)	1.22 ± 0.46	1.02, 1.41
DV(D)	0.70 ± 0.29	0.58, 0.82
ME(D)	−0.18 ± 0.36	−0.33, 0.04
AE(°)	0.85 ± 13.69	−4.80, 6.51
CI	0.88 ± 0.29	0.76, 0.99
FI	0.78 ± 0.25	0.67, 0.88
IOS	0.51 ± 0.19	0.43, 0.59

TIA target-induced astigmatism, *SIA* surgically induced astigmatism, *DV* difference vector, *ME* magnitude of error, *AE* angle of error, *CI* correction index, *FI* flattening index, *IOS* index of success
[a]95% confidence interval

important. Astigmatism can often be managed by toric IOL implantation; several studies have evaluated the success of this technique [13, 14]. However, some patients are unwilling to choose toric IOL implantation because of the high risk of postoperative IOL rotation; alternatively, modifying corneal incisions can be performed to correct preexisting astigmatism.

There is controversy regarding the clinical understanding of various corneal incisions. AK is a technique of creating paired or unpaired partial thicknesses and incisions of a pre-specified length at the steeper corneal meridian, in order to flatten the steep meridian and reduce corneal astigmatism. The traditional manual AK incision is made closer to the corneal center, with a 6.0-mm arc diameter [15]. The traditional AK technique requires

nearly flawless surgical skills and is associated with a high risk of irregular astigmatisms, which are difficult to rectify and are associated with unpredictable complications; thus, the traditional AK technique is often performed to correct only moderate-to-high astigmatisms. With the introduction of FSAK, the precision of this procedure, including arc length, depth, and location, has been greatly enhanced relative to that of manual incisions, making it suitable for low-to-moderate corneal astigmatisms. FSAK creates single or paired arcuate corneal incisions at the steeper axis of astigmatism, through femtosecond laser guidance [16, 17]. The LRIs, also known as peripheral corneal relaxing incisions (PCRIs), are made more peripherally in the cornea. These incisions are easy to create and are associated with a lower risk of irregular astigmatism and unpredictable complications, making them suitable for low-to-moderate corneal astigmatism [18]. In clinical studies of FLACS combined with corneal refractive surgery, FSAK and femtosecond laser LRI (FS-LRI) are often considered as one entity. They are both defined as arcuate corneal incisions of 8.5–9.0-mm arc diameter at the steep axis of astigmatism, made through femtosecond laser assistance. FLACS can also be combined with the femtosecond laser nonpenetrating intrastromal astigmatic keratotomy (ISAK) to correct low-to-moderate astigmatism; in this technique, the incisions are made intrastromally and retain 60–100 μm of corneal tissue anteriorly and posteriorly [19–21].

The femtosecond laser is a pulsed laser with an ultra-short pulse duration in femtoseconds (10^{-15} s) and a

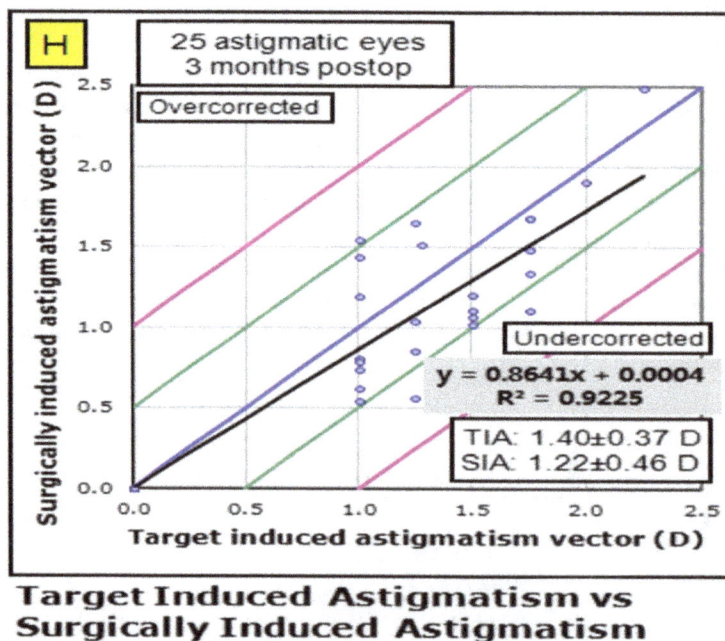

Fig. 2 The scatter plot of target induced astigmatism vs. surgically induced astigmatism

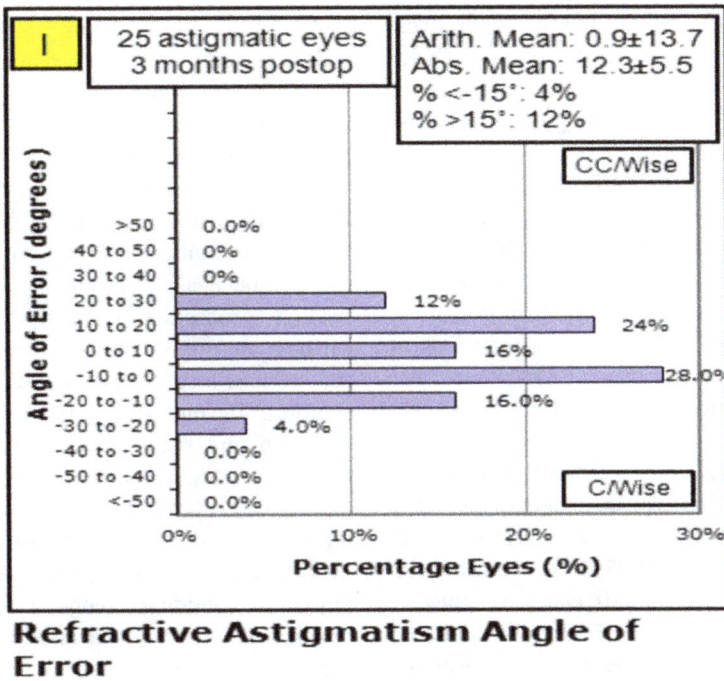

Refractive Astigmatism Angle of Error

Fig. 3 The angle of error was 0.85 ± 13.69°, indicating that the surgically induced astigmatism was counter-clockwise to the target induced astigmatism

near-infrared wavelength of 1030 nm. The femtosecond laser cuts tissue by vaporizing it into carbon dioxide, nitrogen, and other gases. The femtosecond laser hits its target accurately, with no damage to the surrounding tissue. Femtosecond laser-assisted surgery is also called precision medicine or precision surgery. Several clinical studies have demonstrated good refractive outcomes with different kinds of modified corneal incisions in FLACS. However, FSAK created by using a contact system (LenSx) in FLACS remains rare. Our study

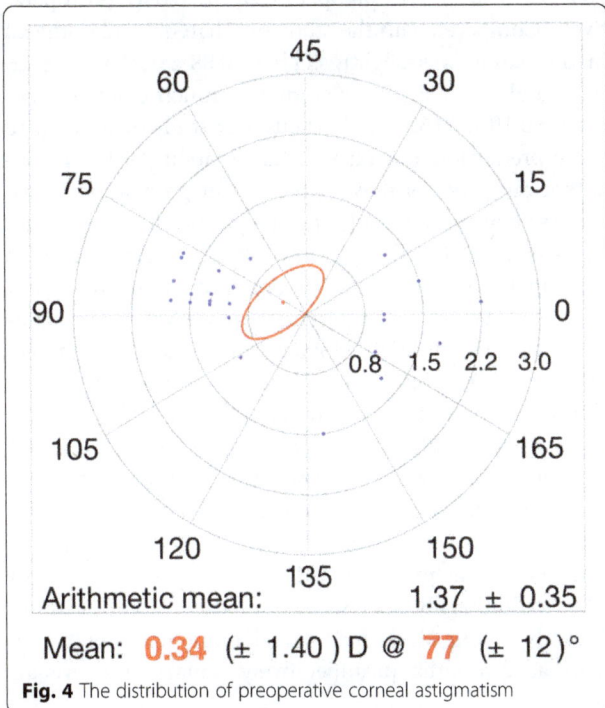

Arithmetic mean: 1.37 ± 0.35

Mean: **0.34** (± 1.40) D @ **77** (± 12)°

Fig. 4 The distribution of preoperative corneal astigmatism

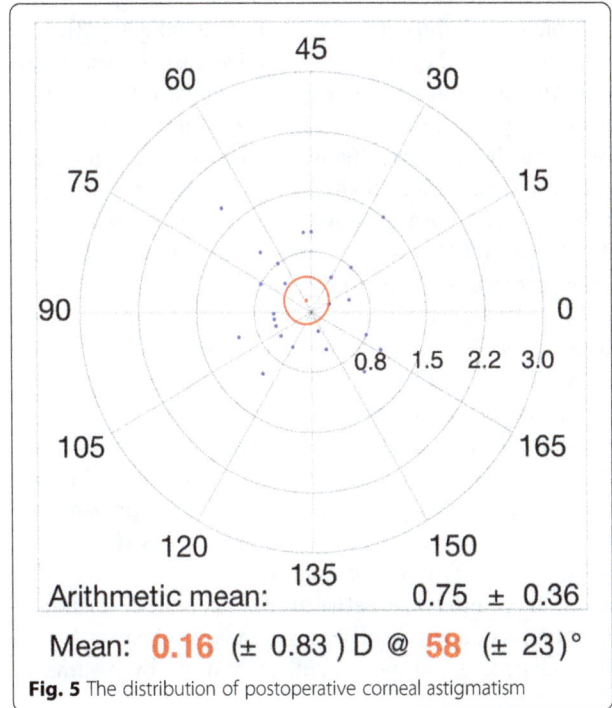

Arithmetic mean: 0.75 ± 0.36

Mean: **0.16** (± 0.83) D @ **58** (± 23)°

Fig. 5 The distribution of postoperative corneal astigmatism demonstrated that refractive astigmatism and corneal astigmatism were significantly reduced postoperatively (1.57D vs. 0.70D and 1.41D vs. 0.69D), concurrent with UDVA and CDVA improvement (logMAR values of 0.72 vs. 0.13 and 0.40 vs. 0.09). The rate of spectacle-wearing also significantly decreased 3 months postoperatively. This shows the effectiveness of FSAK in correcting pre-existing corneal astigmatism in cataract surgery, consistent with other similar studies. Yoo et al. [16] showed that the refractive astigmatism decreased significantly from 1.71D to 0.78D and corneal astigmatism decreased from 1.32D to 0.87D when patients underwent FSAK of the cornea (diameter = 9.0 mm; depth = 85%) to correct post-cataract residual astigmatism by using a 60-kHz IntraLase femtosecond laser. Similar results were reported by Rückl et al. [22]; they reported that the refractive astigmatism and corneal astigmatism both decreased significantly after ISAK, from 1.41D to 0.33D and 1.50D to 0.63D, respectively. ISAK was created for paired arcuate cuts on the steep axis placed completely within the corneal stroma, with a 7.5-mm arc diameter, by an iFS femtosecond laser. At present, the clinical application of manual AK is restricted because of a lack of reproducibility of incision length and depth, a potential for axis misalignment, and wound gape associated with epithelial ingrowth into the incisions. Compared with manual AK, FSAK has many advantages to help improve the accuracy and predictability of cataract surgery. The femtosecond laser can be delivered in a specified pattern and intrastromal depth can be preoperatively set with computer software [16]. FSAK is a more accurate procedure and creates a clearer wound, leading to fewer complications; thus, it is safer than manual AK [23].

Chan et al. [24], in a retrospective case series, evaluated the outcomes of FSAK combined with cataract surgery in eyes with low-to-moderate corneal astigmatism by using the VICTUS (Bausch & Lomb, Inc.) femtosecond laser platform. FSAK showed greater reduction of refractive and corneal astigmatism, 1.33D vs. 0.87D and 1.23D vs. 0.81D; vector analysis demonstrated slight undercorrection. Our study showed that the DV was 0.70 ± 0.29D and ME was − 0.18 ± 0.36D, with a CI of 0.88 ± 0.29. Undercorrection was also detected in our study. The meridian of primary corneal incisions may differ because of patient-specific differences in the steep axis, which may result in a difference between TIA and SIA. Compared with temporal corneal incisions, inferior corneal incisions can cause greater SIA, approximately 0.5D [25]. An unpredictable increase in FSAK incision depth during femtosecond laser pretreatment may also result in a difference between TIA and SIA. Further, it may be related to the offset laser caused by corneal folds or unexpected eye movement. In a study by Nejima et al. [26], anterior segment OCT showed that the depth of FSAK had deepened by 60 μm more than the specified setting. Mayer et al. [27] compared inflammatory cell response and morphological aspects of femtosecond laser-created corneal incisions; they found no differences in corneal inflammatory cell response, but observed a saw-tooth-like cutting edge and a significantly higher cell death rate than in the case of manually performed incisions, indicating an upregulated postoperative wound-healing response [28]. These may affect the healing process and biomechanical action, thereby causing an unpredictable correcting effect. Moreover, the incision location may change slightly due to eyeball rotation. In our study, the patient was seated at a slit-lamp and the corneal limbus was marked to improve accuracy. However, some errors remain in manual limbus marking, which can be resolved by the introduction of a cataract surgery navigation system. This system is the integration of multiple modules and functions, including preoperative measurement, surgery design, intraoperative navigation, and combination with femtosecond laser. In our previous studies, we found that corneal incisions without separation were self-sealing and had little effect on corneal curvature changes. Hence, we suggest that arcuate incisions ought to be separated by blades to achieve better refractive outcomes. However, sufficient quantitative indicators were not available to determine the necessity of FSAK manual separation in the present study: thus, this merits further research.

Our study demonstrated that corneal astigmatism decreased, from 1.41D preoperatively to 0.69D postoperatively. Compared with the study by Chan et al. [24], the CI in our study was slightly higher (0.88 ± 0.29 vs. 0.86 ± 0.52) and the IOS in our study was much closer to zero (0.51 ± 0.19 vs. 0.62 ± 0.45). Thus, our study demonstrated more predictable outcomes. The variability of the inconsistent outcomes of these two different pretreatment procedures may be the result of discrepancies in arc diameter and depth of FSAK incisions. We set parameters of a 9.0-mm arc diameter and 85% depth of corneal thickness, whereas Chan et al. set parameters of 8.5-mm arc diameter and 450-μm depth. Notably, FSAK incisions are deeper and more peripheral. We used a standard arcuate incision combined with only one primary and secondary incision each, rather than two 1.5-mm paired secondary incisions, which could also contribute to the variability in treatment effects. We set 3.0 μJ as the femtosecond laser energy, which was higher than the 1.7 μJ energy used by Chan et al.; this may have led to a stronger laser delivery effect. Additionally, analysis of results at 3 months postoperatively in our study may reveal more stable outcomes than at 2-months postoperatively. Finally, the arcuate keratotomy was separated with blades in our technique, although the duration of wound healing and stabilization remains to be elucidated in further studies.

Conclusions

In conclusion, the use of FSAK in FLACS was effective and promising for eyes with pre-existing corneal astigmatism. However, the combination of FLACS and FSAK can achieve more accurate and consistent outcomes through accurate preoperative topographic measurement and surgical design, sufficient education of patients to improve cooperation during laser pretreatment, adequate surgical experience and skill, and the use of cataract surgery navigation systems, such as the Zeiss Callisto Eye (Carl Zeiss AG, Dublin, CA, USA) and the Alcon Verion Image Guided System (Alcon) [29]. The limitations of the current study are its small sample size and 3-month short-term follow-up. Further work is required to verify the long-term refractive outcomes and refractive stability in large populations of cataract surgery candidates.

Abbreviations

AE: Angle of error; AK: Astigmatic keratotomy; CDVA: Corrected distance visual acuity; CI: Correction index; D: Diopters; DV: Difference vector; FI: Flattening index; FLACS: Femtosecond laser-assisted cataract surgery; FSAK: Femtosecond laser astigmatic keratotomy; IOL: Intraocular lens; IOS: Index of success; ISAK: Intrastromal astigmatic keratotomy; LRIs: Limbal relaxing incisions; ME: Magnitude of error; MRSE: Manifest refraction spherical equivalent; OCCIs: Opposite clear corneal incisions; OCT: Optical coherence tomography; PCRIs: Peripheral corneal relaxing incisions; PI: Patient interface; PIs: Primary corneal incisions; SIA: Surgically induced astigmatism; TIA: Target-induced astigmatism; UDVA: Uncorrected distance visual acuity

Funding

This research was supported by the National Natural Science Foundation of China (grant number 81470617).

Authors' contributions

JW collected the data and wrote the manuscript. JSZ and JYZ were responsible for the clinical management of the patients and the design of the study. JSZ and JX provided critical revision. All authors read and approved the final manuscript.

Competing interests

The authors declare that they have no competing interests.

References

1. Miyake T, Kamiya K, Amano R, Iida Y, Tsunehiro S, Shimizu K. Long-term clinical outcomes of toric intraocular lens implantation in cataract cases with preexisting astigmatism. J Cataract Refract Surg. 2014;40(10):1654–60.
2. Chen W, Zuo C, Chen C, Su J, Luo L, Congdon N, Liu Y. Prevalence of corneal astigmatism before cataract surgery in Chinese patients. J Cataract Refract Surg. 2013;39(2):188–92.
3. Mendicute J, Irigoyen C, Ruiz M, Illarramendi I, Ferrer-Blasco T, Montes-Mico R. Toric intraocular lens versus opposite clear corneal incisions to correct astigmatism in eyes having cataract surgery. J Cataract Refract Surg. 2009;35(3):451–8.
4. Nichamin LD. Treating astigmatism at the time of cataract surgery. Curr Opin Ophthalmol. 2003;14(1):35–8.
5. Amesbury EC, Miller KM. Correction of astigmatism at the time of cataract surgery. Curr Opin Ophthalmol. 2009;20(1):19–24.
6. Fares U, Mokashi AA, Al-Aqaba MA, Otri AM, Miri A, Dua HS. Management of postkeratoplasty astigmatism by paired arcuate incisions with compression sutures. Br J Ophthalmol. 2013;97(4):438–43.
7. Lindstrom RL. The surgical correction of astigmatism: a clinician's perspective. Refract Corneal Surg. 1990;6(6):441–54.
8. Vickers LA, Gupta PK. Femtosecond laser-assisted keratotomy. Curr Opin Ophthalmol. 2016;27(4):277–84.
9. Callou TP, Garcia R, Mukai A, Giacomin NT, de Souza RG, Bechara SJ. Advances in femtosecond laser technology. Clin Ophthalmol. 2016;10:697–703.
10. Alpins NA, Goggin M. Practical astigmatism analysis for refractive outcomes in cataract and refractive surgery. Surv Ophthalmol. 2004;49(1):109–22.
11. Reinstein DZ, Archer TJ, Randleman JB. JRS standard for reporting astigmatism outcomes of refractive surgery. J Refract Surg. 2014;30(10):654–9.
12. Krall EM, Arlt EM, Hohensinn M, Moussa S, Jell G, Alio JL, Plaza-Puche AB, Bascaran L, Mendicute J, Grabner G, et al. Vector analysis of astigmatism correction after toric intraocular lens implantation. J Cataract Refract Surg. 2015;41(4):790–9.
13. Titiyal JS, Khatik M, Sharma N, Sehra SV, Maharana PK, Ghatak U, Agarwal T, Khokhar S, Chawla B. Toric intraocular lens implantation versus astigmatic keratotomy to correct astigmatism during phacoemulsification. J Cataract Refract Surg. 2014;40(5):741–7.
14. Kessel L, Andresen J, Tendal B, Erngaard D, Flesner P, Hjortdal J. Toric intraocular lenses in the correction of astigmatism during cataract surgery: a systematic review and meta-analysis. Ophthalmology. 2016;123(2):275–86.
15. Inoue T, Maeda N, Sasaki K, Watanabe H, Inoue Y, Nishida K, Inoue Y, Yamamoto S, Shimomura Y, Tano Y. Factors that influence the surgical effects of astigmatic keratotomy after cataract surgery. Ophthalmology. 2001;108(7):1269–74.
16. Yoo A, Yun S, Kim JY, Kim MJ, Tchah H. Femtosecond laser-assisted arcuate keratotomy versus toric IOL implantation for correcting astigmatism. J Refract Surg. 2015;31(9):574–8.
17. Ng AL, Chan TC, Jhanji V, Cheng GP. Simple steep-axis marking technique using a corneal analyzer. J Cataract Refract Surg. 2017;43(2):153–5.
18. Muller-Jensen K, Fischer P, Siepe U. Limbal relaxing incisions to correct astigmatism in clear corneal cataract surgery. J Refract Surg. 1999;15(5):586–9.
19. Day AC, Lau NM, Stevens JD. Nonpenetrating femtosecond laser intrastromal astigmatic keratotomy in eyes having cataract surgery. J Cataract Refract Surg. 2016;42(1):102–9.
20. Marino GK, Santhiago MR, Wilson SE. Femtosecond lasers and corneal surgical procedures. Asia Pac J Ophthalmol. 2017;6(5):456–64.
21. Day AC, Stevens JD. Stability of keratometric astigmatism after non-penetrating femtosecond laser intrastromal astigmatic keratotomy performed during laser cataract surgery. J Refract Surg. 2016;32(3):152–5.
22. Ruckl T, Dexl AK, Bachernegg A, Reischl V, Riha W, Ruckhofer J, Binder PS, Grabner G. Femtosecond laser-assisted intrastromal arcuate keratotomy to reduce corneal astigmatism. J Cataract Refract Surg. 2013;39(4):528–38.
23. Kim P, Sutton GL, Rootman DS. Applications of the femtosecond laser in corneal refractive surgery. Curr Opin Ophthalmol. 2011;22(4):238–44.
24. Chan TC, Cheng GP, Wang Z, Tham CC, Woo VC, Jhanji V. Vector analysis of corneal astigmatism after combined femtosecond-assisted phacoemulsification and arcuate keratotomy. Am J Ophthalmol. 2015;160(2):250–255.e252.
25. Rainer G, Menapace R, Vass C, Annen D, Findl O, Schmetterer K. Corneal shape changes after temporal and superolateral 3.0 mm clear corneal incisions. J Cataract Refract Surg. 1999;25(8):1121–6.
26. Nejima R, Terada Y, Mori Y, Ogata M, Minami K, Miyata K. Clinical utility of femtosecond laser-assisted astigmatic keratotomy after cataract surgery. Jpn J Ophthalmol. 2015;59(4):209–15.

27. Mayer WJ, Klaproth OK, Hengerer FH, Kook D, Dirisamer M, Priglinger S, Kohnen T. In vitro immunohistochemical and morphological observations of penetrating corneal incisions created by a femtosecond laser used for assisted intraocular lens surgery. J Cataract Refract Surg. 2014;40(4): 632–8.
28. Hooshmand J, Vote BJ. Femtosecond laser-assisted cataract surgery, technology, outcome, future directions and modern applications. Asia Pac J Ophthalmol. 2017;6(4):393–400.
29. Hura AS, Osher RH. Comparing the Zeiss Callisto Eye and the Alcon Verion image guided system toric lens alignment technologies. J Refract Surg. 2017;33(7):482–7.

6

Antimicrobial efficacy of corneal cross-linking in vitro and in vivo for Fusarium solani: a potential new treatment for fungal keratitis

Ziqian Zhu[1], Hongmin Zhang[1], Juan Yue[1], Susu Liu[1], Zhijie Li[2] and Liya Wang[1]* ⓘ

Abstract

Background: Fungal keratitis is one of the major causes of visual impairment worldwide. However, the effectiveness of corneal collagen cross-linking (CXL) for fungal keratitis remains controversial. In this study, we developed an in vitro and an in vivo models to assess the efficacy of CXL for Fusarium keratitis.

Methods: The effect of in vitro CXL fungicidal was evaluated on the cultures of *Fusarium solani* which were exposed to irradiation for different durations. Viability of fungal was appraised under four conditions: no treatment (control); CXL: UVA (365 nm)/riboflavin; riboflavin and UVA (365 nm). Each batch of sterile plate culture was irradiated for different CXL durations.
The in vivo Therapeutic effect was studied on a mouse keratitis model. The animals were divided randomly into three groups: group A with no treatment (control); Group B with CXL treatment for two minutes and group C with CXL treatment for three minutes. The CXL procedure was performed 24 h post inoculation in each group. All mice with corneal involvement were scored daily for 7 days and 10 days after infection. Corneals were extracted at various time points for quantitative fungal recovery. Histological evaluations were conducted to calculate the number of polymorphonuclear cells.

Results: Viability of fungal decreased significantly in CXL group with 30-min irradiation compared with that in control, riboflavin and UVA groups ($P < 0.01$).
The colony-forming units (CFUs) of fungal solutions in culture significantly decreased with CXL treatment ($P < 0.05$). Clinical scores, corneal lesion, corneal opacity, neovascularization and the depth of ulceration scores in group B and group C were remarkably lower than that in group A ($P < 0.05$, $P = 0.001$, $P = 0.001$, $P = 0.034$ and $P = 0.025$ respectively). Scores of group C were much lower than that in group B. Histological revealed that destruction of corneal collagen fibers and infiltration of inflammatory cells into corneal tissue in group B and group C were much lower than that in group A.

Conclusions: We believe that CXL treatment may be applied to fungal keratitis, therapeutic efficacy will improve with longer treatment duration.

Keywords: Antifungal therapeutic use, Corneal collagen cross-linking, Fungal keratitis, Fusarium solani, Mice

* Correspondence: wangliya_55@126.com
[1]People's Hospital of Zhengzhou University and Henan Provincial People's Hospital, Henan Eye Institute, Henan Eye Hospital, Zhengzhou 450003, China
Full list of author information is available at the end of the article

Background

Fungal keratitis(FK), a major eye disease, is one of the leading causes of severe visual loss. In all cases of infectious keratitis, fungal keratitis accounts for approximately 61.9% in North China [1], 39% in North India [2] and 6–20% in the United States [3]. Filamentous fungi (such as *fusarium solani*) are the key pathogens of fungal keratitis [4]. The overall prevalence of fungal keratitis has a clearly increasing trend in recent years. However, the therapy of fungal diseases of the eye is unsatisfactory due to several reasons: Therapeutic efficacy of traditional treatment such as eye drops is very limited in clinical because of poor bioavailability together with serious side effects [5]. It was also reported that 27% to 66% of patients with FK required surgical intervention [6]. Furthermore, eye banks cannot match demand, which is particularly common in most developing countries. Therefore, a new method of treatment is urgently needed to control the infection process more effectively.

Techniques such as Corneal Collagen Cross-Linking(CXL), a combination treatment with ultraviolet (UVA) light and riboflavin (vitamin B2) were proposed by Wollensak in 2003 [7], which has become an established treatment option for improving the biomechanical stability and resisting the progression of keratoconus. Further indications for the clinical use of CXL emerged rapidly since then, including Fuch's corneal dystrophy [8], pseudophakic bullous keratopathy as well as infectious keratitis [9]. Recently the efficacy of CXL for the treatment was reported [10–12]. Although some cases of fungal keratitis were cured successfully, the efficacy of the CXL procedure in the management of fungal keratitis remains controversial [13–15].

In this study, we developed an in vitro and an in vivo model, to evaluate the inhibitory effects of the designed CXL against *F.solani* growth. We further explored the clinical and histological bio-pathology of mouse model of fungal keratitis to assess the anti-biofilm efficacy.

Methods

Fungi strains

F.solani (No.3.1791) was obtained from China General Microbiological Culture Collection Center (CGMCC, Beijing, China). After two or three subcultures, two milliliters of stroke-physiological saline solution(NS) were added to the slant medium containing well-grown *F. solani*. The fungal hyphae were ground with a sterile glass rod for making the fungal suspension, solution of which was adjusted by turbidimeter to get 0.5 Mx fungal suspension.

In vitro viability test by CXL

Suspension of 10ul was placed to grow in each well of a sterile 96-well plate (Corning Life Science, Lowell, MA, USA) filled with 100 μl of potato dextrose agar (PDA, Beijing Sanyao Technique Development Co. China) per well for 24 h of incubation at 25 °C [16, 17]. The microplate wells have an internal diameter of 6.40 mm, so that the entire area can be exposed to UVA from 7.00 mm diameter light source.

Under sterile conditions, with the mass fraction of 0.1% riboflavin photosensitizer 20ul after 30-min, the cultures of *F.solani* were exposed to irradiation for different durations (respectively two, five, ten, 20 and 30 min). Further, the fungal viability in plate cultures irradiated with UVA (30 min) were evaluated under four conditions: no treatment (control), CXL: UVA (365 nm)/ riboflavin, riboflavin and UVA (365 nm). Each process was repeated three times.

The standard procedure applied in the treatment of progressive keratoconus was followed to assess the antifungal effects of riboflavin and long-wave UVA irradiation. At a distance of 5 cm, fungal was exposed to laser irradiation. The size of the laser beam spot was 7 mm. The UVA (365 nm) has a power density of 45 mW/cm^2 and fungal beyond the irradiation scope was sheltered against light. After irradiation, the culture dishes were placed at 25 °C in an incubator for 48 h, photos of which were taken with a digital camera. Fungal gray values were analyzed by Image J software [18], and then the quantification of fungal cells viability was calculated.

Animals

In total, 150male C57BL/6 J mice, weighing from 24 g to 27 g were used. The animals were fed and handled in strict compliance with the ARVO Statement For the Use of Animals in Ophthalmic and Vision Research. The study was approved by the Henan Eye Hospital Institutional Committee. All mice were anesthetized with an intraperitoneal injection of pentobarbital sodium (80 mg/kg.b.w.) (Sigmae Aldrich, USA) before interventions. Topical anesthetic (1% tetracaine hydrochloride drops) was applied for local anesthesia of corneal. The cornea of each mouse was scarified using a sterile scalpel to create a superficial wound of intersecting marks in a grid pattern, as referred [19]. A sharpened bamboo toothpick (0.30 mm tip diameter, 1.10 mm tip length) was used to scrape along the scratch 2 to 3 times to create a rough surface. The scarified cornea was subsequently smeared with fungi for fungal infection. A positive model was confirmed by an observation from a confocal microscope detection of fungal hyphae and/or spores 24 h post-inoculation.

Corneal CXL treatment

The mice were divided randomly into three groups: group A. control group; group B. treated with CXL for two minutes; group C. treated with CXL for three minutes. Treatment started 24 h after fungal was smeared.

The corneal epithelium of mice was scraped each group of 2-mm fields (which is a standard method). Then group B and group C were initiated CXL treatment. The lesions were instilled immediately with 0.1% riboflavin solution at 5-min intervals until a yellow dye in the aqueous humor were confirmed in the anterior chambers under a slit lamp with a cobalt blue filter. The corneas were continuously exposed to UVA irradiation (365 nm; irradiance 45 mW/cm^2; CCL-365VARIO instrument: guangteng technology xiamen co.LTD).

Clinical examination

All mice were observed under a slit-lamp biomicroscopic and were scored accordance with the Schreiber scoring system [20] daily for 7 days and 10th day after modeling. Corneal lesion, the depth of ulceration, corneal opacity, edema, neovascularization were clinically evaluated on the 10 days. Corneal ulcers were graded as follows [21]: stage 0, no ulcer; stage 1, superficial ulcer; stage 2, medium-depth ulcer; stage 3, deep ulcer; stage 4, descemetocele; and stage 5, corneal perforation.

Corneal fungal plate count

Ten mice were randomly sacrificed in each group in 1, 3, 7, 10 days after modeling respectively, eyes were enucleated for quantitative fungal recovery confirmed by plate counts [22], 0.85% of the stroke-physiological saline solution(NS) was added to the cornea which was grounded with a grinding stick to release the fungus. The suspension was centrifuged at 2000 rpm for 10 min for collecting supernatant, then cultured on potato dextrose agar(PDA) at 25 °C for 2 days, the quantity of colonies was determined in all cultures.

Pathological observation of corneal tissue in mice

On the 10th day after treatment, mice went through cervical dislocation and the corneals were extracted for histopathological examination. The corneas of mice, with the mass fraction of 4% formaldehyde fixed after 24 h. Then the samples were embedded in paraffin and sagittally cut into 5-um-thick sections. Hematoxylin–eosin (HE) staining was used for histomorphological analysis of all groups. Observation was performed with the aid of a Nikon Eclipse E100 light microscope (Nikon, Sendai, Japan) under × 20 magnification. The disposition of collagen fibers, and inflammatory infiltration, were analyzed in terms of the microcorneal slices. Based on a scale of 0 to 4, the previously described inflammation score [23] was modified to the following: 0, no inflammation; 1, minimum change; 2. mild changes; 3. moderate changes; 4. severe changes.

Statistical analyses

Statistical analyses were made by applying the triplicate values of each experimental condition. The data were expressed as the mean ± SD. Fungal gray values for different durations were compared with the control group was determined by T-test. Wilcoxon matched sign rank test for 2 related samples was used to compare the 30-min intra-group values. Clinical score and corneal fungal plate count obtained for each mouse were given One-way ANOVA for multiple comparisons. When homogeneity of variance was detected, the least significant difference (LSD) was used. In all other instances, Tamhane's T2 test was performed. Pearson product correlation analysis was used to study the relationship between clinical score and corneal fungal plate count Nonparametric Kruskal–Wallis 1-way analysis of variance by rank were used for the corneal transformation. $P < 0.05$ was judged to be statistically significant. SPSS21.0 software (IBM, Inc., Chicago, IL, USA) was used for data analysis.

Results

In vitro

The fungal cells density was measured to determine the effect of CXL treatment on Fusarium. The strain under the CXL treatment exhibited a slightly lower growth rate than that without treatment (2 min: $P = 0.168$; 5 min: $P = 0.463$; 10 min: $P = 0.345$; 20 min: $P = 0.037$; 30 min: $P = 0.006$). Antifungal efficiency test of UVA on F. solani showed fungal cells density decreased significantly when the time of UVA irradiation increased (2、5、10、20 and 30 min) (Fig. 1a–c). The effect was maximal at 30 min ($P = 0.006$).

In vivo

Clinical examination

Clinical Schreiber scores obtained after infection indicated that there were statistically significant differences between CXL group and the control group ($P < 0.05$) (Fig. 2a, b). The longer the treatment time, the better keratitis recovered.

Corneal fungal plate count

There is a statistically significant difference between treatmen groups ($P < 0.05$) and Group A. The number of fungal colonies in Group C was much lower than that of the Group B. However, the difference was not statistically significant (Fig. 2c).

In addition, on the 3rd day after infection, pearson correlation analysis showed that the number of colonies in CXL group was positively correlated with the severity of corneal lesion group. A: $r = 0.771$, $P = 0.009$; group B: $r = 0.678$, $P = 0.031$ whereas group C: $r = 0.707$, $P = 0.022$, see (Fig. 2d).

Histological examination

The clinical findings on the 10th day showed that the mean corneal lesion, corneal opacity, neovascularization and the depth of ulceration scores differed greatly

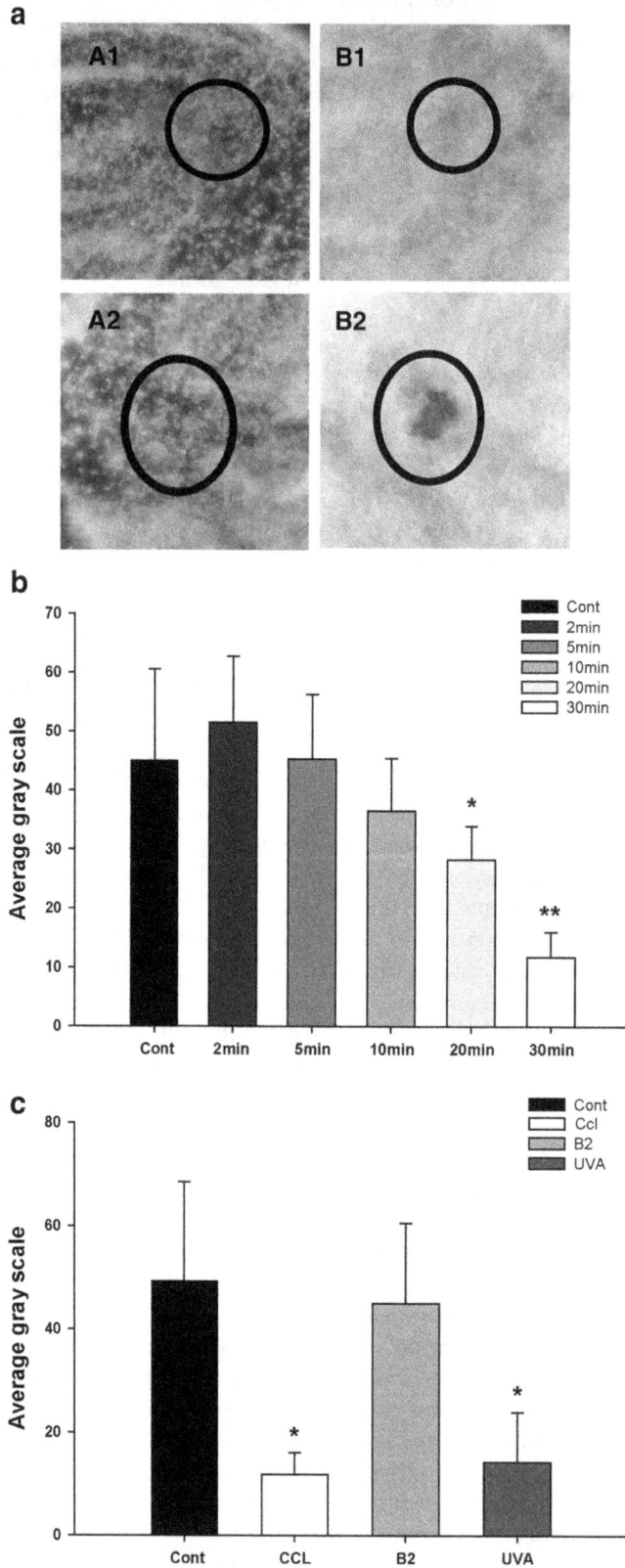

Fig. 1 (See legend on next page.)

(See figure on previous page.)
Fig. 1 a The quantification of fungal cells viability obtained in culture treated with irradiation for 48 h. Black circles represent the radiation area, comparison before and after 10 min and 30 min CXL irradiation. **b** The fungal viability obtained was treated with different CXL time (2, 5, 10, 20 and 30 min). Statistically, there were big decreases in fungal viability with UVA (20, 30 min) compared to the control group, as assessed by the t-test. **c** The fungal viability irradiated with CXL (30 minutes) were evaluated under four conditions. Mean ± SD, $n = 6$, *$p < 0.05$ Vs Cont, **$p < 0.01$ Vs Cont

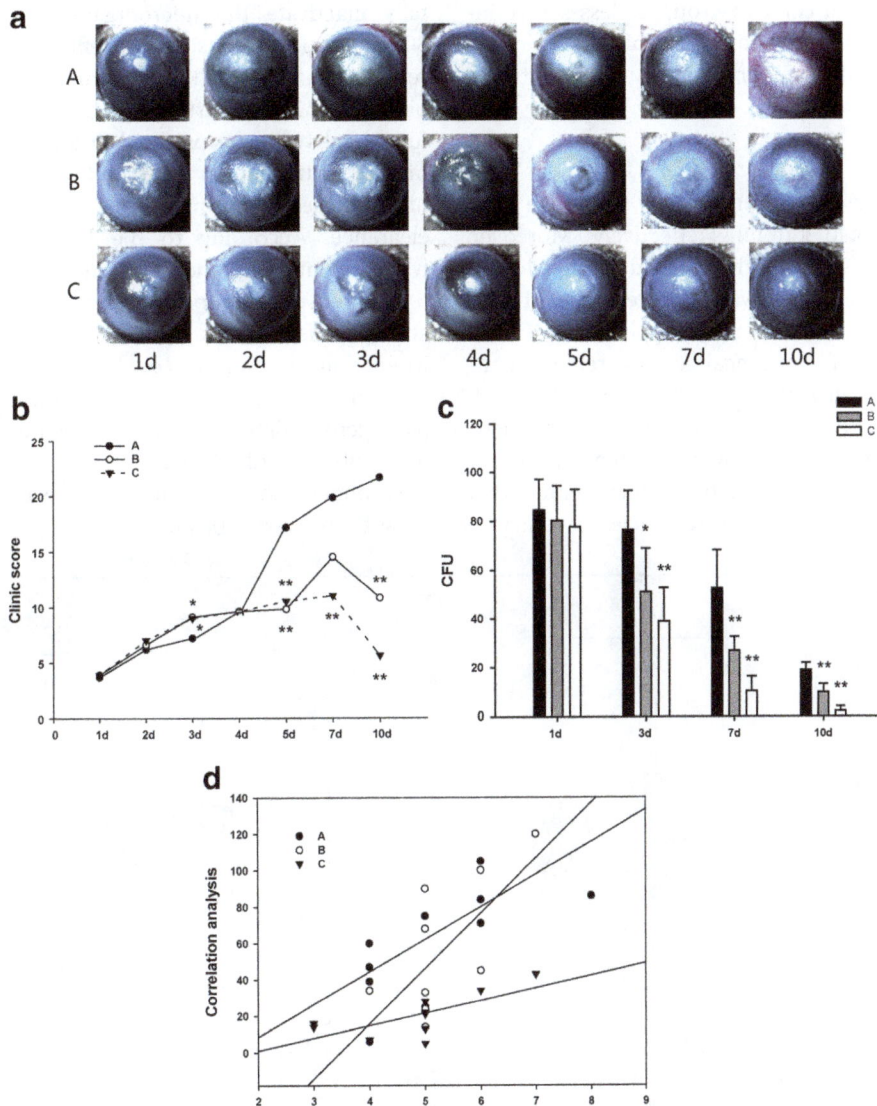

Fig. 2 Eyes from each group after infection. **a** All mice were photographed every 24 h for seven successive days(× 16). **b** Efficacy of each treatment was evaluated under the Schreiber scoring system. There were severe corneal infiltrates, clouding and anterior chamber hypopyon in the group A. Statistically, there were big differences between Group B and Group C compared to Group A. Mean ± SD, $n = 10$, *$p < 0.05$ Vs Cont, **$p < 0.01$ Vs Cont, Group A: no treatment (control); Group B: CXL treatment for two minutes; Group C: CXL treatment for three minutes. **c** The CFUs was obtained in culture from each group, in 1 day, 3, 7,10 days after modeling. There was a statistically significant decrease in CFUs in both group B and group C compared to group A. $n = 10$, *$p < 0.05$ Vs Cont, **$p < 0.01$ Vs Cont, Group A: no treatment (control); Group B: CXL treatment for two minutes; Group C: CXL treatment for three minutes. **d** Scatter plots of correlation between corneal lesions and the fungal colonies in each group of mice. Mean ± SD, $n = 10$, *$p < 0.05$ Vs Cont, **$p < 0.01$ Vs Cont, Group A, control group; Group B, treated with CXL for 2 min; Group C, treated with CXL for 3 min

among the control group($P = 0.001$, $P = 0.001$, $P = 0.034$ and $P = 0.025$ respectively). In addition, group C apparently tended to have lower scores than group B (Fig. 3).

In histological findings, there were severe inflammatory changes in Group A on the 10 days, inflammatory cells, and stromal edema were histologically evident within corneal tissue. Collagen destruction and sequence impairment were evident in the whole stroma, inflammatory cells accounted for 72.65% of the total cells. In group B, collagen impairment was evident at the level of the anterior stroma. The inflammatory cells accounted for 43.67% of the total cells. In group C, less severe inflammatory changes were noted on histopathological examination. The Inflammatory cells in corneal stroma were 13.29%, as shown in (Fig. 4b).

Discussion

Based upon the results of our in vitro study, we conclude that CXL could kill fungi effectively. Moreover, fungal activity was significantly reduced with a longer CXL irradiation time, which was consistent with the results of Jawaher [24]. However, the application of CXL in the therapeutic profile of fungal keratitis remains controversial. In 2013, shiwabuch [16] confirmed that CXL could inactivate Candida albicans in vitro fungal inactivation experiments, but there was no fungicidal effect against fusarium solani. It has been documented that fungal keratitis is caused by over 70 species covering 40

fungal genera [25], in this case, we believe that the sensitivity of the treatment differs, due to a wide variety of fungi species and the differences in their biological behaviors [26]. In addition, treatment sensitivity might also be related to the concentration of the solution. Demidova and Hamblin [27] also found that UVA only had an inactivation effect on the low concentration of Fungi. Furthermore, the treatment sensitivity seems relate to exposure-duration dependent pattern, as Makdoumi [28] revealed, with the energy density of 3 mW/cm^2, the 60 min exposure of bacterial suspension to UVA can totally inactivate the microorganism in solution, while 30 min exposure has limited effect of eradication. It is reported that fungal keratitis infection often exists as a biofilm, which is particularly difficult to clear because fungal cells are encapsulated in a protective and impermeable extracellular matrix (ECM) [4]. Thus, much higher doses of antimicrobials are required for biofilm clearance. According to the Bunsen-Roscoe rule [4], while maintaining the total energy, the absorption of light intensity is proportional to the time of irradiation and the effectiveness would increase with extension of irradiation duration. In conclusion, it could be hypothesized that the effect of CXL on inactivation of fungal pathogens is determined by the total energy provided by ultraviolet and riboflavin.

To obtain more evidence, the effect of CXL on fungal keratitis in vivo was further investigated. As the genes

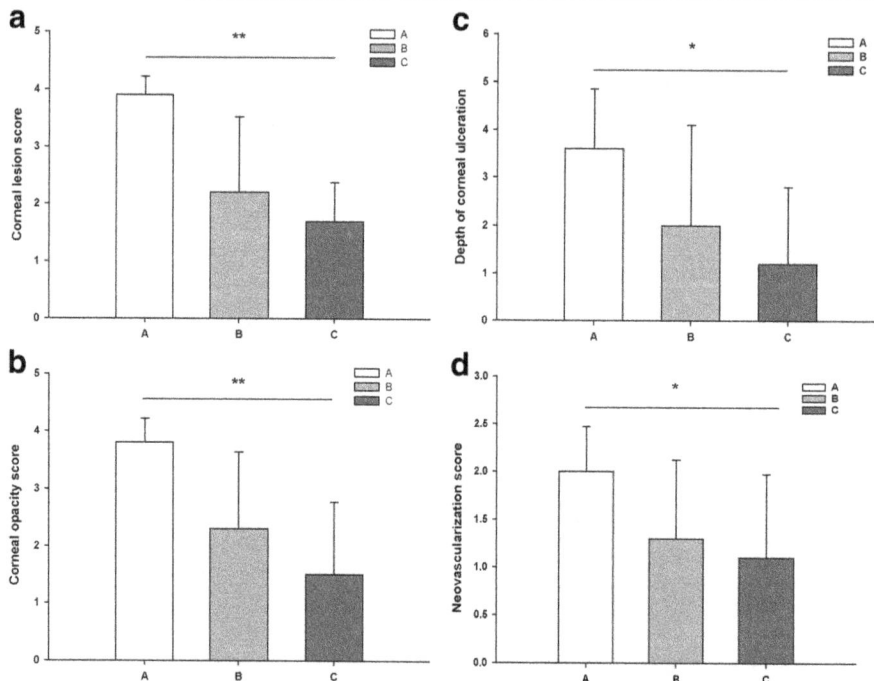

Fig. 3 A comparison of the Clinical Findings on 14 day after treatment. **a** Corneal lesion ($P = 0.001$). **b** Corneal opacity ($P = 0.001$). **c** neovascularization ($P = 0.034$). **d** The depth of ulceration ($P = 0.025$), Mean ± SD, $n = 10$, *$p < 0.05$ Vs Cont, **$p < 0.01$ Vs Cont, Group A, control group; Group B, treated with CXL for 2 min; Group C, treated with CXL for 3 min

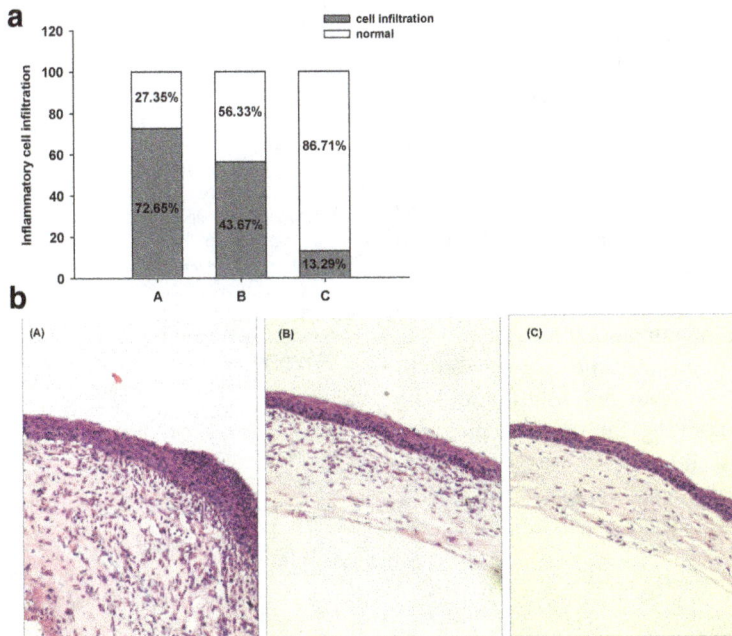

Fig. 4 Histopathology of corneas in each group(× 20). **a** Comparison of inflammation cells infiltration among groups, (**b**). The corneal tissue of mice in each group was subject to HE staining. Group A, control group; Group B, treated with CXL for 2 min; Group C, treated with CXL for 3 min

between mouse and humans are highly homologous, the mouse model is more conducive to assess the efficacy of CXL on fungal keratitis. Our findings suggested that with the increase of CXL time, the fungal colonies in treatment group decreased, the structure of corneal collagen fiber enhanced, the ability of corneal to resist edema increased, the digestion of corneal collagen suppressed, the progress of corneal ulcer delayed, the prognosis of mice better than that of the control group. Meanwhile, the therapeutical effect of CXL on fungal keratitis varied with different treatment time. Although the favorable outcomes obtained in this study are coincident with a certain of other laboratory studies and clinical studies [29], which report that CXL is effective in managing fungal keratitis, there are also studies obtaining contrary results to ours. Vajpayee [30] claimed that the practice of CXL combined with drug therapy did not increase the cure rate. After studying with 41 cases, he found that there was no significant difference between monotherapy on CXL and CXL combined with fungal regimen. Uddaraju [15] evaluated CXL curative effect on deep matrix of fungal keratitis, just to find that CXL group had a higher perforation rate than the control group. Most of the clinical researches aim at drug-resistant infectious keratitis for trial treatment. On account of the different time antimicrobial effects and different level of the keratitis, implement CXL for advanced progressive keratitis, further aggravated the severity of keratitis, late intervention may cut down the effectiveness of CXL treatment.

Basically, the effects of CXL inhibited fungal growth and infection may be related to the following factors: (1). Direct damage of Microorganisms by exposure to UVA radiation [31].(2). Riboflavin, as a photochemical medium, is non-toxic. Studies have shown that although the riboflavin could not inactivated fungi, it can induce the conformational changes of the component structure of fungal cell wall, which appears as the senescence of filamentous cells, decrease its cell size and increase its cytotoxicity [32, 33]. (3) Reactive oxygen species generate when riboflavin absorbs light and interacts with dissolved oxygen in solution damage the pathogen nucleic acids [34] (4). CXL reduce corneal melting and resist to enzymatic digestion, increase the strength and simultaneously reducing its penetrability by fungal hyphae [7, 35, 36]. Furthermore, after scraped corneal epithelium, CXL might entrap the fungal hyphae within the collagen matrix, thereby reducing the growth rate severity.

We found that CXL affected the various complications of fungal keratitis. Studies have suggested that CXL can activate fibroblasts, leading the increasing of ki-67 secretion, thereby increasing the degree of corneal opacity. However, the opacity of the CXL group was no different from that of the control group, which may be due to decreased α-SMA activation of fibroblasts [37]. The process of corneal healing may be associated with varying degrees of corneal neovascularization, thereby reducing the cornea transparency. Corneal neovascularization promotes the migration and recruitment of inflammatory cells into the lesion area, which is not only the key parts of the occurrence and maintenance of the entire inflammatory response, but also accompanying with pathological changes such as corneal neurodegeneration [38]. Chang and Bock [39, 40] believed that CXL can alleviate the pathologic neovascularization in the cornea of a mouse, but there is no research on fungal keratitis.

The results of our study showed that the number of corneal neovascularization and inflammatory cells decreased significantly after CXL. So we speculated that CXL increased the cornea toughness, reduced neovascularization invasion, thereby reducing inflammation response.

We should change the exposure time and wavelength of UVA, the concentration of riboflavin solution and the time of corneal action. Looking for the specificity of CXL for the treatment of different severity of keratitis with different pathological stages, in order to provide minimal side-effects on the healthy cells and tissue of the cornea.

Conclusions

To sum up, the treatment with CXL is effective on inhibiting fusarium growth and causes symptomatic relief. But how can CXL coordinate the various processes and molecular mechanisms of the recovery of fungal keratitis, and further research is needed.

Abbreviations

CXL: Corneal Collagen Cross-Linking; FK: Fungal keratitis; HE: Hematoxylin–eosin; NS: Stroke-physiological saline solution; PDA: Potato dextrose agar; UVA: Ultraviolet

Acknowledgments

We thank Tao Wang Singapore for editing the paper. We thank Henan Key Laboratory of Ophthalmology and Visual Science, National Key Clinical Specialties Construction Program of China for its support.

Funding

This project was supported by the National Natural Science Foundation of China grants (81670827), Henan Province Science and Technology Research Project (No.152102410085) and Zhengzhou City Project for Science and Technology Talents Team Construction Plan Science and Technology Innovation Team (No.131PCXTD620).

Authors' contributions

LYW defined the research theme. LYW and HMZ designed the methods. ZQZ and HMZ interpreted the results. ZQZ, HMZ, JY, SSL, and ZJL performed data collection and interpreted the data. All authors read and approved the final manuscript.

Competing interests

The authors declare that they have no competing interests.

Author details

[1]People's Hospital of Zhengzhou University and Henan Provincial People's Hospital, Henan Eye Institute, Henan Eye Hospital, Zhengzhou 450003, China. [2]Department of Pediatrics, Baylor College of Medicine, Houston, TX, USA.

References

1. Wang L, Sun S, Jing Y, et al. Spectrum of fungal keratitis in central China. Clin Exp Ophthalmol. 2009;37(8):763–71.
2. Chowdhary A, Singh K. Spectrum of fungal keratitis in North India. Cornea. 2005;24(1):8–15.
3. Jurkunas U, Behlau I, Colby K. Fungal keratitis: changing pathogens and risk factors. Cornea. 2009;28(6):638–43.
4. Frei R, Breitbach AS, Blackwell HE. 2-Aminobenzimidazole derivatives strongly inhibit and disperse Pseudomonas aeruginosa biofilms. Angew Chem Int Ed Engl. 2012;51(21):5226–9.
5. Sharma N, Chacko J, Velpandian T, et al. Comparative evaluation of topical versus intrastromal voriconazole as an adjunct to natamycin in recalcitrant fungal keratitis. Ophthalmology. 2013;120(4):677–81.
6. Xie L, Zhong W, Shi W, et al. Spectrum of fungal keratitis in north China. Ophthalmology. 2006;113(11):1943–8.
7. Wollensak G, Sporl E, Seiler T. Treatment of keratoconus by collagen cross linking. Ophthalmologe. 2003;100(1):44–9.
8. Hafezi F, Dejica P, Majo F. Modified corneal collagen crosslinking reduces corneal oedema and diurnal visual fluctuations in Fuchs dystrophy. Br J Ophthalmol. 2010;94(5):660–1.
9. Ghanem RC, Santhiago MR, Berti TB, et al. Collagen crosslinking with riboflavin and ultraviolet-a in eyes with pseudophakic bullous keratopathy. J Cataract Refract Surg. 2010;36(2):273–6.
10. Iseli HP, Thiel MA, Hafezi F, et al. Ultraviolet a/riboflavin corneal cross-linking for infectious keratitis associated with corneal melts. Cornea. 2008;27(5):590–4.
11. Makdoumi K, Mortensen J, Sorkhabi O, et al. UVA-riboflavin photochemical therapy of bacterial keratitis: a pilot study. Graefes Arch Clin Exp Ophthalmol. 2012;250(1):95–102.
12. Price MO, Tenkman LR, Schrier A, et al. Photoactivated riboflavin treatment of infectious keratitis using collagen cross-linking technology. J Refract Surg. 2012;28(10):706–13.
13. Jayesh V, Vaddavalli PK. Cross-linking for microbial keratitis. Indian J Ophthalmol. 2013;61(8):441.
14. Vajpayee RB, Shafi SN, Maharana PK, et al. Evaluation of corneal collagen cross-linking as an additional therapy in mycotic keratitis. Clin Exp Ophthalmol. 2015;43(2):103–7.
15. Uddaraju M, Mascarenhas J, Das MR, et al. Corneal cross-linking as an adjuvant therapy in the Management of Recalcitrant Deep Stromal Fungal Keratitis: a randomized trial. Am J Ophthalmol. 2015;160(1):131–4.e5.
16. Kashiwabuchi RT, Carvalho FR, Khan YA, et al. Assessment of fungal viability after long-wave ultraviolet light irradiation combined with riboflavin administration. Graefes Arch Clin Exp Ophthalmol. 2013;251(2):521–7.
17. Bilgihan K, Kalkanci A, Ozdemir HB, et al. Evaluation of antifungal efficacy of 0.1% and 0.25% riboflavin with UVA: a comparative in vitro study. Curr Eye Res. 2016;41(8):1050–6.
18. López B, González A, Beaumont J, et al. Identification of a potential cardiac antifibrotic mechanism of torasemide in patients with chronic heart failure. J Am Coll Cardiol. 2007;50(9):859.
19. Zhang H, Wang L, Li Z, et al. A novel murine model of fusarium solani keratitis utilizing fluorescent labeled fungi. Exp Eye Res. 2013;110:107–12.
20. Ozturk F, Yavas GF, Kusbeci T, et al. Efficacy of topical caspofungin in experimental fusarium keratitis. Cornea. 2007;26(6):726–8.
21. Karti O, Zengin MO, Cinar E, Tutuncu M, Karahan E, Celik A, Kucukerdonmez C. Effect of 1- and 6-Hour-Delayed Corneal Collagen Cross-Linking on Corneal Healing in a Rabbit Alkali-Burn Model: Clinical and Histological Observations. Cornea. 2016;35(12):1644–9.
22. Choi KS, Yoon SC, Rim TH, et al. Effect of voriconazole and ultraviolet-a combination therapy compared to voriconazole single treatment on fusarium solani fungal keratitis. J Ocul Pharmacol Ther. 2014;30(5):381–6.
23. Kitamura K, Farber JM, Kelsall BL. CCR6 marks regulatory T cells as a colon-tropic, IL-10-producing phenotype. J Immunol. 2010;185(6):3295–304.
24. Alshehri JM, Caballerolima D, Hillarby MC, et al. Evaluation of corneal cross-linking for treatment of fungal keratitis: using confocal laser scanning microscopy on an ex vivo human corneal model. Invest Ophthalmol Vis Sci. 2016;57(14):6367.

25. Thomas PA. Mycotic keratitis—an underestimated mycosis. J Med Vet Mycol. 1994;32(4):235–56.

26. Kuzucu C, Rapino B, McDermott L, et al. Comparison of the semisolid agar antifungal susceptibility test with the NCCLS M38-P broth microdilution test for screening of filamentous fungi. J Clin Microbiol. 2004;42(3):1224–7.

27. Demidova TN, Hamblin MR. Effect of cell-photosensitizer binding and cell density on microbial photoinactivation. Antimicrob Agents Chemother. 2005;49(6):2329–35.

28. Makdoumi K, Backman A, Mortensen J, et al. Evaluation of antibacterial efficacy of photo-activated riboflavin using ultraviolet light (UVA). Graefes Arch Clin Exp Ophthalmol. 2010;248(2):207–12.

29. Vazirani J, Vaddavalli PK. Cross-linking for microbial keratitis. Indian J Ophthalmol. 2013;61(8):441–4.

30. Vajpayee RB, Shafi SN, Maharana PK, et al. Evaluation of corneal collagen cross-linking as an additional therapy in mycotic keratitis. Clin Exp Ophthalmol. 2015;43(2):103.

31. Chan TC, Agarwal T, Vajpayee RB, et al. Cross-linking for microbial keratitis. Curr Opin Ophthalmol. 2016;27(4):348.

32. Spoerl E, Huhle M, Seiler T. Induction of cross-links in corneal tissue. Exp Eye Res. 1998;66(1):97–103.

33. Bartnicki-Garcia S. Cell wall chemistry, morphogenesis, and taxonomy of fungi. Annu Rev Microbiol. 1968;22:87–108.

34. Maisch T, Baier J, Franz B, et al. The role of singlet oxygen and oxygen concentration in photodynamic inactivation of bacteria. Proc Natl Acad Sci U S A. 2007;104(17):7223–8.

35. Tsugita A, Okada Y, Uehara K. Photosensitized inactivation of ribonucleic acids in the presence of riboflavin. Biochim Biophys Acta. 1965;103(2):360–3.

36. Wang T, Peng Y, Shen N, et al. Photochemical activation increases the porcine corneal stiffness and resistance to collagenase digestion. Exp Eye Res. 2014;123:97–104.

37. Wollensak G, Iomdina E, Dittert DD, et al. Wound healing in the rabbit cornea after corneal collagen cross-linking with riboflavin and UVA. Cornea. 2007;26(5):600–5.

38. Mahdy RA, Nada WM, Wageh MM. Topical amphotericin B and subconjunctival injection of fluconazole (combination therapy) versus topical amphotericin B (monotherapy) in treatment of keratomycosis. J Ocul Pharmacol Ther. 2010;26(3):281–5.

39. Pober JS, Sessa WC. Evolving functions of endothelial cells in inflammation. Nat Rev Immunol. 2007;7(10):803–15.

40. Chang JH, Gabison EE, Kato T, et al. Corneal neovascularization. Curr Opin Ophthalmol. 2001;12(4):242–9.

7

Coverage of azithromycin mass treatment for trachoma elimination in Northwestern Ethiopia

Zelalem Tilahun and Teferi Gedif Fenta*

Abstract

Background: Mass drug administration with antibiotics predominantly with azithromycin is one of the four arms of the SAFE strategy. The elimination of ocular chlamydial infection is only achieved as long as the azithromycin mass treatments (AMT) are given frequently enough and at a high enough coverage. This study was conducted to assess the coverage of azithromycin mass treatment and its determinants in Awi Zone, Northwestern Ethiopia.

Methods: House to house survey using a structured questionnaire was done between July 7 to July 25, 2013. Coverage is defined as the proportion of individuals in the eligible population who actually ingested the Azithromycin during the Campaign.

Results: A total of 1267 households were enrolled in the survey in which 5826 eligible members were living in these households. Almost half (54.6%) of the community members who were eligible for all six campaigns had participated in more than three campaigns of azithromycin mass treatment. The overall average self-reported coverage of the azithromycin mass treatment (AMT) in all six campaigns was 62.8% (64% in rural vs. 61.6% urban). On average, each eligible person had taken the drug 3.77 times. The rural residents were significantly more likely to have received treatment during the last round of AMT in 2012 {AOR = 2.35; 95% CI [1.80–3.06]}. Azithromycin uptake status of female household heads was less than the corresponding male household heads {AOR = 0.41; 95% CI [0.24–0.72]}. Household heads' awareness about trachoma (AOR = 2.55; 95% CI [1.19–5.44]) and AMT {AOR = 7.19; 95% CI [3.27–15.82]} had positive association with acceptability.

Conclusion: The overall average AMT coverage was found to be low. There was low coverage of the treatment in the urban community as compared to the rural residents. Misconceptions of household heads about trachoma and azithromycin have negatively affected the coverage. Further work on why female household heads are associated with higher risk of non-participation in AMT is warranted. Strengthening awareness creation and consideration of additional campaigns is essential.

Keywords: Azithromycin mass treatment, Coverage, Trachoma elimination, Northwest Ethiopia

* Correspondence: tgedif@gmail.com; teferi.gedif@aau.edu.et
Social and Adminstrative Pharmacy Working Group, Departement of Pharmaceutics and Social Pharmacy, College of Health Sciences, Addis Ababa University, P.O.Box 1176, Addis Ababa, Ethiopia

Background

"Trachoma, a neglected tropical disease, is the world's leading infectious cause of blindness" [1]. Globally, 1.2 billion people live in trachoma endemic areas; of these, 48.5% of the global burden is concentrated in Ethiopia, India, Nigeria, Sudan and Guinea [2]. In Ethiopia, approximately 67 million people are at risk for trachoma [3]. The Amhara National Regional State (ANRS) of Ethiopia was the most trachoma-endemic regional states in Ethiopia. Awi zone is one of the trachoma endemic zones among the 10 zonal administrations in ANRS with a TF and TT prevalence of 38.9 and 5.4%, respectively [3, 4].

For many years, topical agents such as tetracycline were used as a treatment of choice for ocular infection with *C.trachomatis* because it is devoid of systemic side effects in children [5]. However, effective treatment requires that the drug be taken every day for four to six weeks [6]. Moreover because of its oily base, its use may be associated with blurred vision. Due to these reasons, compliance with these agents is poor [7].

Many randomized control trials indicated that azithromycin is the treatment of choice for ocular infection with *C.trachomatis* [2, 8–10]. Azithromycin is also associated with a short-term reduction in diarrheal morbidity in children [11, 12]. It is easy to administer and higher coverage may be possible as compared to tetracycline topical treatment [13].

The World Health Assembly passed a resolution to eliminate blinding trachoma by implementing the "SAFE" (S = surgery, A = antibiotic, F = facial cleanliness and E = environmental improvement) strategy [14]. In Ethiopia the first strategic plan for trachoma control was developed in 2005 after a pilot trial of the SAFE strategy in four districts of ANRS. Then, ANRS Health Bureau partnering with the Lions Club of Ethiopia and the Carter Center had expanded trachoma control efforts from the four pilot districts to all districts with the SAFE strategy [3].

Mass drug administration with antibiotics predominantly with azithromycin is one of the four arms of the SAFE strategy. WHO had recommended community-wide distribution of oral azithromycin when the prevalence of trachomatous inflammation follicular (TF) is greater than 10% in children aged 1–9 years, and trichiasis prevalence exceeding 1% in persons aged over 14 years [15]. Full participation is necessary for maximizing the impact of trachoma control programs [16]. Antibiotic distribution teams should offer azithromycin to all individuals over the age of six months in eligible communities. Overall coverage should be as high as possible, but treatment of 80% of the resident population should be the minimum target [17].

Unlike patient oriented treatments that are commonly self-initiated, there may not be full acceptance of the community for drugs that are given in the form of campaign due to different reasons [18, 19]. In Ethiopia, even if there are many studies addressing the effectiveness of azithromycin mass treatment (AMT) for trachoma control, its acceptability and determinants has not been well explored. This study was therefore conducted to assess the acceptability of the azithromycin mass treatment and its determinants in Awi zone, Northwestern Ethiopia.

Methods

Study area and design

A community based cross sectional survey was conducted following 6 AMT rounds in both urban and rural *kebeles* (the smallest administrative units in the government structure) of Injibara town and Adjacent Banja districts from July 7 to July 25, 2013.

Study participants

All individuals living in Injibara town and Banja districts were taken as source population. The study population was all individuals who live in the selected two urban and six rural kebeles. All family members who lived more than 8 months in that household during the time of the survey were included. All children who were older than 6 months during 2012 AMT program were also taken as study participants.

Sample size determination

The number of households to be involved in the survey was determined using the single proportion formula [20]. The sample size was calculated with the assumption that the level of coverage was 0.5 and the absolute sampling error to be tolerated as 0.04 with 95% confidence interval. Taking the experiences of similar African Studies the design effect of 2 was considered to calculate the sample size [21]. Adding 10% for non-responses, a total of 1321 households were included.

Sampling method

The number of households covered in urban and rural *kebeles* were allocated based on proportionate to the size of population established in 2007 CSA census (28% Urban and 72% Rural) [22]. Accordingly, six rural and two urban *kebeles* were randomly selected. Finally, the number of households in each kebele was determined proportionate to the size of households in each *kebele* and specific households were selected using a systematic random sampling technique.

Operational definition

Coverage

Coverage is defined as the proportion of individuals in the sampled population who actually ingested the Azithromycin during the Campaign.

Azithromycin mass treatment (AMT)

It is an annual mass administration of azithromycin to all eligible community members (children less than 6 months old are excluded) for the purpose of trachoma elimination. Six rounds of mass distribution were conducted by Health Extension Workers in the Districts and the last campaign was in November 2012.

Serious adverse effects

An adverse experience following AMT that results in death, life threatening condition, in-patient hospitalization, disability and/or birth defects.

Data collection instruments

Adult household members were interviewed with a pretested structured questionnaire (attached as Additional file 1) by 13 trained data collectors. The structured questionnaire was translated to Amharic (official language) and most of the interview was done using Amharic. For those participants who couldn't speak and understand Amharic, interview was done using the local language. The head of each household was interviewed about himself and eligible children less than 18 years old as well as for family members who were absent during the data collection time. Data collectors with health background were carefully selected and given training on how to administer the questionnaire to avoid possible interviewer bias.

Data analysis and interpretation

Data was coded and entered into Epi Info version 3.5.3 by three trained data entry clerks. Then, the data was transferred to SPSS version 20.0 and analyzed. Socio-demographic variables including sex, age, marital status, educational status, occupation and place of residence, and awareness about AMT were considered as independent variables and frequency of self reported AMT coverage as outcome variable. In addition to simple descriptive statistics, chi square test, correlation and logistic regression analysis were conducted to show possible associations. P-value< 0.05 was considered as statistically significant.

Results

A total of 1321 households were enrolled in the survey. Complete questionnaires were obtained from 1267 households; making a response rate of 96%. All members in the 1267 households who fulfilled the inclusion criteria were included and hence a total of 5826 eligible household members were considered in the subsequent analysis. Among these, 5266 (90.4%) were greater than or equal to 7 years old at the time of the survey and anticipated as eligible for all six rounds.

Socio-demographic characteristics

Among the total 1267 households included in the study, 897 (70.8%) of them were from rural areas. Most of the household heads 973 (76.8%) were males. The mean age of household heads was 46.3 ± 14.2. The mean age of the AMT eligible participants was 25.1 ± 17.64. More than half of the participants were less than 20 years (Table 1).

Household heads' awareness and perception about trachoma

Among the total 1267 household heads, 1203 (94.9%) had ever heard about trachoma. The main information source for most of the household heads about trachoma was health professionals 1076 (89.44%) followed by neighbors 87 (7.23%). Poor environmental sanitation was mentioned by 717 (59.6%) of them as a cause of trachoma. Among 1203 household heads who had ever heard about trachoma, 428 (35.6%) mentioned fly as a way of transmission; 401 (33.3%) of them did not know the way of trachoma transmission whereas 22 (1.8%) household heads believed that trachoma is a non-communicable disease. But a sizable proportion 1084 (90%) believed that trachoma is a preventable disease. However, 77 (7.1%) of them did not know any prevention methods for trachoma.

Household heads' awareness and perception about AMT

From the total household heads participated in the survey, 1234 (97.4%) of them had ever heard about AMT administrated for the elimination of trachoma. Among these, 1117 (90%) had heard about it from health professionals. Almost all of them 1263 (99.7%) reported that mass drug treatment had ever been given in their *kebeles* even though some of them were not aware about the treatment and its purpose. Of the total respondents, 150 (11.8%) believed that the drug was not given based on free will. Among the total household heads participated in the study, 1204 (95%) reported that they would volunteer to participate in the mass treatment if it was to be continued in the future. The most frequently mentioned reasons to end their participation to AMT by the rest of 63 (5%) household heads were fear of illness and death by the drug, serious side effect in previous campaign, having chronic illness, and absence of change to their eye health.

Self-reported azithromycin mass treatment coverage

In 1240 (97.9%) of the households, it was reported that at least one member had ever participated in any rounds of the campaign and the rest 27 (2.1%) claimed that none of the members had ever taken AMT. Being absent from home during the campaigns, health problems, and fear of the severe side effects were the major reasons mentioned for non-participation in AMT.

Table 1 Socio demographic distribution of the study participants, Injibara town and Banja districts of Awi zone, Northwestern Ethiopia, July 2013

Socio demographic variables N = 5826	Urban residents	Rural residents	Total n (%)
1. Sex			
Male	706	2172	2878 (49.4)
Female	804	2144	2948 (50.6)
2. Age			
1–5 years	135	318	453 (7.8)
6–10 years	208	608	813 (14)
11–15 years	207	727	934 (16)
16–20 years	224	696	920 (15.8)
21–40 years	537	1066	1603 (27.5)
41–60 years	169	671	840 (14.4)
> 60 years	30	233	263 (4.5)
3. Occupation			
Student	635	1679	2314 (39.7)
Farmer	51	1791	1842 (31.6)
Merchant	100	45	145 (2.5)
Government employee	245	36	281 (4.8)
House wife	182	181	363 (6.2)
Jobless	56	32	88 (1.5)
Others[a]	241	552	793 (13.6)
4. Religion			
Orthodox	1497	4276	5773 (99.1)
Muslim	0	8	8 (0.13)
Protestant	13	1	14 (0.24)
Others[b]	0	31	31 (0.53)
5. Educational Status			
Unable to read and write[c]	336	1970	2306 (39.6)
Able to read and write	97	322	419 (7.2)
Grade 1–4	167	604	771 (13.2)
Grade 4–8	356	964	1320 (22.6)
Grade 9–12	261	412	673 (11.6)
College and Above	293	44	337 (5.8)
6. Marital Status			
Single[d]	871	2562	3433 (58.9)
Married	573	1562	2135 (36.7)
Divorced	32	86	118 (2.0)
Widowed	34	106	140 (2.4)

[a] Children < 5 years, daily laborer, handicraft, local beer maker, monk, tailor
[b] Catholic, paganism
[c] (This category includes preschool children)
[d] (This category includes children)

From the total 5266 (90.4%) household members who were eligible for all campaigns, only 2876 (54.6%) of them claimed to have participated more than three times out of the six rounds of AMT campaigns. The overall average self-reported coverage of the AMT in all six campaigns was 62.8% (64% rural and 61.6% urban). On average, each eligible person participated 3.77 times. From the total 560 children who were not eligible for all campaigns, 75 children were less than 1 year old and expected to participate in the campaign once. Of these, only 54 (72%) were taken the treatment. From 1510 AMT urban household members enrolled in the study, 1344 (89%) were eligible for all campaigns. Of these 78 (5.8%) of them had never participated and only 72 (27.7% completed the six rounds of AMT (Fig. 1).

The self-reported AMT coverage of the 2012 campaign was 92.9%; whereas a report obtained from District Health Office indicated that the coverage was close to 96%.

Out of the total 1227 household heads who had ever taken azithromycin, 1166 (95%) believed that AMT was beneficial. Among those who said AMT is beneficial, 978 (83.9%) related the benefit to eye health; 481 (41.3%) for eradicating intestinal worm; and 15 (1.3%) for improving the general health. Other benefits such as treatment for hemorrhoid and stimulating appetites were mentioned by 5 (0.4%) of the respondents.

Reported side effects with AMT use

From the total 1227 household heads who had ever taken the drug, 538 (43.9%) reported to have had side effects of azithromycin. Anal burning sensation, diarrhea, and heartburn were the three most prevalent side effects reported (Fig. 2).

Out of the total 538 household heads who had ever encountered side effects of azithromycin, 83 (15.4%) had claimed that they experienced with serious adverse effects of the drug. In addition, 296 (23.4%) of the household heads had heard other persons complaining about the drug's side effects. Of which, 88 (29.7%) of them reported that they had ever heard about serious adverse effects of the drug such as birth defect, inpatient hospitalization and disability. From this, 38 (43.2%) of them reported that they knew persons who encountered with at least one of the serious adverse effects of the drug.

From the total 1227 household heads who had ever participated in AMT, 66 (5.4%) of them used the drug for different purposes other than trachoma such as for treating intestinal worms, promote animal fertilization and for the relief of abdominal pain.

Determinants of the 2012 azithromycin mass treatment coverage

The 2012 Azithromycin uptake was not found to be influenced by socio demographic characteristics, except job. Students' participation in the mass treatment

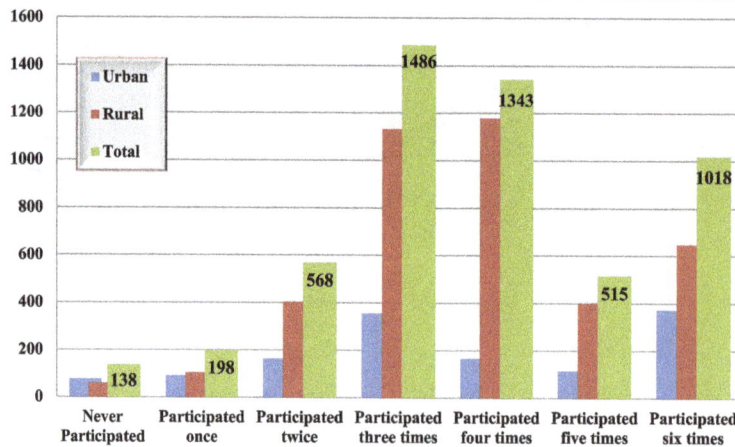

Fig. 1 Frequency of AMT self-reported uptake among urban and rural household members in Injibara town and Banja districts of Awi Zone, July 2013

was higher as compared to farmers, merchants and others. Place of residence affects the drug uptake status. In this regard, the proportion of eligible rural residents who took AMT more than three times was 56.7% and for urban residents, it was 48.7%. This difference was statistically significant {AOR = 2.35, 95% CI [1.80–3.06]}.

There was a significant difference between the rural residents and urban residents in the number of times they took azithromycin. Higher number of rural residents had taken azithromycin more than 3 times as compared to urban residents {AOR = 1.69; 95% CI [1.44–1.98]}. There was no significant difference in frequency of AMT uptake between males and females. There was a significant difference in the frequency of AMT uptake among children ages between 7 to 10 years compared to other age groups. In this regard, the proportion of adults with age between 16 and 20 years who

took azithromycin more than 3 times was higher than in children with age between 7 to 10 years {AOR = 2.77; 95% CI [2.15–3.57]}. Similarly, the study participants who were older than 20 years were at better enactment in taking azithromycin more than 3 times as compared to children less than 15 years. There was also a positive correlation between the number of times they took azithromycin and age ($r = 0.235$; 95%CI, $p = 0.01$). As age increased, participation in AMT increased but being literate had no effect in participation rate (Table 2).

Factors associated with participation in the 2012AMT

The self-reported participation rate of rural household heads in the 2012 mass treatment was higher than their urban counterparts (AOR = 2.33; 95% CI [1.07–5.10]). Azithromycin uptake status of female household heads was significantly less than the corresponding male

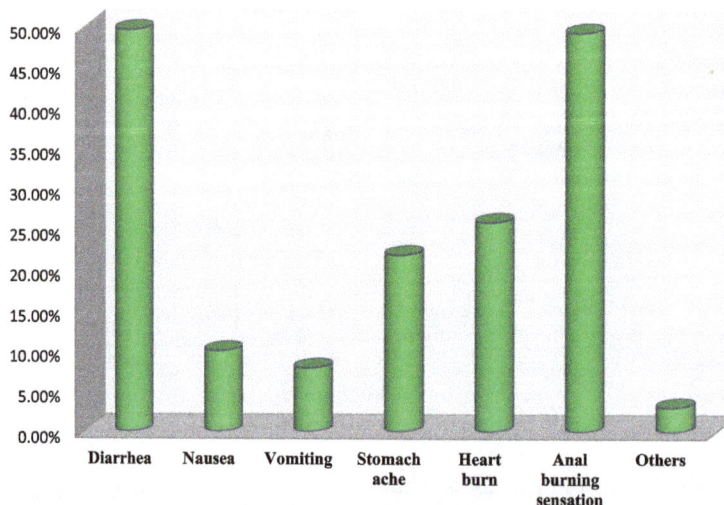

Fig. 2 Types of side effects reported by household heads after they took AMT in Injibara town and Banja districts of Awi zone, July 2013 ($N = 538$)

Table 2 Socio demographic factors associated with the frequency of AMT uptake among eligible participants to all campaigns, in Injibara town and Banja districts of Awi zone, July 2013

Socio demographic variables [N = 5266]	Frequency of AMT uptake		95% Confidence Interval	
	> 3 Times	≤ 3 Times	COR	AOR
Residence				
Rural	2222	1700	1.37 [1.22–1.56]	1.69 [1.44–1.98]
Urban	654	690	1.00	
Sex				
Female	1450	1217	0.98 [0.88–1.09]	0.92 [0.82–1.04]
Male	1426	1173	1.00	
Age				
> 60 years	165	98	3.70 [2.75–4.97]	4.40 [2.96–6.56]
41–60 years	532	309	3.78 [3.06–4.67]	4.71 [3.38–6.58]
21–40 years	968	634	3.35 [2.78–4.04]	4.04 [3.01–5.42]
16–20 years	543	377	3.16 [2.47–3.89]	2.77 [2.15–3.57]
11–15 years	447	487	2.01 [1.64–2.47]	1.76 [1.40–2.22]
7–10 years	221	485	1.00	1.00
Job				
Farmer	1074	734	1.45 [1.28–1.64]	1.04 [0.81–1.33]
Merchant	83	62	1.32 [0.94–1.86]	1.03 [0.70–1.52]
Government employee	156	125	1.23 [0.96–1.58]	0.94 [0.62–1.43]
Housewife	234	129	1.79 [1.42–2.26]	1.49 [1.08–2.06]
Jobless	48	40	1.19 [0.77–1.82]	1.00 [0.63–1.58]
Others	140	173	0.80 [0.630.28–1.04]	0.77 [0.58–1.03]
Student	1141	1127	1.00	1.00
Educational Status				
College and above	183	154	0.87 [0.69–1.10]	1.26 [0.85–1.85]
Grade 9–12	416	257	1.19 [0.99–1.43]	1.78 [1.39–2.28]
Grade 4–8	712	607	0.86 [0.75–0.99]	1.21 [0.98–1.50]
Grade 1–4	288	449	0.47 [0.40–0.56]	0.62 [0.49–0.78]
Able to read and write	240	162	1.09 [0.87–1.36]	1.01 [0.79–1.28]
Unable to read and write	1037	761	1.00	1.00
Marital Status				
Married	1277	853	1.51 [1.35–1.69]	1.41 [1.15–1.74]
Divorced	79	39	2.05 [1.38–3.02]	1.89 [1.21–2.94]
Widowed	88	52	1.71 [1.20–2.43]	1.54 [1.02–2.34]
Single	1432	1446	1.00	1.00

household heads {AOR = 0.41 95% CI [0.24–0.72]}. Occupation, educational status and marital status of household heads did not affect their uptake status. However, their participation was influenced by their awareness and perception about AMT. For example, those household heads who had ever heard about AMT were more likely participated in the 2012 campaign as compared to those who were unaware {AOR = 7.19;95% CI [3.27–15.82]}. In addition, the proportion of household heads who believed that AMT was given on free will and had participated in 2012 mass campaign was more than the proportion of those who considered AMT as an obligation {AOR = 2.93; 95% CI [1.77–4.86]} (Table 3).

Discussion

The 2012 self reported azithromycin mass treatment coverage was 92.9%. This was higher than 80%, the minimum attainable coverage set by WHO [17]. This finding was also higher than 76% taken from the mass treatment

Table 3 Association between awareness about AMT and self-reported uptake status of household heads in 2012, Awi Zone, July 2013

Variables	Took 2012 AMT		95% Confidence Interval	
	Yes	No	COR	AOR
Heard about AMT				
Yes	1125	109	10.97 [5.39–22.32]	7.19 [3.27–15.82]
No	16	17	1.00	
Did they Know why AMT given in free?				
Yes	764	79	1.21 [0.82–1.77]	0.97 [0.63–1.48]
No	377	47	1.00	1.00
Was the treatment given to those willing to take?				
Yes	1024	93	3.11 [2.0–4.83]	2.93 [1.77–4.86]
No	117	33	1.00	1.00
Did they think that the drug is beneficial for trachoma?				
Yes	1100	87	12.03 [7.37–19.63]	7.33 [4.13–13.02]
No	41	39	1.00	1.00
Did they experience any side effects' of the drug?				
Yes	495	43	1.00	1.00
No	646	43	1.31 [0.84–2.02]	1.40 [0.87–2.26]
Had they got SAE of the drug?				
Yes	75	8	0.78 [0.35–1.75]	0.87 [0.35–2.12]
No	419	35	1.00	1.00
Heard drug's side effects from other Persons?				
Yes	257	39	1.00	1.00
No	884	87	1.54 [1.03–2.31]	1.34 [0.78–2.32]
Did they know a person with SAE of the drug?				
Yes	32	6	1.02 [0.32–3.22]	1.16 [0.24–5.57]
No	42	8	1.00	
Did treatment providers provide any information?				
Yes	852	40	3.39 [2.17–5.29]	2.49 [1.53–4.08]
No	289	46	1.00	
Willingness to take the drug in the future				
Yes	1113	91	15.29 [8.90–26.26]	5.78 [2.44–13.68]
No	28	35	1.00	

SAE Serious adverse effect

coverage in Tanzania [19]; and the mean treatment coverage in 48 eligible communities in four Gambian districts taken at baseline, and after one and two years [21].

The overall self-reported coverage of AMT for the six campaigns in the study area was estimated based on the number of times that each eligible household member had taken the treatment. In this regard, the proportion of eligible household members for all campaigns who took azithromycin more than three times out of the six rounds was 54.6%. The reported mean number of times that each person had taken azithromycin was 3.77 ± 1.51. Even though the self-reported coverage

might be liable to recall bias, the 2012 AMT data obtained from the official records of the district health office was higher than the self-reported coverage for the same year (96% vs. 92.8%). A similar type of discrepancy was observed in a study conducted in Plateau State of Nigeria, in which only 60.3% of the participants reported to have received azithromycin or tetracycline eye ointment during mass drug administration but the coverage report taken from administrative data was 75.8% [23]. The reasons for such differences should be explored in the future.

There was a report from the community that the drug manifested side effects. Consequently, even all the community members who had received the drug might have not taken it; resulting a decrease in the overall actual coverage below the minimum WHO target [17]. This may have negative impact in the program success as intended elimination can only occur if the mass treatment is given frequently enough and at a high coverage. This is due to the fact that treatment of few persons in endemic areas may result in reinfection from family or neighborhood sources unless the treatment is more widespread [24–26]. Therefore, the present study finding is an indicative of the need for determining the prevalence of TF and consider additional campaigns of AMT in the studied communities.

This study also showed that the proportion of eligible rural residents who took azithromycin more than three times in the six campaigns was higher as compared to urban residents (AOR = 1.69; 95% CI [1.44–1.98]). Better acceptance and coverage of the program in the rural community is more appreciable since the prevalence of trachoma in the rural population showed a fourth fold increase as compared to the urban [4].

Older age groups were more likely to participate in AMT than the younger age group. A bivariate correlation analysis also showed that there is positive correlation between the number of times they participated in AMT campaigns and age. It was also noted that low uptake among children in the present study was in contrary to widely advocated goal that high coverage should be attained in children less than 15 years [16, 17]. This is due to the fact that the average duration of trachoma infection at younger ages is long since tears and secretions infected with chlamydia are easily and frequently swapped among the young preschool children and their caretakers, which leads to repeated episodes of reinfection [27, 28].

Out of the total 1227 household heads who had ever taken the drug, 538 (43.9%) of them reported to have experienced side effects of azithromycin. Among these, 83 (15.4%) of them claimed that they had serious adverse effect of the drug. Another study conducted in Ethiopia reported that the prevalence of adverse events ranged

4.9–7.0% in children of 1–9 years of age and 17.0–18.7% in persons ≥10 years of age [29]. As it is pointed out in a recent study, patients taking azithromycin had an increased risk of cardiovascular death as compared to those who didn't take [30, 31]. Another very recent meta-analysis of observational studies of 5 cohorts evidenced that azithromycin use was not associated with higher risk of death particularly in younger population whereas older population might be at higher risk of death (HR = 1.64 (CI, 1.232.19), I = 4%) [32]. Giving careful consideration on the safety impact of the mass treatment in special population such as elderly and patients with co-morbidity is mandatory [33].

Prior awareness of household heads' about AMT has a positive association with the drug uptake (AOR = 7.19; 95% CI [3.27–15.82]). Household heads who thought that the mass treatment is beneficial were more likely to take the treatment as compared to those who believed the opposite (AOR = 7.33; 95% CI [4.13–13.02]). Another study documented that increased knowledge about the drugs given in mass treatment and their side effects may result in a better perception of its benefits than its barriers [34]. Hence adequate health education as well as awareness creation programs should precede the mass treatment campaigns for better coverage and acceptability of the treatment program.

Limitations of the study
The study depended on the report of household heads on the participation of himself or herself and other eligible household members in the six rounds of AMT campaigns. The accuracy of the response therefore depends on the ability of the respondents to recall. Hence our study was liable to recall bias. In addition the focus group discussion we had before the survey showed that there was a great public concern on the adverse effect of azithromycin in the first round of the campaigns. This public concern could have affected how respondents answered the survey, especially with regards to adverse events.

Conclusion
The overall average self-reported coverage of AMT in all six campaigns was low. There is low coverage and acceptability of the treatment in the urban community as compared to the rural residents. Being female and urban resident and low awareness about trachoma and azithromycin have negatively affected the acceptability of the AMT by household heads and hence the coverage. Awareness creation and health education programs about trachoma and AMT are needed for effective implementation of trachoma elimination programs. Further work on why female household heads are associated with higher risk of non-participation in AMT is also warranted.

Abbreviations
AMT: Azithromycin mass treatment; ANRS: Amhara National Regional States; AOR: Adjusted odds ratio; COR: Crude odds ratio; TF: Trachomatous inflammation follicular; TT: Trachomatous trichiasis

Acknowledgements
The authors acknowledge Graduate Program of Addis Ababa University for funding this research project. We are also thankful to the Staffs of Carter Center (Ethiopia Office) for their technical assistance and data collectors and data entry clerks for their devoted work.

Funding
Graduate Program of Addis Ababa University funded the research. The funders had no role in study design, data collection and analysis, decision to publish, or preparation of the manuscript.

Authors' contributions
Both ZT and TGF designed the research. ZT supervised the data collection process, analyzed the data and drafted the report. TGF critically reviewed the report. Both Authors approved the manuscript.

Competing interests
All authors declared that there are no competing interests.

References
1. WHO. WHO Alliance for Global Elimination of Blinding Trachoma by 2020: Weekly epidemiological record 2014; 39(89):421–428.
2. Mariotti SP, Pascolini D, Rose-Nussbaumer J. Trachoma: global magnitude of a preventable cause of blindness. Br J Ophthalmol. 2009;93:563–8.
3. Carter Center. Summary Proceedings: Eleventh Annual Trachoma Control Program Review; Planning for Trachoma Elimination, District by District; 2010.URL: http://www.cartercenter.org/resources/pdfs/news/health_publications/trachoma/trachreview_final_eng2010.pdf (Accessed on December 2012).
4. FMOH. National survey on blindness, Low Vision and Trachoma in Ethiopia; 2006. http://pbunion.org/Countriessurveyresults/Ethiopia/Ethiopian_National_Blindness_and_trachoma_survey.pdf (Accessed on 05 DeC 2012).
5. Darougar S, Jones BR, Viswalingam M, et al. Topical therapy of hyper endemic trachoma with rifampicin, oxytetracycline or spiramycin eye ointments. Br J Ophthalmol. 1980;64:37–42.
6. Dawson CR, Daghfous T, Hoshiwara I, et al. Trachoma therapy with topicaltetracycline and oral erythromycin: a comparative trial. Bull World Health Organ. 1982;60:347–55.
7. West SK, Solomon AW. Azithromycin for control of trachoma. Community Eye Health. 1999;12:55–6.
8. Bailey RL, Arullendran P, Whittle HC, Mabey DC. Randomized controlled trial of single-dose azithromycin in treatment of trachoma. Lancet. 1993;342:453–6.
9. Solomon AW, Holland MJ, Alexander NDE, Massae PA, Aguirre A, Natividad-Sancho A, Molina S, Safari S, Shao JF, Courtright P, Peeling RW, West SK, Bailey RL, Foster A, Mabey DC. Mass treatment with single dose azithromycin for trachoma. N Engl J Med. 2004;351:1962–71.
10. Solomon AW, Harding-Esch E, Alexander ND, Aguirre A, Holland MJ, Bailey RL, Foster A, Mabey DC, Massae PA, Courtright P, Shao JF. Two doses of azithromycin to eliminate trachoma in a Tanzanian community. New Engl J Med. 2008;358:1870 1.
11. Coles CL, Seidman JC, Levens J, Mkocha H, Munoz B, West S. Association of Mass Treatment with azithromycin in trachoma-endemic communities with short-term reduced risk of diarrhea in young children. Am J Trop Med Hyg. 2011; https://doi.org/10.4269/ajtmh.2011.11-0046.
12. Keenan JD, Ayele B, Gebre T, Zerihun M, Zhou Z, House JI, Gaynor BD, Porco TC, Emerson PM, Lietman TM. Childhood mortality in a cohort treated with mass azithromycin for trachoma. Clin Infect Dis. 2011;52:883–8.
13. Fraser-Hurt N, Bailey RL, Cousens S, Mabey D, Faal H, Mabey DCW. Efficacy of oral azithromycin versus topical tetracycline in mass treatment of endemic trachoma. Bull World Health Organ. 2001;79:632–40.

14. WHO. World Health Assembly Resolution 51.11 Global Elimination of blinding trachoma; 1998. http://www.who.int/neglected_diseases/mediacentre/WHA_51.11_Eng.pdf. Accessed 30 Nov 2012.

15. WHO-ITI. Joint Research Agenda Meeting for the Elimination of Blinding Trachoma. Geneva: World Health. Organization; 2004.

16. Ssemanda EN, Levens J, Mkocha H, Munoz B, West SK. Azithromycin Mass Treatment for Trachoma Control: Risk Factors for Non-Participation of Children in Two Treatment Rounds. PLoS Negl Trop Dis. 2012; https://doi.org/10.1371/journal.pntd.0001576.

17. Melese M, Chidambaram JD, Alemayehu W, Lee DC, Yi EH, Cevallos V, Zhou Z, Donnellan C, Saidel M, Whitcher JP, Gaynor BD, Lietman TM. Feasibility of eliminating ocular chlamydia trachomatis with repeat mass antibiotic treatments. Jama. 2004;292:721–5.

18. University of Twente. Health Belief Model; 2013. https://www.utwente.nl/en/bms/communication-theories/sorted-bycluster/Health%20Communication/Health_Belief_Model/. Accessed 28 June 2013.

19. Desmond N, Solomon AW, Massae PA, Lema N, Anemona A, Foster A, Mabey DW. Acceptability of azithromycin for the control of trachoma in northern Tanzania. Trans R Soc Trop Med Hyg. 2005;99:656–63.

20. Lwanga SK, Lemeshow S. Sample size determination for health studies: a practical manual. Geneva: World Health Organization; 1991. p. 1–5.

21. Harding-Esch EM, Sillah A, Edwards T, Burr SE, Hart JD, Joof H, Laye M, Makalo P, Ahmed M, Molina S, Sarr-Sissoho I, Quinn TC, Lietman T, Holland MJ, Mabey D, West SK, Robin B. Mass treatment with azithromycin for trachoma: when is one round enough? Results from the PRET Trial in the Gambia. PLoS Negl Trop Dis. 2013;7:e2115. https://doi.org/10.1371/journal.pntd.0002115.

22. Central Statistics Authority. Summary and Statistical Report of the 2007 Population and Housing Census. 2008, Addis Ababa. https://searchworks.stanford.edu/view/8650186. Accessed 12 Dec 2012.

23. Cromwell EA, King JD, McPherson S, Jip FN, Patterson AE, Mosher AW, Evans DS, Emerson PM. Monitoring of mass distribution interventions for trachoma in plateau state, Nigeria. PLoS Negl Trop Dis. 2013;7:e1995. https://doi.org/10.1371/journal.pntd.0001995.

24. Malaty RR, Zaki SS, Said ME, Vastine DW, Dawson DW, Schachter J. Extra ocular infections in children in areas with endemic trachoma. J Infect Dis. 1981;143:853.

25. Blake IM, Burton MJ, Bailey RL, Solomon AW, West S, Munoz B, Holland MJ, Mabey DCW, Gambhir M, Basanez MG, Grassly NC. Estimating household and community transmission of ocular chlamydia trachomatis. PLoS Negl Trop Dis. 2009;3:e401. https://doi.org/10.1371/journal.pntd.0000401.

26. Lakew T, House J, Hong KC, Yi E, Alemayehu W, Melese M, Zhou Z, Ray K, Chin S, Romero E, Keenan J, Whitcher JP, Gaynor BD, Lietman TM. Reduction and return of infectious trachoma in severely affected communities in Ethiopia. PLoS Negl Trop Dis. 2009;3:e376. https://doi.org/10.1371/journal.pntd.0000376.

27. Grassly NC, Ward ME, Ferris S, Mabey DC, Bailey RL. The natural history of trachoma infection and disease in a Gambian cohort with frequent follow-up. PLoS Negl Trop Dis. 2008;2:e341. https://doi.org/10.1371/journal.pntd.0000341.

28. Taylor KI, Taylor HR. Distribution of azithromycin for the treatment of trachoma. Br J Ophthalmol. 1999;83:134–5.

29. Ayele B, Gebre T, House JI, Zhou Z, McCulloch CE, Porco TC, Gaynor BD, Emerson PM, Lietman TM, Keenan JD. Short report: adverse events after mass azithromycin treatments for trachoma in Ethiopia. Am J Trop Med Hyg. 2011;85:291–4.

30. FDA. United states Food and Drug Administration safety announcement; 2013. https://www.fda.gov/downloads/Drugs/DrugSafety/UCM343347.pdf. Accessed Dec 2013.

31. Ray WA, Murray KT, Hall K, Arbogast PG, Stein CM. Azithromycin and the Risk of Cardiovascular Death. N Engl J Med. 2012; https://doi.org/10.1056/NEJMoa1003833.

32. Bin Abdulhak AA, Khan AR, Garbati MA, Qazi AH, Erwin P, Kisra S, Aly A, Farid T, ElChamiM WAP. Azithromycin and risk of cardiovascular death: a Meta analytic review of observational studies. Am J Ther. 2015; https://doi.org/10.1097/MJT.0000000000000138.

33. Alemayehu D, Andrews EN, Glue P, Knirsch CA. Considerations for the design and conduct of a pharmacovigilance study involving mass drug Administration in a Resource-Constrained Setting. PLoS Negl Trop Dis. 2010; https://doi.org/10.1371/journal.pntd.0000564.

34. Amarillo MLE, Belizario VY, Sadiang-abay JT, Sison SAM, Dayag AMS. Factors associated with the acceptance of mass drug administration for the elimination of lymphatic filariasis in Agusan del Sur, Philippines. Parasit Vectors. 2008;1:14. https://doi.org/10.1186/1756-3305-1-14.

8

Comparison of the MyoRing implantation depth by mechanical dissection using PocketMaker microkeratome versus Melles hook via AS-OCT

Shiva Pirhadi[1], Neda Mohammadi[2], Seyed Aliasghar Mosavi[3], Hashem Daryabari[4], Hossein Aghamollaei[3] and Khosrow Jadidi[4*]

Abstract

Background: This paper seeks to evaluate the depth and outcomes of MyoRing implantation using two mechanical dissection procedures including: PocketMaker microkeratome in opposition to the Melles hook method.

Methods: This retrospective study was carried out on 39 eyes of 38 keratoconus patients (28 male and 10 female) with the mean age of 28.97 ± 10.37 years and had undergone MyoRing implantation by the two mentioned methods. The MyoRing was inserted into the corneal pocket which was made manually in 18 eyes (Melles hook group) or with PocketMaker microkeratome in 21 eyes (PocketMaker group). The mean follow up time was 9.81 ± 3.7 months with pre-operative and post-operative ophthalmic examination including uncorrected visual acuity (UCVA), best-corrected visual acuity (BCVA), keratometry readings and central corneal thickness measurement. AS-OCT (Casia, SS-1000, Tomey, Nagoya, Japan) imaging was used to measure MyoRing insertion depth, exactly.

Results: Pre-operative and post-operative UCVA (LogMAR) mean change for the PocketMaker and Melles hook groups were recorded at 0.75 ± 0.32 and 0.78 ± 0.33, respectively. Similarly, BCVA (LogMAR) mean change were 0.27 ± 0.22 and 0.23 ± 0.22. Mean keratometry (Kmean) change were 6.06 ± 4.18 and 6.56 ± 3.55 respectively. UCVA change ($P = 0.767$), BCVA change ($P = 0.77$) and Kmean change ($P = 0.693$) showed that there was no statistically significant difference between both groups for any parameter. Depth measurements achieved from AS-OCT images showed that there was no statistically significant difference in pocket depth between two methods of MyoRing implantation ($P = 0.413$).

Conclusions: The results of Myoring implantation outcomes using mechanical dissection via PocketMaker microkeratome as against Melles hook are comparable.

Keywords: Cornea, Keratoconus, Intracorneal rings, PocketMaker microkeratome, Melles hook

* Correspondence: kh.jadidi@gmail.com
[4]Department of Ophthalmology, Baqiyatallah University of Medical Sciences, Tehran, Iran
Full list of author information is available at the end of the article

Background

Keratoconus is a non-inflammatory disease of the cornea and it manifests by progressive steepening, thinning and ectasia of the cornea [1]. This condition negatively affects patient's visual function. There are several ways to manage different stages of this disease. These stages include the use of contact lens, corneal collagen cross-linking (CXL), intracorneal ring implantation, lamellar and penetrating keratoplasty [2–6].

The intracorneal ring is made of synthetic material that can be inserted into the corneal stroma to reshape the cornea. Cornea remodeling, using this device can result to modification of cornea curvature and improvement of visual acuity [7]. Intraocular corneal rings available in the market include incomplete and complete rings. The incomplete rings include: Intacs (Addition Technology Inc.), Ferrararings (Ferrara Ophthalmic Ltd.), and Keraring (Mediphacos Ltd.). MyoRing (Dioptex GmbH, Austria), as a complete ring, is a new method that can be safe and effective in the treatment of Keratoconus [7–12]. The ring is inserted into an intrastromal pocket, which is created by femtosecond laser [11, 13] or a microkeratome Pocket-Maker (Dioptex GmbH, Austria) [8]. It can also be inserted mechanically using the Melles hook approach. In previous studies, the depth of the corneal pocket was suggested to be 300 μm [11, 12].

Different depths of ring insertion may have different visual outcomes. The implantation depth of intracorneal ring has been measured by scheimpflug [14, 15] or anterior segment optical coherence tomography (AS-OCT) images in previous studies [16–19]. In some of these studies, actual versus intended insertion depth were assessed whereas others evaluated visual outcomes relative to intracorneal ring depth. In addition, pocket creation for intracorneal ring implantation using femtosecond laser and Pocket-Maker has been compared in several studies [20–23]. However, to the best of our knowledge, there are no reports on the MyoRing implantation depth measurement using AS-OCT images and comparison of its insertion by two methods including PocketMaker and Melles hook. This study fixed MyoRing at a depth of 300 μm by these two different methods. Thereafter, the exact inserted depth was determined using high-resolution AS-OCT postoperatively to determine if the MyoRing was implanted at the same depth by the two methods. Also, a comparison was made between the visual and refractive outcomes of MyoRing implantation by Pocket-Maker microkeratome against the Melles hook method.

Methods

In this study, 39 eyes of 38 keratoconus patients were registered between July 2011 to April 2015 at Bina Eye Hospital, Tehran. The inclusion criteria involves factors such as patients with keratoconus, poor visual acuity with

glasses, contact lens intolerance, a clear central cornea, a minimum corneal thickness of 400 μm, and a maximum keratometry reading of less than 60 diopters (D). Keratoconus grading was determined based on the Krumeich classification [24]. MyoRing is available in 5- or 6-mm both in diameter and in thickness ranging from 200 to 320 μm (in 20 μm increments). The appropriate MyoRing was selected based on an innovative nomogram, previously described in detail [25]. The Corneal pocket was made using PocketMaker microkeratome in 21 eyes and manually using Melles hook in 18 eyes. The eyes were assigned for pocket creation by PocketMaker microkeratome or Melles hook based on the corneal steep meridian. The PocketMaker method was employed if the steep meridian was in the temporal area in the range of − 30 to +30 degrees. If the steep meridian was out of this range or in the superior area, the mechanical method would be selected. All patients were required to sign an informed consent form before treatment upon explanation of the purpose and procedures of the surgery. Afterwards, written informed consent forms were obtained from all participants.

All procedures performed in this study are in accordance with the ethical standards of the institutional research committee and with the 1964 Helsinki declaration and its later amendments.

Surgical procedure

All surgical procedures were performed by the same experienced surgeon (Kh.J) in a general operating room using a surgical microscope under topical anesthesia with 0.5% proparacaine hydrochloride solution. MyoRing implantation in all surgeries was performed by the steep meridian. In order to mark the steep point of the cornea, keratometry and keratoscopy were used in a sterilized situation.

Mechanical dissection using PocketMaker microkeratome

Mechanical dissection using PocketMaker microkeratome procedure for MyoRing implantation included the creation of pocket within corneal stroma at 8 or 9 mm diameter (based on MyoRing diameter) and 300 μm in depth using a PocketMaker microkeratome (Dioptex GmbH). After determining the correct position of the blade, the micro-vibrating diamond blade was set at 300 μm of the measured corneal thickness and a single 0.5 mm radial incision was made at the steepest meridian. Thereafter, the ring was inserted into the created pocket and its position was adjusted intraoperatively using a keratoscope.

Mechanical dissection using Melles hook

Mechanical dissection using the Melles hook procedure of Myoring implantation involved making an incision in the steep axis of the cornea with 0.5 mm length (smaller than MyoRing diameter) using a diamond blade. Afterward, a dissection in 300 μm depth with 3 mm (bigger than MyoRing diameter) was created using a Melles hook. Subsequently, the MyoRing was inserted into the pocket, which was mechanically created in the cornea, and its proper centration was determined using a keratoscope.

In both surgical methods, it was observed that the created pocket was capable of self-sealing and did not require any suture. Eventually, a bandage contact lens (Bausch & Lomb) was placed on the cornea and MyoRing implantation surgery was completed using chloramphenicol (Sinadaru Laboratories, Iran) eye drops. The bandage contact lens was removed 1 day after surgery. Four drops per day of chloramphenicol and betamethasone (Sinadaru Laboratories, Iran) and six drops per day of preservative-free artificial tears (Artelac Rebalance, Bausch & Lomb, Inc., USA) were prescribed postoperatively. The chloramphenicol drop was interrupted 1 week after surgery while the betamethasone dosage was tapered off during 4–6 weeks. Also, Artelac was continued 6 times a day for 1 month.

Patient evaluation

Preoperative and postoperative ophthalmic examinations in PocketMaker and manual groups included uncorrected visual acuity (UCVA), best-corrected visual acuity (BCVA) with a standard Snellen chart, corneal thickness, thinnest corneal point, anterior chamber depth (ACD) and keratometry readings by scanning-slit topography (Orbscan II), manifest spherical and cylindrical refraction and spherical equivalent (SE). For statistical analysis, decimal Snellen UCVA and BCVA were converted to LogMAR values.

After surgery, AS-OCT (Casia, SS-1000, Tomey, Nagoya, Japan) images were used to measure MyoRing

insertion depth, exactly. AS-OCT imaging was performed by one technician. The MyoRing depth and the depth of the intracorneal pocket were measured in horizontal and vertical axes at temporal, nasal, inferior and superior positions. Figure 1 shows 12 measured distances in two axes at 4 different sites in AS-OCT images. In each axis, distances between the anterior ring surface and the anterior corneal surface (AA), the posterior ring surface and the posterior corneal surface at ring sites (PP) and distances between the pocket depth and the anterior corneal surface (PDA) were measured at pocket sites (Fig. 1). Since an intracorneal ring was inserted into the cornea, it usually compressed the corneal lamella. Therefore, a decision was made to measure the PDA distance as the depth of the created pocket. For evaluating the MyoRing depth, nine parameters were defined as follows:

1) $AA_{0-180} = (AA_T + AA_N)/2$

Mean of AA distance at temporal and nasal sites in the 0–180 axis.

2) $AA_{90-270} = (AA_S + AA_I)/2$

Mean of AA distance at superior and inferior sites in the 90–270 axis.

3) $AA_{total} = (AA_{0-180} + AA_{90-270})/2$

Mean of AA distance in the horizontal and vertical axes.

4) $PP_{0-180} = (PP_T + PP_N)/2$

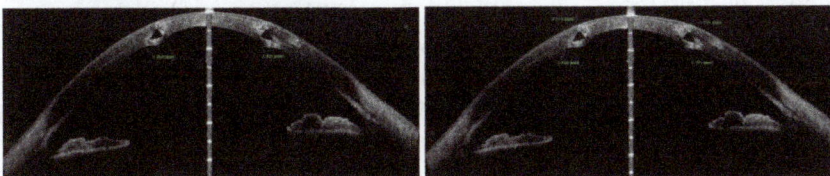
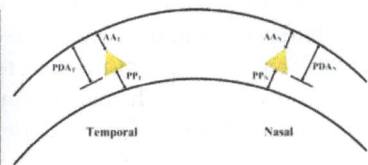
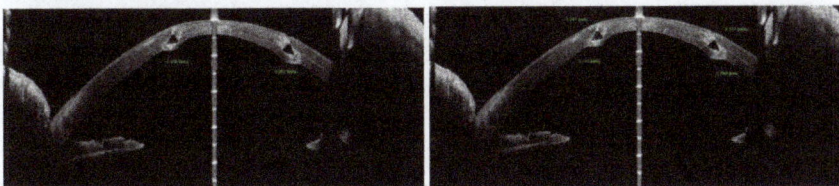
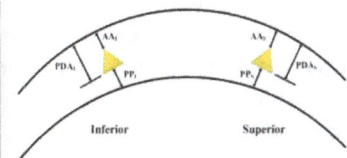

Fig. 1 The distances between the pocket depth to the anterior corneal surface (Left), the anterior ring surface and the anterior corneal surface, the posterior ring surface and the posterior corneal surface (middle) and the schematics of AS-OCT images (Right) in horizontal (**a**) and vertical axes (**b**) after MyoRing implantation. In each axis 3 parameters defined: distances between the anterior ring surface and the anterior corneal surface (AA), the posterior ring surface and the posterior corneal surface (PP) and distances between the pocket depth and the anterior corneal surface (PDA). These parameters measured for temporal and nasal, inferior and superior sites for 0–180 and 90–270 axes, respectively

Mean of PP distance at temporal and nasal sites in the 0–180 axis.

5) $PP_{90-270} = (PP_S + PP_I)/2$

Mean of PP distance at superior and inferior sites in the 90–270 axis.

6) $PP_{total} = (PP_{0-180} + PP_{90-270})/2$

Mean of PP distance in horizontal and vertical axes.

7) $PDA_{0-180} = (PDA_T + PDA_N)/2$

Mean of PDA distance at temporal and nasal sites in the 0–180 axis.

8) $PDA_{90-270} = (PDA_S + PDA_I)/2$

Mean of PDA distance at superior and inferior sites in the 90–27 axis.

9) $PDA_{total} = (PDA_{0-180} + PDA_{90-270})/2$

Mean of PDA distance in the horizontal and vertical axes.

All distances with 0–180 index compared with the same ones in the 90–270 axis intragroup for Pocket-Maker and manual groups. The total indices of other parameters were compared between groups.

Statistical analysis

Statistical analysis was performed using SPSS software for Windows (version 24; SPSS Inc., Chicago, IL, USA). To compare the same distances at different axes in each group, the t-paired test was used. The t-test or if necessary, its replace test, nonparametric Mann-Whitney, was used to compare the depth parameters with total indices between two groups. The paired t-test was used to compare visual, refractive, keratometric and corneal thickness variables before and after ring insertion by the method of insertion used; and the non-parametric Wilcoxon test was used in its place wherever required. The two groups were compared in terms of these variables before ring implantation using the independent t-test, and the non-parametric Mann-Whitney test (where necessary). After ring implantation, these variables were also compared between groups using the independent t-test and the non-parametric Mann-Whitney test (where necessary). The difference between these variables before and after ring insertion was measured as the mean changes, and the independent t-test was used to compare the mean changes obtained by the Melles hook method and the PocketMaker mikrokeratome.

Results

This study evaluated 39 eyes of 38 keratoconus patients with a mean age of 28.97 ± 10.37 years (Range 17–55 years). The Corneal pocket was made using Pocket-Maker in 21 eyes and manually using Melles hook in 18 eyes. The mean follow-up period was 9.81 ± 3.7 months in the PocketMaker group and 9.89 ± 3.3 months in the Melles hook group. MyroRing with 5- and 6-mm diameter were fixed at 12 and 9, 10 and 8 eyes in the Pocket-Maker and Melles hook groups, respectively. The mean MyoRing thickness was 298.1 ± 36.27 and 302.22 ± 36.87 in the PocketMaker and Melles hook groups, respectively. There were no statistically significant differences between 2 groups in the mean follow-up ($P > 0.999$), patients' ages ($P = 0.6$) and ring thickness ($P = 0.41$). Moreover, preoperative keratoconus grades were determined in each group (Table 1). No significant difference was found in the distribution of grades between both groups ($P = 0.715$, chi-square test).

All AA, PP and PDA depth parameters were compared between the 0–180 and 90–270 axes in each group (Table 2). There were no statistically significant differences in depth parameters between the two axes in the Pocket-Maker group. In the Melles hook group, only PP parameter had a significant difference between the two axes ($P = 0.001$) which means that the corneal thickness below the ring in the 0–180 axis is lower compared to the other axis. The parameters with total indices between groups were also compared (Table 3). There were no significant differences in these variables. Moreover, a correlation analysis was performed to evaluate the effect of MyoRing thickness on depth parameters. No correlation was found between MyoRing thickness and AA_{total} ($r = -0.11$, $P = 0.636$), PP_{total} ($r = 0.011$, $P = 0.961$), and PDA_{total} ($r = -0.031$, $P = 0.892$) parameters in the PocketMaker group. Also, there were no correlations between Myoring thickness and AA_{total} ($r = -0.156$, $P = 0.536$), PP_{total} ($r = 0.027$, $P = 0.914$), and PDA_{total} ($r = -0.026$, $P = 0.918$) parameters in the mechanical group.

The visual, refractive, keratometric, corneal thickness and ACD variables were assessed before and after the operation in each group and compared between the two groups (Table 4). The results showed a significant improvement in UCVA, BCVA, sphere, cylinder, SE, Sim-K,

Table 1 Keratoconus grading based on Krumeich classification

Grade of KCN	Eyes, n (%)	
	Mechanical	PocketMaker
1	3 (16)	6 (28)
2	7 (38)	9 (42)
3	1 (5)	1 (4)
4	7 (38)	5 (23)

Table 2 Comparison of depth parameters at horizontal and vertical axes between Manual group and PocketMaker group

| Variables | Type of surgery | | | | | |
| | Mechanical | | | PocketMaker | | |
	N	Mean ± SD	P-value	N	Mean ± SD	P-value
AA_{0-180}	18	206.33 ± 48.68	0.07	21	199.14 ± 36.77	0.227
AA_{90-270}	18	196.22 ± 49.83		21	216.95 ± 66.59	
PP_{0-180}	18	208.86 ± 33.76	0.001	21	230.64 ± 54.87	0.364
PP_{90-270}	18	226.64 ± 38.4		21	234.81 ± 51.02	
PDA_{0-180}	18	341.14 ± 42.58	0.447	21	347.6 ± 36.19	0.548
PDA_{90-270}	18	334.58 ± 53.15		21	351.38 ± 52.45	

AA_{0-180}: Mean of AA distance at temporal and nasal sites in 0–180 axis, AA_{90-270}: Mean of AA distance at superior and inferior sites in 90–270 axis, PP_{0-180}: Mean of PP distance at temporal and nasal sites in 0–180 axis, PP_{90-270}: Mean of PP distance at superior and inferior sites in 90–270 axis, PDA_{0-180}: Mean of PDA distance at temporal and nasal sites in 0–180 axis, PDA_{90-270}: Mean of PDA distance at superior and inferior sites in 90–27 axis

astigmatism as well as the maximum, minimum and mean keratometry in each group. Corneal thickness and the thinnest corneal point increased in both groups after the operation, and this increase was significant in the Melles hook group. ACD reduced after the operation in both groups, but not significantly. There were no significant differences between the two groups in these variables before the operation. However, after the operation, the two groups differed significantly only in terms of the cylinder variable.

Discussion

The MyoRingintracorneal implantation has been presented in order to treat keratoconus as well as improve visual and refractive outcomes. Three techniques were suggested to make a pocket for MyoRing insertion. The-Pocket can be created using a femtosecond laser [11, 13], using a PocketMaker microkeratome (Dioptex GmbH, Austria) [8] and manually, using the Melles hook approach. The present study is the first to compare the Melles hook method and the PocketMaker in terms of both the pocket depth created, the refraction as well as the visual outcomes.

Daxer et al. compared two methods of MyoRing implantation, including the Femtosecond laser-assisted

Table 3 Comparison of depth total parameters between manual group and PocketMaker group

variables	Type of surgery	N	Mean ± SD	P-value
AA_{total}	Manual	18	201.2778 ± 47.99	0.644
	PocketMaker	21	208.0476 ± 42.68	
PP_{total}	Manual	18	217.75 ± 34.96	0.307
	PocketMaker	21	232.7262 ± 51.97	
PDA_{total}	Manual	18	337.8611 ± 44.72	0.413
	PocketMaker	21	349.4881 ± 42.76	

method and the PocketMaker. They did not assess the pocket depth created by the two methods and thus was insufficient to compare their fraction and visual outcomes between the two groups [23].

The PocketMaker is an expensive device and its delicate blades may be damaged in the autoclaving process or during the operation, and repairing damaged blades requires a high expenditure of time and money. In manual ring insertion, only Melles hooks are required, which are inexpensive and easy to use. The present study was conducted to compare the creation of pockets using the PocketMaker and Melles hooks in terms of the depth of implant, refraction and visual outcomes in order to determine if the Melles hook method can be used in places where the PocketMaker is unavailable, provided the outcomes are similar. The MyoRing was therefore inserted to the same depth (300 μm) using these two different methods. Thereafter, Casia AS-OCT was used to measure the precise post-operative ring implantation depth created in the two methods. The post-operative ring implantation depth was measured in horizontal and vertical axes in temporal, nasal, superior and inferior positions.

In the present study, in the Melles hook group, the mean distance from the posterior part of the ring to the posterior part of the cornea was 208.86 ± 33.76 μm in the nasal and temporal regions and 226.64 ± 38.4 μm in the superior and inferior regions, which is statistically significant ($P = 0.001$). Nonetheless, no significant differences were observed in the PocketMaker group ($P = 0.364$). In the Melles hook group, the ring was implanted 18 μm deeper in the horizontal axis, and the uneven movement of the hook in the Melles hook method may have caused this difference. However, in the PocketMaker group, the eye pressure increased to 70 mmHg, and the incision was created on a smooth surface. Despite this difference, measuring the mean distance in all the four regions in the two groups and comparing it with each group showed no significant differences. In addition, the mean distance between the anterior part of the ring and the anterior part of the cornea was also measured in the four regions and no significant differences were observed between the two groups ($P = 0.664$). It can thus be concluded that the mean depth of ring implantation at the distance from the anterior part of the ring to the anterior part of the cornea and from the posterior part of the ring to the posterior part of the cornea is the same in both methods.

In one study, Koussai et al. compared Intacs implant depth in mechanical and Femtosecond laser-assisted methods using AS-OCT. The mean difference between the depth expected before the operation and the final implant depth was 76.64 μm in the mechanical group

Table 4 Comparison of refractive, keratometric, thickness and visual outcomes between manual group and PocketMaker group

Variables	Mean ± SD		
	Manual	PocketMaker	P-value
UCVA (*LogMAR*)			
Pre	1.18 ± 0.25	1.03 ± 0.28	0.083
Post	0.39 ± 0.25	0.27 ± 0.17	0.106
Mean change	0.78 ± 0.33	0.75 ± 0.32	0.767
P-value	< 0.001	< 0.001	
BCVA (*LogMAR*)			
Pre	0.56 ± 0.34	0.48 ± 0.2	0.791
Post	0.26 ± 0.19	0.21 ± 0.13	0.512
Mean change	0.23 ± 0.22	0.27 ± 0.22	0.77
P-value	< 0.001	< 0.001	
Sphere (*D*)			
Pre	−7.89 ± 4.42	−7.5 ± 2.97	0.754
Post	−1.49 ± 3.46	−0.37 ± 1.6	0.394
Mean change	−6.4 ± 4.79	−7.13 ± 3.5	0.584
P-value	< 0.001	< 0.001	
Cylinder (*D*)			
Pre	−5.58 ± 2.1	−4.36 ± 1.33	0.053
Post	−2.65 ± 1.44	−1.46 ± 0.77	0.006
Mean change	−2.93 ± 2.55	−2.89 ± 1.46	0.954
P-value	< 0.001	< 0.001	
SE (*D*)			
Pre	−10.68 ± 4.26	−9.68 ± 2.93	0.407
Post	−2.82 ± 3.42	−1.1 ± 1.51	0.11
Mean change	−7.86 ± 4.7	−8.58 ± 3.51	0.59
P-value	< 0.001	< 0.001	
Sim k astigmatism(*D*)			
Pre	−5.81 ± 1.858	−5.1 ± 2.56	0.336
Post	−2.54 ± 1.4642	−2.2 ± 1.46	0.364
Mean change	−3.26 ± 2.45	−2.89 ± 2.29	0.633
P-value	< 0.001	< 0.001	
Kmax (*D*)			
Pre	55.73 ± 5.43	53.14 ± 5.96	0.213
Post	47.84 ± 3.31	45.85 ± 3.14	0.192
Mean change	7.89 ± 4.14	7.29 ± 5.06	0.692
P-value	< 0.001	< 0.001	
Kmin (*D*)			
Pre	51.12 ± 5.54	48.48 ± 4.11	0.097
Post	45.34 ± 3.54	43.64 ± 2.85	0.106
Mean change	5.77 ± 4.81	4.83 ± 3.75	0.495
P-value	< 0.001	< 0.001	
Kmean (*D*)			

Table 4 Comparison of refractive, keratometric, thickness and visual outcomes between manual group and PocketMaker group (*Continued*)

Variables	Mean ± SD		
	Manual	PocketMaker	P-value
Pre	53.26 ± 5.05	50.81 ± 4.86	0.192
Post	46.56 ± 3.46	44.75 ± 2.91	0.174
Mean change	6.56 ± 3.55	6.06 ± 4.18	0.693
P-value	< 0.001	< 0.001	
Corneal thickness (*μm*)			
Pre	421.06 ± 45.58	452.52 ± 60.42	0.078
Post	447.78 ± 27.85	467.67 ± 44.61	0.099
Mean change	−26.72 ± 41.99	−15.14 ± 56.6	0.479
P-value	0.015	0.234	
Thinnest corneal point (*μm*)			
Pre	394.44 ± 57.76	431.67 ± 68.43	0.077
Post	425.33 ± 31.05	441.05 ± 45.8	0.226
Mean change	−30.89 ± 52.66	−9.38 ± 62.49	0.257
P-value	0.023	0.499	
ACD (mm)			
Pre	3.7106 ± 0.59	3.59 ± 0.48	0.508
Post	3.3975 ± 0.42	3.39 ± 0.39	0.773
Mean change	0.31 ± 0.49	0.21 ± 0.25	0.397
P-value	0.023	0.001	

UCVA Uncorrected visual acuity, *BCVA* Best-corrected visual acuity, *Sphere* manifest spherical refraction, *Cylinder* manifest cylindrical refraction, *SE* Spherical equivalent, *K* keratometric power, *ACD* Anterior chamber depth

and 85.85 μm in the Femtosecond-assisted group, with no significant differences between the two groups. Their study showed that shallower Intacs implant depths had been created in both methods compared to the expected depth [20]. Gorgun et al. measured anterior stromal thickness from the Ferrara segment apex after ring implantation using a Femtosecond laser along with an AS-OCT and found that the Ferrara segments were implanted 97 μm shallower on average [16]. In another study, Barbara et al. measured the final implant depth and the expected depth after Intacs insertion in the mechanical method using an AS-OCT. It was discovered that the Intacsimplant depth created was 153 μm shallower than the expected depth [19]. In the present study, the pocket depths created in the PocketMaker and Melles hook groups were compared to the target depth of 300 μm. The measurements showed that the mean pocket depth created in the horizontal and vertical axes was 349.48 μm in the PocketMaker group and 337.86 μm in the Melles hook group. Although the depth created was 50 μm deeper in the PocketMaker group and 38 μm in the Melles hook group compared to the expected depth, no significant differences were observed between both groups ($P = 0.413$). Thus, both the PocketMaker and the Melles hook method can be said to have created similar pocket depths for MyoRing implantation.

The surgeon's skill, however, is a noteworthy point. Although surgical skills are required to achieve the correct depth in ring implantation in both methods, these skills are twice as important as in the Melles hook method, because the surgeon's lack of skills in the Melles hook method can lead to complications such as anterior or posterior corneal perforation, superficial ring placement and ring extrusion. In the present study, no intraoperative or postoperative complications were observed in either group.

As already discussed, an 18-μm difference was observed in the Melles hook group between the horizontal and vertical axes at the distance from the posterior part of the ring to the posterior part of the cornea, indicating uneven hook movement. Although this 18-μm difference can be overlooked, an uneven pocket can affect visual outcomes. The hypothesis in the present study was that the sharper and more regular pocket made by the PocketMaker compared to the Melles hook method, the better the visual outcomes of the PocketMaker. The two groups were therefore compared in terms of SE, UCVA, BCVA and keratometric parameters.

Daxer et al. compared refraction and visual outcomes after MyoRing implantation using a PocketMaker and the Femtosecond method and obtained similar outcomes in the two methods [23]. The present findings showed improvements in both groups in UCVA, BCVA, SE and keratometric parameters, with no significant differences between the two groups. It can thus be concluded that the created pocket did not affect the final outcomes in either method.

The limitations of this study include the small sample of treated eyes and the short follow up period. However, due to the difference in the indications of selected patients for MyoRing, and since only one study has assessed the two methods of MyoRing implantation (Daxer et al.), in which only 14 eyes were examined, it appears that the comparison of 39 eyes in the present study is reasonable.

Conclusions

In conclusion, the MyoRing implant depths created by the PocketMaker and the Melles hook may be considered similar. On the other hand, if the surgeon is adequately skilled, the mechanical method using Melles hook can produce similar outcomes with fewer costs. However, large comparative multicenter studies are recommended to verify and further clarify these results.

Abbreviations
AA: Distances between the anterior ring surface and the anterior corneal surface; ACD: Anterior chamber depth; AS-OCT: Anterior segment optical coherence tomography; BCVA: Best-corrected visual acuity; Kmax: Maximum keratometry reading; Kmean: Mean keratometry reading; Kmin: Minimum keratometry reading; LogMAR: Logarithm of the minimum angle of resolution; PDA: Distances between the pocket depth and the anterior corneal surface; PP: Distance between the posterior ring surface and the posterior corneal surface; SD: Standard deviation; SE: Spherical equivalent; UCVA: Uncorrected visual acuity

Acknowledgements
The authors would like to acknowledge the staffs of eye clinic in Bina Eye Hospital for their valuable help during the entire process of this study.

Funding
The whole study was performed without any funding.

Authors' contributions
KJ, SP, SAM and HD were responsible for the conception and design of the study. SP acquired the data. KJ, SP, NM and HA analyzed and interpreted the data. SP wrote the draft. KJ, SP, SAM and HD revised the manuscript critically. All authors have read and approved the final manuscript.

Competing interests
The authors declare that they have no competing interests.

Author details
[1]Department of Biomedical Engineering, Tehran Science and Research Branch, Islamic Azad University, Tehran, Iran. [2]Department of Epidemiology and Biostatistics, School of Public Health, Tehran University of Medical Sciences, Tehran, Iran. [3]Vision Health Research Center, Semnan University of Medical Sciences, Semnan, Iran. [4]Department of Ophthalmology, Baqiyatallah University of Medical Sciences, Tehran, Iran.

References
1. Ertan A, Colin J. Intracorneal rings for keratoconus and keratectasia. J Cataract Refract Surg. 2007;33(7):1303–14.
2. Barnett M, Mannis MJ. Contact lenses in the management of keratoconus. Cornea. 2011;30(12):1510–6.
3. Vega-Estrada A, Alió JL, Puche AB, Marshall J. Outcomes of a new microwave procedure followed by accelerated cross-linking for the treatment of keratoconus: a pilot study. J Refract Surg. 2012;28(11):787–92.
4. Colin J, Cochener B, Savary G, Malet F. Correcting keratoconus with intracorneal rings. J Cataract Refract Surg. 2000;26(8):1117–22.
5. Snibson GR. Collagen cross-linking: a new treatment paradigm in corneal disease–a review. Clin Exp Ophthalmol. 2010;38(2):141–53.
6. Busin M, Scorcia V, Zambianchi L, Ponzin D. Outcomes from a modified microkeratome-assisted lamellar keratoplasty for keratoconus. Arch Ophthalmol. 2012;130(6):776–82.
7. Piñero DP, Alio JL. Intracorneal ring segments in ectatic corneal disease–a review. Clin Exp Ophthalmol. 2010;38(2):154–67.
8. Daxer A. Adjustable intracorneal ring in a lamellar pocket for keratoconus. J Refract Surg. 2010;26(3):217–21.
9. Daxer A, Mahmoud H, Venkateswaran RS. Intracorneal continuous ring implantation for keratoconus: one-year follow-up. J Cataract Refract Surg. 2010;36(8):1296–302.
10. Mahmood H, Venkateswaran RS, Daxer A. Implantation of a complete corneal ring in an intrastromal pocket for keratoconus. J Refract Surg. 2011;27(1):63–8.
11. Alio JL, Piñero DP, Daxer A. Clinical outcomes after complete ring implantation in corneal ectasia using the femtosecond technology: a pilot study. Ophthalmology. 2011;118(7):1282–90.
12. Jabbarvand M, SalamatRad A, Hashemian H, Khodaparast M. Continuous corneal intrastromal ring implantation for treatment of keratoconus in an Iranian population. Am J Ophthalmol. 2013;155(5):837–42.
13. Jabbarvand M, SalamatRad A, Hashemian H, Mazloumi M, Khodaparast M.

Continuous intracorneal ring implantation for keratoconus using a femtosecond laser. J Cataract Refract Surg. 2013;39(7):1081–7.

14. Ertan A. Measurement of depth of Intacs implanted via femtosecond laser using Pentacam. J Refract Surg. 2009;25(4):377–82.

15. Sadigh AL, Aali TA, Sadeghi A. Outcome of intrastromal corneal ring segment relative to depth of insertion evaluated with scheimpflug image. J Curr Ophthalmol. 2015;27(1):25–31.

16. Gorgun E, Kucumen RB, Yenerel NM, Ciftci F. Assessment of intrastromal corneal ring segment position with anterior segment optical coherence tomography. Ophthalmic Surg Lasers and Imaging Retina. 2012;43(3):214–21.

17. Lai MM, Tang M, Andrade EM, Li Y, Khurana RN, Song JC, Huang D. Optical coherence tomography to assess intrastromal corneal ring segment depth in keratoconic eyes. J Cataract Refract Surg. 2006;32(11):1860–5.

18. Hashemi H, Yazdani-Abyaneh A, Beheshtnejad A, Jabbarvand M, Kheirkhah A, Ghaffary SR. Efficacy of IntacsIntrastromal corneal ring segment relative to depth of insertion evaluated with anterior segment optical coherence tomography. Middle East Afr J Ophthalmol. 2013;20(3):234–8.

19. Barbara R, Barbara A, Naftali M. Depth evaluation of intended vs actual intacsintrastromal ring segments using optical coherence tomography. Eye. 2016;30(1):102–10.

20. Kouassi FX, Buestel C, Raman B, Melinte D, Touboul D, Gallois A, Colin J. Comparison of the depth predictability of intra corneal ring segment implantation by mechanical versus femtosecond laser-assisted techniques using optical coherence tomography (OCT Visante (®)). J Fr Ophtalmol. 2012; 35(2):94–9.

21. Kubaloglu A, Sari ES, Cinar Y, Cingu K, Koytak A, Coşkun E, Özertürk Y. Comparison of mechanical and femtosecond laser tunnel creation for intrastromal corneal ring segment implantation in keratoconus: prospective randomized clinical trial. J Cataract Refract Surg. 2010;36(9):1556–61.

22. Kubaloglu A, Sari ES, Cinar Y, Koytak A, Kurnaz E, Özertürk Y. Intrastromal corneal ring segment implantation for the treatment of keratoconus. Cornea. 2011;30(1):11–7.

23. Daxer B, Mahmood H, Daxer A. MyoRing treatment for keratoconus: DIOPTEX PocketMakervsZiemer LDV for corneal pocket creation. Int J Keratoconus Ectatic Corneal Dis. 2012;1(3):151–2.

24. Sinjab MM. Classifications and Patterns of Keratoconus and Keratectasia. In: Quick Guide to the Management of Keratoconus. Berlin Heidelberg: Springer; 2012. p. 13–58.

25. Jadidi K, Nejat F, Mosavi SA, Naderi M, Katiraee A, Janani L, Aghamollaei H. Full-ring intrastromal corneal implantation for correcting high myopia in patients with severe keratoconus. Med Hypothesis Discov Innov Ophthalmol. 2016;5(3):89–95.

9

Assessment of meibomian glands using a custom–made meibographer in dry eye patients in Ghana

Eugene Appenteng Osae[1,2*] (iD), Reynolds Kwame Ablorddepey[1], Jens Horstmann[2,3], David Ben Kumah[1] and Philipp Steven[2,3]

Abstract

Background: Meibomian Gland Dysfunction (MGD) is a leading cause of evaporative Dry Eye Disease (DED). This makes non-invasive meibography an important procedure in the clinical evaluation of DED patients. Our purpose was to conduct a lead-off investigation focused on the practicality of performing meibography in a developing country, with limited access to complex ophthalmic imaging systems, using a custom meibographer, as a step to future comparative studies on meibomian glands and DED in Africa.

Methods: Meibomian glands(MG) in 76 upper eyelids (UL) and 49 lower eyelids (LL) in 1 eye each of 125 patients randomly selected from a patient population presenting with subjective DED symptoms at a clinic were photographed using a custom meibographer. Single frames were captured, and the MG area determined by intensity threshold segmentation and area calculation using Image J software. MG loss (MGL) was quantified by outlining its area and expressing it as a percentage of the total MG per Pult's grading scheme. Dry eye measures included Tear Film Break Up - Time (TUBT), Schirmer's test and Ocular Surface Staining (OSS). Symptoms were evaluated using the SPEED II questionnaire. Correlations between MGL and age, ocular signs and symptoms were analyzed by Pearson's. Differences between comparable groups were analyzed by Mann - Whitney test; $p < 0.05$ was considered significant.

Results: Overall mean MGL was 32.10% ± 25.0% (26.25% ± 22.40% for UL and 40.33% ± 26.70% for LL). MGL correlated significantly with age [$r = 0.91$, $p = 0.001$], SPEED scores [$r = 0.90$, $p = 0.001$], OSS [$r = 0.75$, $p = 0.001$] and TBUT [$r = -0.81$, $p = 0.001$]. MGL scores were significantly higher in the UL than LL [$U = 1293.5$ $p = 0.004$].

Conclusion: This study for the first time presents data on the status of Meibomian glands in Africa. It furthermore suggests that it is feasible to examine Meibomian glands using a custom meibographer in developing countries with limited access to complex imaging systems. It also demonstrates the benefit and cost-effectiveness of a simple device by the observed significant relations between meibomian gland loss and DED in these patients.

Keywords: Dry eye disease, Meibomian gland dysfunction, Ocular surface, Meibographer, Tear film

* Correspondence: osaeappen@gmail.com
This work was presented as a poster at the 2016 Association for Research in Vision and Ophthalmology (ARVO) Annual Meeting in Seattle, USA.
[1]Department of Optometry and Visual Science, Kwame Nkrumah University of Science and Technology, PMB, Kumasi, Ghana
[2]Department of Ophthalmology, Faculty of Medicine, University of Cologne, Cologne, Germany
Full list of author information is available at the end of the article

Background

Dry eye disease (DED), synonymous to dysfunctional tear syndrome (DTS) or dysfunction of the lacrimal functional unit (LFU) is a multifactorial disease of the tears and ocular surface which results in symptoms of discomfort, visual disturbance and tear film instability with potential damage to the ocular surface [1, 2]. DED can broadly be classified as evaporative and aqueous – deficient DED or overlapping forms. In evaporative DED, there is decreased stability of the tear film due to abnormality in its lipid component. Aqueous – deficient DED on the other is linked to a reduced volume of the aqueous component of the tear film [3, 4].

The tear film lipids are produced by modified sebaceous glands in the eye lids, located within the tarsal plates [5]. These glands are called Meibomian glands (MG). Their secretion, also called meibum, is produced within these glands. It is secreted via ductal systems which open at the lid margin where it forms a thin layer on top of the aqueous and mucin tear components on the surface of the eye, preventing fast evaporation of tears and enhancing the lubricant properties of tears [5, 6]. A dysfunction of these glands is clinically referred to as Meibomian gland dysfunction (MGD). In MGD, there is poor quality and/or reduced volume of meibum – it is these alterations which lead to evaporative DED [7]. Different forms of MGD are distinguished as recently defined in the International Workshop on MGD Report. In particular low delivery and high delivery forms are distinguished that are related to dermatological diseases such as rosacea, systemic cicatrizing diseases such as pemphigoid or induced by drugs such as retinoids [2] .

Comparable to most developed countries, DED is a growing significant clinical problem in developing countries and emerging economies. Early studies conducted in these regions of the world have reported associations between DED and infectious disease like Trachoma and forms of malnutrition like vitamin A deficiency [8–13]. However, the current patterns of industrialization, modernization, urbanization and general socioeconomic transformations – including significant successes achieved at combating these infectious diseases and malnutrition in these areas could mean a present shift to other forms and causes of DED [14–22], such as MGD induced by aging, androgen deficiency, skin diseases, contact lens wear, etc.

It is widely known that MGD causes DED by altering the tear film lipids, destabilizing the entire tear film structure by disrupting the cohesivity between the various components. This causes tears to evaporate from the eye leading to reduced lubricity of the ocular surface therefore dryness at the ocular surface. Thus, assessment of the MG [5] is a crucial component in the comprehensive clinical evaluation and successful management of DED patients. The International Workshop on MGD suggests assessing for MGD in people by evaluating eyelid morphology, MG mass, MG expressibility, tear film lipid layer and MG drop-out or loss by meibography [7, 22].

Meibography is an imaging technique that provides an in - vivo means to assess the structure of the MG and makes it possible to view and quantify loss of glandular tissue (MGL) using a device called meibographer [24]. This is achievable because the technique allows for photographic documentation of Meibomian glands under specialized illumination situations. Meibography has undergone remarkable evolution but presently exists in two main forms – transillumination of the everted eye lids and direct illumination of the everted eyelids [24, 25]. The latter form is also called the non-contact (NCT) meibography, which has previously been described in different reports [23, 24].

NCT meibography comprises a slit lamp equipped with an infrared – charge coupled device with a video camera and infrared transmitting filter which makes it possible to view the glands in the everted lid non-invasively - without touching the eyelids. NCT meibography is believed to be a comfortable procedure for most patients compared to the transillumination method [25] but commercially existing NCT meibographers are expensive and thus may not be readily obtainable by most clinics especially those in developing countries.

Herein, we investigated the feasibility of conducting meibography in a developing country using a custom-made meibographer.

Methods

Construction of the customized meibographer

Following Pult's suggestions [26], We obtained a simple infra – red video camera (Sunluxy SL – C221, Shen Zhen, China) and adapted it for near field imaging by an additional + 20 dioptre lens (Fig. 1). In addition, we blocked the light sensor of this camera to permanently cause it to image in dark or low levels of illumination – a condition which allows for the maximal illumination of the lids by the light source from the infrared diodes. The video camera is connected to a computer via a video –to – high speed serial bus converter / Logilink®V-GA0001A (2direct GmbH, Schalksmühle, Germany).

Clinical measurements and subject inclusion

Meibomian glands (MG) in one eye (overall 76 UL and 49 LL) of 125 patients, randomly selected from a patient pool presenting with subjective dry eye symptoms at a private practice in Kumasi Ghana, were photographed with the custom-made meibographer. Single frames were captured, and the MG area was determined. Additionally, a thorough slit lamp examination was conducted, and 2% topical fluorescein was applied to the ocular surface to measure Tear Film Break – Up Time (TBUT).

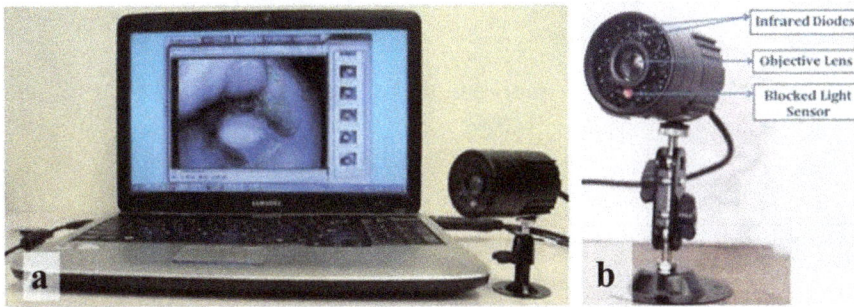

Fig. 1 a Computer - meibographer set up. **b** Picture of meibographer with major components labelled

We also graded Ocular Surface Staining (OSS) in 95 subjects using the Oxford Grading Scheme described by Bron et al. [27] using a Wratten # 12 filter (Kodak, New Jersey, USA). Symptoms of DED were evaluated using the SPEED II Questionnaire.

None of subjects included in the study had a history of ocular surgery including lid correction, neither did any report use of systemic drugs like isotretinoin [28] that could impair MG function. Further, none of the subjects had ever received treatment for MGD prior to the study.

Meibomian gland evaluation

Meibography images were evaluated by intensity threshold segmentation and area calculation with Image J software [29]. In detail, Meibomian Gland Loss (MGL) was determined by outlining the meibomian gland area present and expressing the area as a percentage of the total tarsal area as described by Pult's et al. [26]. MGL was assigned grade 0 when there was approximately no (0%) glandular loss. Grades 1, 2, 3 and 4 represented ≤ 25%, 26–50%, 51–75% and > 75% of glandular loss (MGL) respectively. Representative images are shown in Fig. 2.

Statistical analysis

Data was analyzed using SPSS version 20 (SPSS Inc., Chicago, USA). Normality was assessed using a graphical approach (visual inspection) method and the appropriate statistical testing performed subsequently. Relationship between MGL, age and ocular signs and symptoms were evaluated by Pearson's Correlation. The differences between comparable categorical groups were investigated by performing the Mann – Whitney U test. Chi-square test was performed on certain distributions. $p < 0.05$ was considered significant.

Ethical considerations

We adhered to the Declaration of Helsinki. Ethical approval was granted by the Committee on Human Research, Publication and Ethics at the School of Medical Sciences, Kwame Nkrumah University of Science and Technology/ Komfo Anokye Teaching Hospital, Ghana (CHRPE/ AP/448/16).

Results

The summary of results of the major parameters of interests are represented in Table 1.

Meibomian gland loss

As many as 84% of the patients studied showed some degree of Meibomian gland loss. The distribution of MGL based on Pult's grading scheme is cross-tabulated in Table 2 for gender groups and eyelids. A Chi test revealed a statistically meaningful difference in the distribution of MGL between eyelid types (UL and LL) and between genders, $\chi 2(12, N = 125) = 28.49$, $p = 0.0047$ We observed a significant difference in MGL between the UL (mean MGL = 26.25% ± 22.40) MGL and LL (mean MGL = 40.33% ± 26.70); $[U = 1293.5$, $p = 0.004]$ but no significant difference between males (mean MGL =

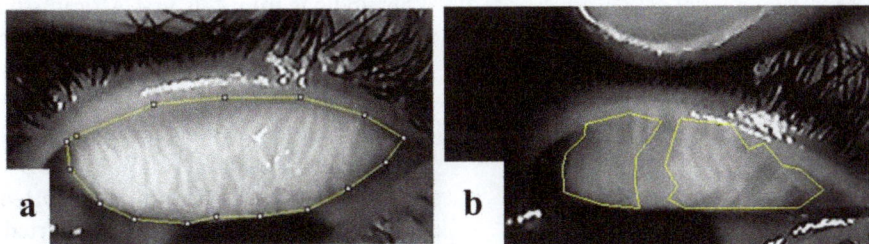

Fig. 2 Meibographs of (**a**) an upper eyelid with ≈ 0%MGL (grade 0) (**b**) an upper eyelid with ≈50% MGL (grade 2)

Table 1 Overview of results

Parameter	Mean ± SD	N	Range
Age [yrs]	46.20 ± 17.42	125	18.0–80.0
MGL [%]	32.10 ± 25.0	125	0.0–100.0
SPEED Scores	6.7 ± 3.9	125	2.0–6.0
TBUT Scores [sec]	6.2 ± 3.5	125	0.0–13.0
Oxford Grade of OSS	0.65 ± 0.75	95	0.0–2.0

SD Standard Deviation, *n* Number of patients/eyes, *MGL* Meibomian Gland Loss, *TBUT* Tear Break – Up Time, *OSS* Ocular Surface Staining

32.56% ± 26.50) and females (mean MGL = 30.98% ± 23.70); [U = 1934. 5, p = 0.927] (Fig. 3a, b).

Tear film stability and ocular surface staining
There was a general reduced tear film stability among the study subjects. The overall mean TBUT was 6.5 s ± 3.5. Tear film stability scores among male patients were similar to that among females. Mean TBUT among males was 6.4 s ± 3.6 and that of females was 6.03 s ± 3.6; (U = 1813, p = 0.488).

The mean OSS value (for 95 subjects) was 0.65 ± 0.79. The difference in OSS between gender groups was not significant. We detected similar grades of ocular surface staining across male versus female groups. For males, mean OSS was 0.71 ± 0.85 and for females, mean OSS was 0.59 ± 0.74; (U = 1190 p = 0.609).

Dry eye symptoms
The severity and frequency of dry eye symptoms was measured with the SPEED II questionnaire. An item on the questionnaire is graded a 0–4 Likert-type scale; where 0 means no symptoms and 4 means intolerable symptom. The composite score on the SPEED questionnaire ranges from 0 to 28 where 0 means and 28 would very severe and frequent symptoms. Average SPEED scores were similar between gender groups; males (6.65 ± 3.74) and females (6.81 ± 4.05); (U = 1943.0, p = 0.960).

Table 2 Distribution of MGL grades between gender groups and eyelids

Pult's Grades	Upper eyelids [n = 76]	Lower Eyelids [n = 49]	Males [n = 62]	Females [n = 63]
Grade 0	19	10	14	16
Grade 1	40	27	42	28
Grade 2	25	24	16	34
Grade 3	13	32	22	21
Grade 4	3	7	6	1
Total %	100	100	100	100

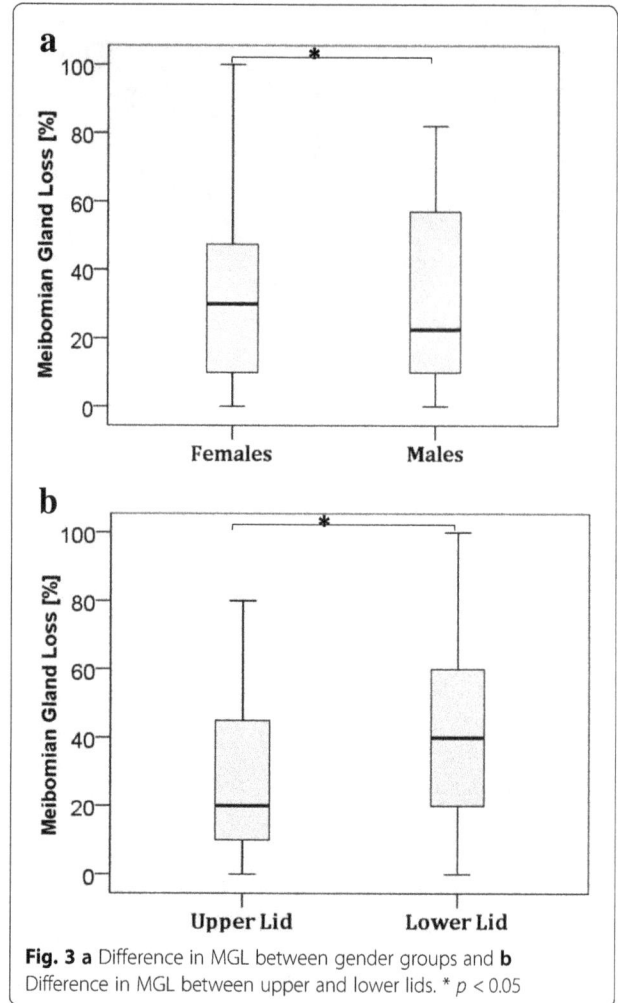

Fig. 3 a Difference in MGL between gender groups and **b** Difference in MGL between upper and lower lids. * p < 0.05

Relationship meibomian gland loss and age, speed, TBUT and OSS scores
We detected a strong positive correlation between MGL and age [r = 0.91, p = 0.001]. A similar correlation was also found between MGL and SPEED scores [r = 0.90, p = 0.001] and between MGL and Ocular Surface Staining [r = 0.75, p = 0.001]. There was a strong negative correlation between MGL and TBUT [r = – 0.81, p = 0.001]. (Fig. 4a,b) and (Fig. 5a,b).

Discussion
Our findings from this first African study on meibomian glands and dry eye disease underscore Meibomian gland dysfunction as a major underlying cause of dry eye disease in this region of the world. Our findings hereby demonstrate a greater percentage (84%) of the total number of the subjects showed MGD of various degree or severity. While there is no reported absolute prevalence of MGD in Africa, our reported value is slightly higher than the 69.3% reported in the Beijing Eye Study [30] and 61.9% in the Japanese Studies [31]. It however,

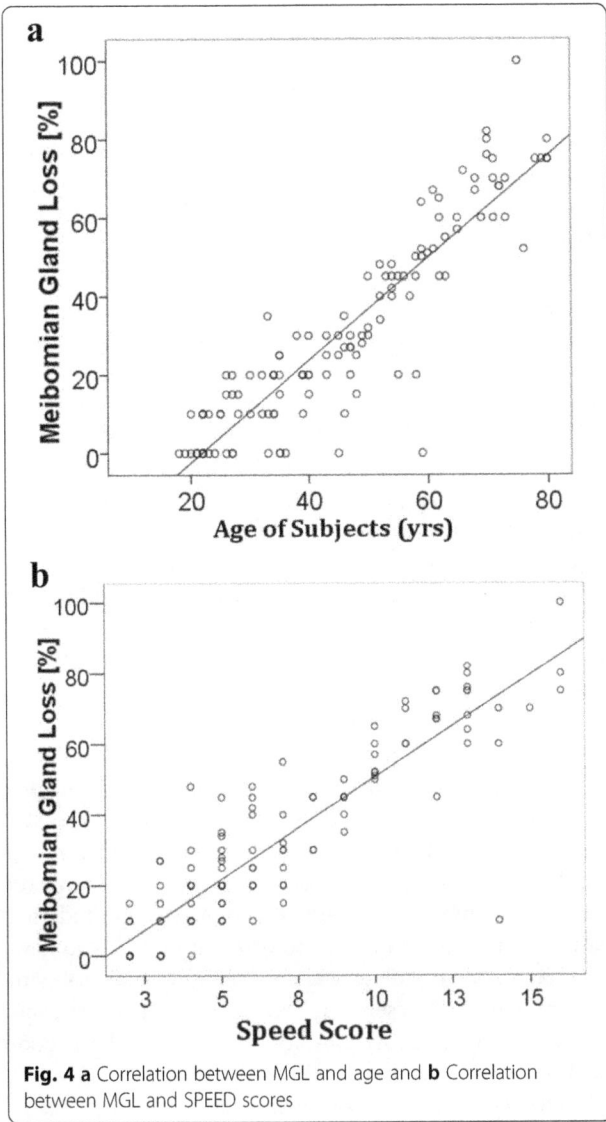

Fig. 4 a Correlation between MGL and age and **b** Correlation between MGL and SPEED scores

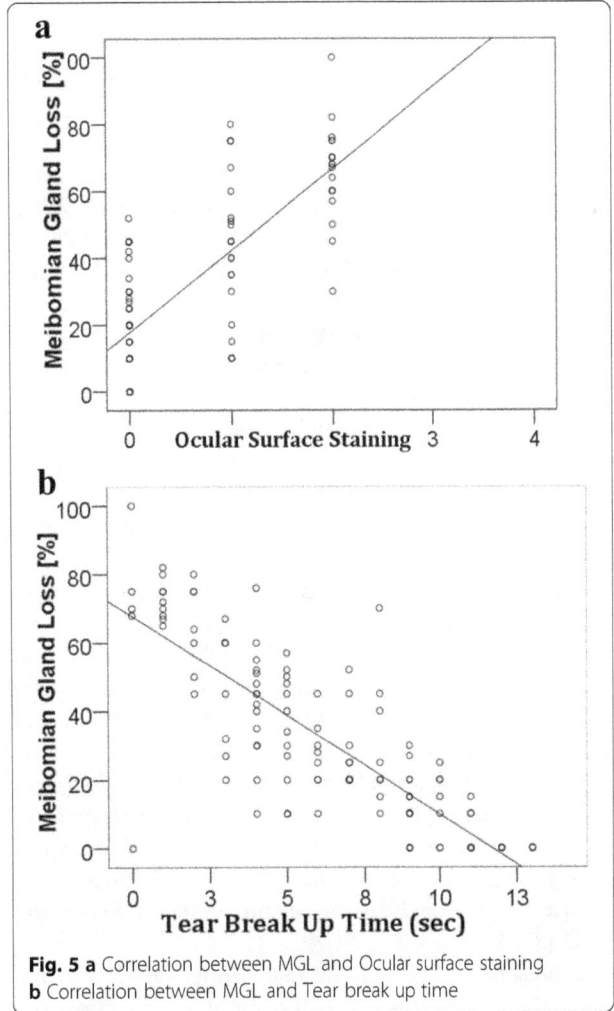

Fig. 5 a Correlation between MGL and Ocular surface staining **b** Correlation between MGL and Tear break up time

very high than 3.5% reported in the Salisbury Eye Evaluation Study [32] and 19.9% in the Melbourne Visual Impairment [33, 34].

The current understanding is that the prevalence of MGD is seemingly higher from studies conducted in Asian population compared to Caucasian populations [33]. As first-time study, our finding does not provide a complete picture of the prevalence of MGD among Africans; this warrants future studies necessary for knowing how MGD distributes on the Continent. It is important to state that these different studies report variable prevalence values due to differences in study design, especially variations in the diagnostic criterion for MGD. However, all of our study patients presented with subjective complaints of DED, suggesting a potential contribution of MGD to the dry eye disease process. Several different studies have also reported the presence of dysfunctional Meibomian glands in DED cohorts [35, 36].

It is understood that, MGD can lead to diffuse and specific changes in the gland itself resulting in reduced quality and volume of meibum [36]. MGD may present as hyposecretory action of the Meibomian gland, inspissation of meibum, change in colour and consistency of meibum, change in meibum oils composition and overall atrophy of the glands [4, 7, 36]. These changes prohibit the tear lipid layer from playing its normal role of preventing faster evaporation and enhancing the lubrication property of the tear film.

While the link between MGD and DED is well understood, the exact pathomechanism underlying MGD itself is poorly understood. Some experimental studies conducted to understand the disease process in MGD suggests the potential involvement of keratinization of the Meibomian gland ductal epithelium, chronic infection of the eyelids and inflammation [37, 38]. Others have also suggested the role of ageing, use of certain medications, dyslipidemia, and hyperosmolar stress at the ocular surface [39–42].

Additionally, it has been frequently reported that there is high prevalence of MGD among contact lens wearers [43, 44] even though the role of contact lens in the development of MGD is not completely understood yet. None of the subjects reported a history of contact lens wear but this does not preclude the likely role of other factors that could influence MGD-related DED. What draws our attention is that, infectious diseases (Trachoma) and malnutrition (vitamin A deficiency) have effectively being controlled (with some reports of successful eradication) in this region of Africa by global health interventional programmes like the World Health Organization's SAFE strategy [S = surgery for trichiasis, A = Antibiotics F = Facial cleanliness, E = Environmental improvement] for trachoma control. Vitamin A supplementation programs have also seen significant success in these parts of the world [12–14, 18, 19]. We thus believe there are other risk factors and causes influencing DED - especially there may be greater role of environment and lifestyle in development of DED [13].

Higher temperatures and low humidity are believed to influence MGD and DED. Ghana like many other Africa countries have these characteristic climatic conditions and these may indirectly impact ocular surface health. Low humidity, dusty environment, high ventilation flow, prolonged use of computers and longer hours spent in air-conditioned environment among other factors can lead to ocular surface "injury" and inflammatory responses which mediate the vicious cycle of MGD and DED [33, 45].

In present day Ghana and many other developing nations, there is increased use of computers in schools and offices, many buildings and cars used in these hot climate regions are also air conditioned now. Much of the formerly agrarian settlements have also become heavily industrialized. This comes with alterations in the natural environment due increased construction of roads, factories, houses, and offices – all of which can cause concomitant increase in environmental pollution - directly or indirectly impacting health and disease including ocular surface health [13, 22, 45, 46].While this present study did not look at the potential contributions of these environmental factors to MGD and MGD-related dry eye, future studies should look at these factors may modulate MGD and MGD -related dry eye.

We found a significantly higher MGL in the UL than LL. This contradicts the findings of the Pult et al. who rather found greater MGL in the LL than UL [47]. While there is no definite explanation to this, earlier and current reports document a generally high number of glands in the UL than LL [5, 37]. In terms of morphology however, they report that LL MGs appeared more wider and shorter than UL MGs. We realize, this configuration may due to the relatively small physical space in the LL fornix; this perhaps makes it less easy to perform meibography on LL MGs than on UL MGs. We also think that; the upper eyelids do the greater part of movement during blinking and so its MGs are bound to experience mechanical (friction) forces that could affect its morphology and function and the overall development of MGD later in life – particularly in contact lens wearers [44, 48].

Further, we observed no significant difference in MGL between males and females. Our study is only a cross-sectional observational study with a limited number of participants. Therefore, the statistical interpretation of our findings should be considered in the same context. Several other studies suggest differences in phenotypes of MGD and therefore DED between male and female subjects [22, 33]. The function of the entire lacrimal functional unit, particularly the Meibomian glands is said to be regulated by sex - specific steroids [49–51] .

As has been frequently reported in other studies, we found a generally reduced tear film stability – measurable as low TBUT. A TBUT value less than the clinical average normal of 15 s is indicative of dry eye [52]. An overall of mean 6.2 ± 3.5 s was recorded in this study population, suggesting a general presence of DED population [53]. TBUT scores further correlated with meibomian gland dropout. This indicates the observed changes in the meibomian glands could be influencing the DED situation in our subjects. While correlations do not mean causations, several studies have reported that patients with meibomian gland dropout or MGD in general have issues with tear film instability. Patients with evaporative DED essentially have tears which dry away quickly from the ocular surface because they have poor quality and low volume meibum because of MGD [49, 54]. Dryness at the ocular surface can excite cascades of inflammatory response – including the expression inflammatory cytokines. Matrix metalloproteinase 9 (MMP9) is one of such expressed inflammatory factors – this is known to cause destruction of ocular surface integrity. MMP9s can slough off epithelial tight junctions of the conjunctival and cornea [55].

This causes irregularity in the cornea and conjunctiva. In the cornea, this can impair optical transmission of light resulting in blur or reduced visual acuity in most DED patients [56]. We detected such a change on slit lamp examination as ocular surface staining of various degrees following topical application of 2% fluorescein.

Dry eye patients may or may not be symptomatic. According to the SPEED scores we obtained, the subjects experienced one form or the other of DED -related symptoms. These may include pain, itchiness, redness, tearing, burning sensation, blur and itchiness [57, 58]. Different questionnaires for assessing dry eye symptoms demonstrate different degrees of sensitivity. The SPEED questionnaire was used in this population because it was simple to interpret, in the local Twi language, to some of patients when necessary. It also contained fewer items making it time - efficient to administer. Additionally, a previous study conducted in another region of Ghana concluded that SPEED questionnaire proves useful as valid measure of DED symptoms in the population [59]. We reported an average SPEED score of 6.7 ± 3.9 and a range of 2–6, comparable to the SPEED score of asymptomatic, mild, moderate and severe dry eye groups respectively reported in this other Ghanaian study [59]. Furthermore, it appeared useful but redundant to use a symptom assessment tool like the Ocular Surface Disease Index (OSDI) questionnaire because not many people in this Ghanaian community operated an ATM or drove a car [60]. This limitation presents an opportunity to design and validate region - specific questionnaire for evaluating DED patients in Ghana and other developing countries [13].

It is important to mention that, the clinical signs and symptoms of DED do not always correlate. Our findings however showed that MGL correlated well with age, DED symptoms (SPEED scores), tear film instability (TBUT) and ocular surface damage (OSS) among the subjects of this study. Atrophy of the Meibomian gland is known to increase with ageing. Plausible reasons offered to explain to this phenomenon include reduced cell cycling of MG acinar basal cells, reduced proliferative potential, hyperkeratinization and age-related co-morbidities [39, 40, 58]. Regarding relation between MGL, TBUT and OSS, there is a defined clear connection. When MGL occurs, volume and quality of meibum decreases, tear film evaporates faster from the ocular surface – inflammation may set in causing damage to ocular surface – which in turn causes and or exacerbates symptoms of dryness, pain and general ocular discomfort [57, 58].

Conclusion

To summarize, this study for the first time presents data on the status of Meibomian glands in Africa. The observed results show that there is presently a potential link between DED and other factors (like MGD) other than infectious diseases and malnutrition in these regions. We have also demonstrated the feasibility of conducting meibography in DED patients using a custom-made meibographer in a developing country where there is limited access of complex imaging systems.

Abbreviations

DED: Dry Eye Disease; LFU: Lacrimal Functional Unit; LL: Lower Lid; MG: Meibomian Gland; MGD: Meibomian Gland Dysfunction; MGL: Meibomian Gland Loss; NCT: Normal Contact; OSDI: Ocular Surface Disease Index; OSS: Ocular Surface Staining; SPEED: Standardized Patient Evaluation of Eye Dryness; TBUT: Tear Break Up Test; UL: Upper Lid

Acknowledgements

Dr. Kwadwo Amoah and Dr. Angela Ofeibea Amedo, both faculty at the Department of Optometry at the Kwame Nkrumah University of Science and Technology, Kumasi, Ghana supported data collection.

Funding

As of the time of the study, Philipp Steven had a Deutsche Forschungsgemeinschaft Forschergruppe FOR2240, DFG STE 1928/4–1 grant.

Authors' contributions

PS and EAO conceived the project idea. JH with support from PS provided technical expertise including the construction, testing and training for using the custom meibographer. PS provided EAO with further training in dry eye diagnostics. EAO and RKA coordinated data collection and analysis. Finally, PS and DBK provided overall supervision for the project. EAO composed the final manuscript with the support of PS. All authors read and approved the final manuscript.

Competing interests

The authors declare that they have no competing interests.

Author details

[1]Department of Optometry and Visual Science, Kwame Nkrumah University of Science and Technology, PMB, Kumasi, Ghana. [2]Department of Ophthalmology, Faculty of Medicine, University of Cologne, Cologne, Germany. [3]Cluster of Excellence: Cellular Stress Response in Aging – associated Diseases (CECAD), University of Cologne, Cologne, Germany.

References

1. Stern ME, Schaumburg CS, Pflugfelder SC. Dry eye as a mucosal autoimmune disease. Int Rev Immunol. 2013;32(1):19–41.
2. Nelson JD, Shimazaki J, Benitez-del-Castillo JM, Craig JP, McCulley JP, Den S, et al. The international workshop on Meibomian gland dysfunction: report of the definition and classification subcommittee. Invest Ophthalmol Vis Sci. 2011;52(4):1930–7.
3. Gayton JL. Etiology, prevalence, and treatment of dry eye disease. Clin Ophthalmol. 2009;3(1):405–12.
4. Phadatare SP, Momin M, Nighojkar P, Askarkar S, Singh KK. A comprehensive review on dry eye disease: diagnosis, medical management, recent developments, and future challenges. Adv Pharm. 2015;2015
5. Knop E, Knop N, Millar T, Obata H, Sullivan DA. The international workshop on Meibomian gland dysfunction: report of the subcommittee on anatomy, physiology, and pathophysiology of the Meibomian gland. Invest Ophthalmol Vis Sci. 2011;52(4):1938–78.
6. Bron A, Tiffany J, Gouveia S, Yokoi N, Voon L. Functional aspects of the tear film lipid layer. Exp Eye Res. 2004;78(3):347–60.
7. Tomlinson A, Bron AJ, Korb DR, Amano S, Paugh JR, Pearce EI, et al. The international workshop on Meibomian gland dysfunction: report of the diagnosis subcommittee. Invest Ophthalmol Vis Sci. 2011;52(4):2006–49.
8. West KP. Extent of vitamin a deficiency among preschool children and women of reproductive age. J Nutr. 2002;132(9):2857S–66S.
9. Moore DB, Shirefaw W, Tomkins-Netzer O, Eshete Z, Netzer-Tomkins H, Ben-Zion I. Prevalence of xerophthalmia among malnourished children in rural Ethiopia. Int Ophthalmol. 2013;33(5):455–9.
10. Schémann J-F, Malvy D, Sacko D, Traore L. Trachoma and vitamin a deficiency. Lancet. 2001;357(9269):1676.
11. Moss SE, Klein R, Klein BE. Prevalence of and risk factors for dry eye syndrome. Arch Ophthalmol. 2000;118(9):1264–8.
12. Abrahams C, Ballard R, Sutter E. The pathology of trachoma in a black south African population. Light microscopical, histochemical and electron microscopical findings. South Afr Med J. 1979;55(27):1115–8.
13. Osae A, Gehlsen U, Horstmann J, Siebelmann S, Stern M, Kumah D, et al. Epidemiology of dry eye disease in Africa: the sparse information, gaps and opportunities. Ocular Surface. 2017;15(2):159-68.

14. Thylefors B, Dawson CR, Jones BR, West SK, Taylor HR. A simple system for the assessment of trachoma and its complications. Bull World Health Organ. 1987;65(4):477.

15. Dawson CR, Jones BR, Tarizzo ML. Guide to trachoma control in programmes for the prevention of blindness. Geneva: The World Health Organization; 1981.

16. Negrel A, Mariotti S. WHO alliance for the global elimination of blinding trachoma and the potential use of azithromycin. Int J Antimicrob Agents. 1998;10(4):259–62.

17. Stevens GA, Bennett JE, Hennocq Q, Lu Y, De-Regil LM, Rogers L, et al. Trends and mortality effects of vitamin a deficiency in children in 138 low-income and middle-income countries between 1991 and 2013: a pooled analysis of population-based surveys. Lancet Glob Health. 2015;3(9):e528–e36.

18. Mayo-Wilson E, Imdad A, Herzer K, Yakoob MY, Bhutta ZA. Vitamin a supplements for preventing mortality, illness, and blindness in children aged under 5: systematic review and meta-analysis. BMJ. 2011;343:d5094.

19. Burki T. The broad benefits of trachoma elimination. Lancet Infect Dis. 2016; 16(5):530.

20. Fund. TUNCs. In: Vitamin A Supplementation; a Statistical Snapshot; 2016.

21. Bureau TPR. World population data sheet and press release. 2015.

22. Nichols KK, Foulks GN, Bron AJ, Glasgow BJ, Dogru M, Tsubota K, et al. The international workshop on Meibomian gland dysfunction: executive summary. Invest Ophthalmol Vis Sci. 2011;52(4):1922–9.

23. Wise RJ, Sobel RK, Allen RC. Meibography: a review of techniques and technologies. Saudi J Ophthal. 2012;26(4):349–56.

24. Arita R, Itoh K, Inoue K, Amano S. Noncontact infrared meibography to document age-related changes of the meibomian glands in a normal population. Ophthalmology. 2008;115(5):911–5.

25. Arita R. Validity of noninvasive meibography systems: noncontact meibography equipped with a slit-lamp and a mobile pen-shaped meibograph. Cornea. 2013;32:S65–70.

26. Pult H, Riede-Pult B. Non-contact meibography: keep it simple but effective. Contact Lens Anterior Eye. 2012;35(2):77–80.

27. Bron AJ, Evans VE, Smith JA. Grading of corneal and conjunctival staining in the context of other dry eye tests. Cornea. 2003;22(7):640–50.

28. Moy A, McNamara NA, Lin MC. Effects of isotretinoin on meibomian glands. Optom Vis Sci. 2015;92(9):925–30.

29. Abràmoff MD, Magalhães PJ, Ram SJ. Image processing with ImageJ. Biophoton Int. 2004;11(7):36–42.

30. Jie Y, Xu L, Wu Y, Jonas J. Prevalence of dry eye among adult Chinese in the Beijing eye study. Eye. 2009;23(3):688.

31. Uchino M, Dogru M, Yagi Y, Goto E, Tomita M, Kon T, et al. The features of dry eye disease in a Japanese elderly population. Optom Vis Sci. 2006; 83(11):797–802.

32. Schein OD, MUÑO B, Tielsch JM, Bandeen-Roche K, West S. Prevalence of dry eye among the elderly. Am J Ophthalmol. 1997;124(6):723–8.

33. Schaumberg DA, Nichols JJ, Papas EB, Tong L, Uchino M, Nichols KK. The international workshop on Meibomian gland dysfunction: report of the subcommittee on the epidemiology of, and associated risk factors for, MGD. Invest Ophthalmol Vis Sci. 2011;52(4):1994–2005.

34. McCarty CA, Bansal AK, Livingston PM, Stanislavsky YL, Taylor HR. The epidemiology of dry eye in Melbourne, Australia 1. Ophthalmology. 1998; 105(6):1114–9.

35. Viso E, Gude F, Rodríguez-Ares MT. The association of meibomian gland dysfunction and other common ocular diseases with dry eye: a population-based study in Spain. Cornea. 2011;30(1):1–6.

36. McCulley JP, Shine WE. Meibomian gland function and the tear lipid layer. Ocular Surface. 2003;1(3):97–106.

37. Obata H. Anatomy and histopathology of human meibomian gland. Cornea. 2002;21:S70–S4.

38. Mathers WD, Shields WJ, Sachdev MS, Petroll WM, Jester JV. Meibomian gland dysfunction in chronic blepharitis. Cornea. 1991;10(4):277–85.

39. Nien CJ, Massei S, Lin G, Nabavi C, Tao J, Brown DJ, et al. Effects of age and dysfunction on human meibomian glands. Arch Ophthalmol. 2011;129(4):462–9.

40. Jester JV, Parfitt GJ, Brown DJ. Meibomian gland dysfunction: hyperkeratinization or atrophy? BMC Ophthalmol. 2015;15(1):156.

41. Braich PS, Howard MK, Singh JS. Dyslipidemia and its association with meibomian gland dysfunction. Int Ophthalmol. 2016;36(4):469–76.

42. Bron AJ, Yokoi N, Gaffney EA, Tiffany JM. A solute gradient in the tear meniscus. II. Implications for lid margin disease, including meibomian gland dysfunction. Ocular Surface. 2011;9(2):92–7.

43. Chia EM, Mitchell P, Rochtchina E, Lee AJ, Maroun R, Wang JJ. Prevalence and associations of dry eye syndrome in an older population: the Blue Mountains eye study. Clin Exp Ophthalmol. 2003;31(3):229–32.

44. Villani E, Ceresara G, Beretta S, Magnani F, Viola F, Ratiglia R. In vivo confocal microscopy of meibomian glands in contact lens wearers. Invest Ophthalmol Vis Sci. 2011;52(8):5215–9.

45. Fenga C, Aragona P, Cacciola A, Spinella R, Di Nola C, Ferreri F, et al. Meibomian gland dysfunction and ocular discomfort in video display terminal workers. Eye. 2008;22(1):91–5.

46. Rooney MS, Arku RE, Dionisio KL, Paciorek C, Friedman AB, Carmichael H, et al. Spatial and temporal patterns of particulate matter sources and pollution in four communities in Accra. Ghana Sci Total Env. 2012;435:107–14.

47. Pult H, Riede-Pult BH, Nichols JJ. Relation between upper and lower lids' meibomian gland morphology, tear film, and dry eye. Optom Vis Sci. 2012; 89(3):E310–E5.

48. Arita R, Itoh K, Inoue K, Kuchiba A, Yamaguchi T, Amano S. Contact lens wear is associated with decrease of meibomian glands. Ophthalmology. 2009;116(3):379–84.

49. Green-Church KB, Butovich I, Willcox M, Borchman D, Paulsen F, Barabino S, et al. The international workshop on meibomian gland dysfunction: report of the subcommittee on tear film lipids and lipid–protein interactions in health and disease. Invest Ophthalmol Vis Sci. 2011;52(4):1979–93.

50. Sullivan DA, Jensen RV, Suzuki T, Richards SM. Do sex steroids exert sex-specific and/or opposite effects on gene expression in lacrimal and meibomian glands? Mol Vision. 2009;15:1553–72.

51. Sullivan DA, Sullivan BD, Evans JE, Schirra F, Yamagami H, Liu M, et al. Androgen deficiency, meibomian gland dysfunction, and evaporative dry eye. Ann N Y Acad Sci. 2002;966(1):211–22.

52. Tiffany JM. The normal tear film. In: Surgery for the Dry Eye. 41: Karger Publishers; 2008. p. 1–20.

53. Abelson MB, Ousler GW, Nally LA, Welch D, Krenzer K. Alternative reference values for tear film break up time in normal and dry eye populations. In: Lacrimal Gland, Tear Film, and Dry Eye Syndromes 3: Springer; 2002. p. 1121–5.

54. McCulley JP, Shine WE. The lipid layer of tears: dependent on meibomian gland function. Exp Eye Res. 2004;78(3):361–5.

55. Solomon A, Dursun D, Liu Z, Xie Y, Macri A, Pflugfelder SC. Pro-and anti-inflammatory forms of interleukin-1 in the tear fluid and conjunctiva of patients with dry-eye disease. Invest Ophthalmol Vis Sci. 2001;42(10):2283–92.

56. Goto E, Yagi Y, Matsumoto Y, Tsubota K. Impaired functional visual acuity of dry eye patients. Am J Ophthalmol. 2002;133(2):181–6.

57. Nichols KK, Nichols JJ, Mitchell GL. The lack of association between signs and symptoms in patients with dry eye disease. Cornea. 2004;23(8):762–70.

58. Begley CG, Chalmers RL, Abetz L, Venkataraman K, Mertzanis P, Caffery BA, et al. The relationship between habitual patient-reported symptoms and clinical signs among patients with dry eye of varying severity. Invest Ophthalmol Vis Sci. 2003;44(11):4753–61.

59. Asiedu K, Kyei S, Mensah SN, Ocansey S, Abu LS, Kyere EA. Ocular surface disease index (OSDI) versus the standard patient evaluation of eye dryness (SPEED): a study of a nonclinical sample. Cornea. 2016;35(2):175–80.

60. Schiffman RM, Walt JG, Jacobsen G, Doyle JJ, Lebovics G, Sumner W. Utility assessment among patients with dry eye disease. Ophthalmology. 2003; 110(7):1412–9.

10

Characteristics of keratoconic patients at two main eye centres in Palestine

Yousef Shanti[1,2*], Ithar Beshtawi[3], Sa'ed H. Zyoud[4], Ahlam Abu-Samra[2], Areen Abu-Qamar[2], Reem Barakat[2] and Reham Shehada[2]

Abstract

Background: Keratoconus (KC) is a multifactorial, degenerative ectatic condition of the cornea. It usually manifests during late adolescence or the early twenties. A painless disease, KC may end with severe visual loss. The prevalence of KC in middle-eastern countries is much higher than in other regions of the world. This may be due to genetic and environmental risk factors and consanguinity. The goal of this study is to explore the demographic profile of Palestinian keratoconic patients.

Methods: A retrospective study was conducted in two ophthalmology centres (Tertiary Ophthalmic Centre of An-Najah National University Hospital and An-Noor Centre at the Specialized Arab Hospital). All medical charts of keratoconic patients attending both centres over the period from 2009 to 2016 were reviewed. These patients were diagnosed by ophthalmologists depending on history, examination and Pentacam. Severity was determined using the k median index from the Pentacam map. Data analysis was carried out using SPSS Version 22.

Results: The medical files of 936 keratoconic eyes of 505 keratoconic patients were reviewed. Their mean age at the time of diagnosis was 23.3 ranging from 8 to 62 years. Approximately 70.1% of them presented after the age of 20 years, and younger age groups were more likely to develop a severe disease stage than older ones ($P = 0.001$, $r = -0.108$). There was a nearly equal distribution of patients between the two sexes (49.5% male, 50.5% female). On initial evaluation, the best-corrected visual acuity (BCVA) was recorded as ≥6/12 in most affected eyes (71.5%). Regarding severity, 62% presented in a mild form, while 9.9% were at a severe stage. About 88.2% presented with bilateralism.

Conclusions: Most of the patients in their twenties presented with a mild bilateral form of the disease. This result is compatible with published international reports. It is recommended that the results of this study be considered when establishing a screening program in Palestine. Subsequently, patients will be identified at an appropriate time where action can be taken before disease progression take place.

Keywords: Keratoconus, Demographic, Palestine

* Correspondence: yousef.isam.shanti@gmail.com; yousef.shanti@najah.edu
[1]Department of Ophthalmology, An-Najah National University Hospital, 44839 Nablus, Palestine, Palestine
[2]Department of Medicine, College of Medicine and Health Sciences, An-Najah National University, 44839 Nablus, Palestine, Palestine
Full list of author information is available at the end of the article

Background

Keratoconus (KC) has been traditionally classified as a non-inflammatory, degenerative ectatic condition of the cornea in which the cornea assumes an irregular conical shape. The visual consequences range from blurred vision to blindness if the condition is not treated [1]. In recent years, there has been an increasing amount of literature supporting the classification of KC as quasi-inflammatory (inflammatory-related) due to some biochemical changes [2–4]. It is likely to be a multifactorial, multigenic disorder with complex inheritance patterns, and environmental factors probably play an equally important role in disease causation [5–7]. Associations have been identified between KC and systemic conditions such as trisomy 21, Turner's syndrome, cardiovascular diseases, various collagen vascular disorders and Marfan's syndrome [6, 8].

Based on the literature as well as medical and ophthalmological expertise, it is noticed that KC is a major and common eye disease among the Palestinian population compared with other countries. This might be due to genetic and environmental risk factors, such as sun exposure (ultraviolet exposure) and nicotine [9]. Another factor associated with an increase in the risk of KC is consanguinity [10], which is prevalent in our country. Hence, the goal of this study is to determine the epidemiological characteristics of this disease in order to initiate a screening program based on well-organized data collected from our patients' medical files.

Methods

The medical files of 505 keratoconic patients were reviewed. The study participants were patients attending either the ophthalmology Centre of An-Najah National University Hospital (ANNUH) or the An-Noor Centre at the Specialized Arab hospital over the period from September 1, 2009 to January 1, 2016. They were presented as outpatients complaining of various visual symptoms. The diagnosis of KC was confirmed by the ophthalmologists depending on history, thorough slit lamp examination and, most importantly, Pentacam (Pentacam HR, Type 70,900, OCULUS, Germany). Subsequently, the appropriate management strategy was applied to each patient, ranging from spectacles and soft contact lenses to corneal transplantation, focusing on improving visual acuity to the greatest extent possible. Their epidemiological data at the time of diagnosis were collected and analysed, including residency, age at diagnosis, gender, best-corrected visual acuity (BCVA), severity and bilaterality of the disease. Disease severity was determined using the k median index (mean curvature power), which is widely used as a classification method in many studies [11], obtained from the Pentacam map. Thus, mild KC was defined as mean k < 48 diopters, moderate

as 48–54 diopters and severe as > 54 diopters [12]. Regarding BCVA, eyes were classified into three main categories: the first one included eyes reported to have BCVA of ≤6/60 (20/200), the third category included those presenting with BCVA of ≥6/12 (20/40) and the second one in between [12]. According to BCVA and k readings, the data on the affected eyes only were included. Residency was categorized into city, village, and Palestinian refugee camps. It is worth mentioning that all keratoconic patients presenting to either centre in the targeted period were included in the study, so none were excluded. Before conducting the study, Institutional Review Board (IRB) approval was obtained from An-Najah National University ethics committee, and the required permission from both centres was obtained.

Statistical analysis

Statistical analysis of the data was carried out using IBM SPSS V.20. Nominal variables were described using frequencies and percentages, while continuous variables were described by mean and standard deviation. Descriptive statistics, the chi-square test, independent-sample t-test, one-way ANOVA and Pearson's correlation coefficient were used to analyse the data. Results were considered statistically significant at $P \leq 0.05$.

Results

The medical reports of 505 keratoconic patients, including 936 keratoconic eyes, included in our study were saved from 2009 to 2016; 61.6% of the patients presented in the last year, and the remaining 38.4% attended previously. This increase is explainable by the fact that ANNUH ophthalmic centre was established at the end of 2013.

Residency

Depending on their residency, the patients were distributed among three groups (city, village and camp). The highest percentage, 67.9% (343/505), came from the city, while the lowest contribution, around 1.6% (8/505), was found to be from Palestinian refugee camps, and the remaining 30.1% (152/505) were villagers. As shown in Table 1, the residency for two patients was not recorded. A significant difference in k readings was detected between patients from cities, villages and Palestinian

Table 1 Geographical distribution of the sample ($n = 505$)

	Frequency	Percentage (%)
Residency		
City	343	67.9
Village	152	30.1
Palestinian refugee camps	8	1.6
Missing	2	0.4
Total	505	100

refugee camps ($p = 0.041$), reflecting that patients from villages were reported to have higher mean k readings than patients from cities and Palestinian refugee camps.

Distribution by age group at the time of diagnosis

The age range variable was divided into a set of categories, each 5 years in length. The age at presentation ranged from 8 to 62 years, with a mean (SD) age of 23.33 (7.37) years. It is worth mentioning that around 75% of them presented between 16 and 30 years of age with high prevalence rate among this age group (21–25), to which around 32.3% of patients belonged, followed by the age groups 16–20 and 26–30, with 26.5% and 16.4%, respectively. A dramatic decrease was noticed at both age margins, especially when patients aged (Fig. 1).

Sex distribution, BCVA, severity and bilaterality of KC at the time of diagnosis

There was a nearly equal distribution of patients between the two sexes (49.5% males, 50.5% females). On initial evaluation, the BCVA was recorded as ≥6/12 in the majority of affected eyes, around 71.5% (670/936). On the other hand, only 2.4% (21/936) presented with ≤6/60 BCVA, and the rest 16.5% (155/936) were determined to have > 6/60 to < 6/12 BCVA. BCVA data were missing in 9.6% (90/936) of cases. Regarding severity, most of the affected eyes, 62% (580/936), presented with the mild form, while only 9.9% (93/936) had the severe form and an intermediate percentage, 28.1% (263/936) had the moderate form. About 88.2% presented with bilateralism.

Demographic characteristic of patients in relation to sex

Generally, it is worth mentioning that the only significant difference in the epidemiological parameters (age at presentation, severity and bilaterality of KC, BCVA) between the two sexes was detected in severity ($P = 0.030$), with female being more vulnerable to presenting with severe and moderate forms. Otherwise, no significant differences in the rest of parameters were found between the two sexes. For both sexes, the highest contribution was that of the mild form and was higher among males than females (66% vs 58.1%). On the other hand, the lowest contribution was that of the severe form for both sexes and was higher among females than among males (10.7% vs 9.20%). A closer examination of each parameter in turn revealed that the mean (SD) ages of the male and female groups were 22.98 (7.53) and 23.37 (7.15) years, respectively. Around 70% of patients presented at an age of ≥20 years between both sexes. According to BCVA at the time of diagnosis, in both sexes most diseased eyes detected had BCVA ≥6/12, around 72.1% of male eyes compared with 71.1% of female eyes. Meanwhile, the lowest contribution in each sex was by those with BCVA ≤6/60: around 2.6% of males and 1.9% of females. Regarding bilateralism, around 88.4% of males and 88.1% of females were found to have KC in both eyes (Table 2).

Correlation between different demographic parameters

Application of the chi-square test indicated that there was no statistically significant association between sex and the BCVA ($P = 0.665$, $\chi^2 = 0.815$). Using Pearson's correlation, a statistically significant mild correlation was found between K average readings (severity of KC) and age ($P = 0.001$, $r = -0.108$), in which patients who presented at earlier ages had a more severe form of KC than did older patients. Furthermore, a statistically significant moderate negative correlation was found between severity of KC and the BCVA ($P = 0.004$, $r = -0$.

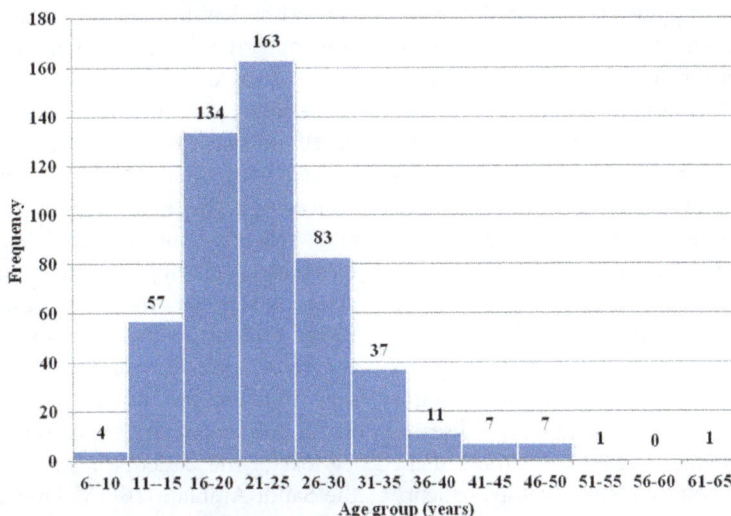

Fig. 1 Sample distribution among age groups at the time of diagnosis ($n = 505$)

Table 2 Demographic characteristics of the study population in relation to sex

Variable	Total n = 505 (%)	Male n = 250 (%)	Female n = 255 (%)	P value[a]
Mean age (year) ± SD	23.33 ± 7.37	22.98 ± 7.53	23.37 ± 7.15	0.548[e]
Age at presentation (year)[b]				
< 20	151(29.9)	79(31.6)	72 (28.2)	0.408[f]
≥20	345 (70.1)	171(68.4)	183(71.8)	
Bilateralism				
Yes	443(88.2)	221 (88.4)	222(88.1)	0.916[f]
No	62 (11.8)	29 (11.6)	33(11.9)	
Severity of KC at presentation[c]				
Severe (k > 54)	93 (9.9)	42(9.2)	51(10.7)	0.030[f]
Moderate (k = 48–54)	263 (28.1)	114(24.3)	149 (31.2)	
Mild (k < 48 D)	580 (62)	303 (66)	277 (58.1)	
BCVA[c, d]				
≤6/60	21(2.4)	12 (2.6)	9 (1.9)	0.975[f]
> 6/60 to < 6/12	155 (16.5)	73(15.9)	82 (17.3)	
≥6/12	670(71.5)	331(72.1)	339(71.1)	

Abbreviations: SD standard deviation, *KC* Keratoconus, *BCVA* best-corrected visual acuity
[a]The *P*-value is bold where it is less than the significance level cut-off of 0.05
[b]20 years is used as the cut-off point as in most of the studies [12]
[c]Values of non-diseased eyes were not entered
[d]Missing data for 90 patients
[e]Statistical significance of differences calculated using the independent-samples *t*-test
[f]Statistical significance of differences calculated using the Pearson's chi-squared test

602); thus, as the severity of the disease increased, the BCVA that could be achieved by the patient decreased.

Discussion

Keratoconus is a serious and common eye disease among the Palestinian population compared with those of other countries; this may be due to genetic and environmental risk factors, such as sun exposure (ultraviolet exposure), as well as consanguinity [8]. It usually manifests during late adolescence or the early twenties, with a gradually slowing progression for 10–20 years from diagnosis [13]. It is a painless disease that, in cases of late diagnosis and management, may end with severe visual loss due to the associated high short-sightedness and irregular astigmatism [14]. Therefore, it is worthwhile to highlight this issue by studying the epidemiological characteristics of all keratoconic patients attending two major ophthalmology centres (at ANNUH and an-Noor centre at the Specialized Arab hospital) in the West Bank, Palestine over the period from September 1, 2009 to January 1, 2016. This, in turn, may help in establishing a screening program for this widespread and serious disease, based on well-organized data collected from these main ophthalmic centres in our country. Subsequently, patients will be identified at an appropriate time when action can be taken before disease progression takes place.

This study found a mean age at the time of diagnosis of around 23.33 ± 7.37 years, and no significant difference was found in the mean age between sexes (P = 0. 548). Our result was nearly consistent with a Malaysian study, where the mean age of disease onset was 20.9 ± 5. 6 years [15]. Meanwhile, in Saudi Arabia, the mean age at diagnosis was slightly lower than in our study, about 17.7 years for males and 19.0 years for females [16]. On the other hand, a higher mean age, around 27 years, was detected in Caucasian populations, suggesting a later disease onset [16], which is also seen in Macedonia, as the mean age at the time of disease detection was 26.81 ± 1.25 [17]. In general, our results agreed with those of internationally published studies concerning the early age of onset [18]. Several possible reasons could be cited here to explain these differences, including genetics and environmental and geographical factors, such as consanguineous marriages and ultraviolet exposure, which are considered the main risk factors for KC development and thus may explain the much earlier age of onset in the Saudi Arabian study compared with other studies.

Most of the patients in this study, as well as those in the Saudi Arabian [16], Malaysian [15] and Macedonian [17] studies presented with the mild disease form at the time of diagnosis, for example, in this study, 62% had the mild form, 28.1% had moderate KC and 9.9% of the total patients' eyes had severe KC. Moreover, in Malaysia 37.6%, were stage I, 30.1% stage II, 4.4% stage III and 27.8% stage IV at the time of diagnosis [15]. Also, in Saudi Arabia it was found that 39.2% were in the early stage, 42.5% in the moderate stage and 18.3% in the advanced one [16]. Finally, In Macedonia 52.08% were in the mild stage, 36.45% were in the moderate stage and 11.57% were in the late stage [17]. In general, most of the patients in the four studies had a mild to moderate form of the disease at the time of diagnosis, with some variability. This finding can be explained by several factors: firstly, this might be due to ophthalmologists' awareness concerning KC, as they have a low threshold for investigation to capture early-stage patients. Secondly, it could be due to an accidental discovery during a routine check-up of visual acuity or when changing glasses, since most KC patients are already myopic and must change their glasses frequently due to changes in refractive error. Finally, the increasing trend towards refractive surgeries in myopic patients raises the likelihood of KC discovery, as preoperative assessment by Pentacam is mandatory for all patients before these surgeries.

As detected in this study, there is a significant mild negative correlation between the mean k readings and the age at which the patient presented with KC ($P = 0.001$, $r = -0.108$); therefore, the younger age group is more likely to develop a severe disease stage than the older one. Our result was consistent with those found in the Saudi Arabian study [16] and Collaborative Longitudinal Evaluation of Keratoconus (CLEK) Study [19]. As stated in the CLEK study, age is considered a key factor in severity-related outcomes in KC, as persons diagnosed with KC at a younger age are more vulnerable to needing penetrating keratoplasty in a shorter time compared with older patients, as disease progression will be faster [19]. Thus having a disease in the early years of life means entering a very rapid progression to an early very severe form of the disease; meanwhile, a gradual regression in severity was noticed as the patients aged, which justifies that developing a disease at a later age offers a greater possibility of a very slow disease progression and subsequently remaining in the mild to moderate stages and less likely to progress to the severe form. In general, our results were consistent with the fact that KC progresses slowly and then gradually stops in the 10–20 years following diagnosis [13].

Our results indicated significant differences between male and female groups regarding the severity of KC ($P = 0.030$). Thus, male patients are more likely to present with mild disease than females. Sex-based differences regarding KC might be due to hormonal changes during pregnancy, which induce KC progression.

In addition, females tend to delay visiting the physician, frequently complaining of being busy all the time; thus, males will be identified more often in the milder form than females. Additionally, resistance to wearing glasses, as they are considered to be a social stigma for them, and prevents them from visiting ophthalmology clinics until the late stage.

Most of the eyes in this study (71.2%) had BCVA of ≥6/12; this result was similar to those of the Saudi Arabian study, in which 100% of the eyes achieved a corrected VA 6/12 or better, and 33% of eyes achieved 6/6 or better with glasses [16]. As well, BCVA was 6/9 in the Malaysian study [15]. This study also found a significant negative correlation between severity of KC and the best spectacle visual acuity achieved ($P < 0.005$, $r = -0.602$). The clear majority of the patients in these three studies have a better chance of correcting their visual acuity at the time of diagnosis. This may be due to the above-mentioned results, as most of these study patients have a mild form of the disease at the onset of diagnosis and subsequently less vision deterioration and a better chance of achieving vision correction. In fact, KC progression negatively affects many important aspects of life besides visual deterioration, such as educational and employment opportunities.

Many keratoconic cases start unilaterally but eventually affect the contralateral eye [20], although this may occur years after the initial disease detection [14]. The prevalence of unilateral KC ranges from 14.4% to 41% [12]. This was apparent in our results, as bilateral disease was found in 87.7% of patients, with no significant association between gender and bilaterality of the disease ($P = 0.916$). This was consistent with other studies, as the bilateral appearance of KC at the moment of diagnosis was present in 84.4% of patients in the Macedonia study [17], and around 77% of cases were bilateral in the Malaysia study [15, 16]. Having these high percentages of bilaterality in these three studies at the time of diagnosis might be a result of missdiagnosis of the disease in the very early stages; thus, it was discovered late enogh to be developed in the fellow undiseased eye and present as being bilateral at the time of diagnosis. Whatever the cause, the end result justifies the importance of examination and Pentacam assissment of both eyes with regular follow-up to avoid missing the disease in the fellow undiseased eye.

Regarding residency, a significant difference in k readings between residents of cities and villages were found, with villagers having a higher probability of presenting at a late stage of KC; this result should prompt us to give more attention to villagers regarding awareness and implementation of a screening program.

Strengths and limitations

To the best of our knowledge, this is the first study to describe the characteristics of keratoconic patients in Palestine. Even though the main objective of our study, which was to studying the epidemiological characteristics of keratoconic patients, was achieved, as any study, it has certain points of limitation. The first one concerns generalizability, since the data were only drawn from two centres; however, we believe this was not a serious concern because these centres are the major ones in our country and receive most of the patients. Secondly, missing data can occur with any retrospective study. However only a few epidemiological and demographic characteristics—sex, bilaterality and residency—were presented and evaluated in the study. Including other epidemiological factors, such as family history, consanguinity, associated systemic diseases, history of atopic disease and eye rubbing, would have provided more valuable information and is recommended for future studies.

Conclusions

Most of the patients presented with a bilateral mild stage of the disease in their second decade. Male patients are more likely to present with a mild stage of the disease than females. In addition, the younger age group has a higher probability of progressing rapidly to the severe stage. These results require our urgent attention to employ a well-organized, accessible and inexpensive screening program at early ages, for example, at school and university and, most importantly, to increase public awareness regarding this issue by several methods, including conducting lectures and printing brochures, among vulnerable people.

Abbreviations

ANNUH: An-Najah National University Hospital; BCVA: best-corrected visual acuity; IRB: Institutional Review Board; KC: Keratoconus

Authors' contributions

RB, AA, AA and RS designed the study, collected data, performed the analyses, searched the literature and drafted the manuscript. RS was the major responsible of designing, writing and editing the article till it is completed in addition to the above mentioned. YS and IB supervised and took responsibility for the integrity of the data and participated in the conception, design data interpretation and manuscript revision. SZ provided critical advice on the design; coordinated, supervised and took responsibility for the data analysis; critically reviewed the manuscript and the interpretation of the results, reanalyzed the data in the preparation of the revised manuscript, and assisted in the final write-up of the revised manuscript. All authors read and approved the final manuscript.

Competing interest

The authors declare that they have no competing interests.

Author details

[1]Department of Ophthalmology, An-Najah National University Hospital, 44839 Nablus, Palestine, Palestine. [2]Department of Medicine, College of Medicine and Health Sciences, An-Najah National University, 44839 Nablus, Palestine, Palestine. [3]Department of Optometry, College of Medicine and Health Sciences, An-Najah National University, 44839 Nablus, Palestine, Palestine. [4]Department of Clinical and Community Pharmacy, College of Medicine and Health Sciences, An-Najah National University, 44839 Nablus, Palestine, Palestine.

References

1. Sinjab MM. Quick guide to the management of keratoconus: a systematic step-by-step approach. Springer- Verlag Berlin Heidelberg: New York, NY; 2012.
2. Galvis V, Sherwin T, Tello A, Merayo J, Barrera R, Acera A. Keratoconus: an inflammatory disorder? Eye (Lond). 2015;29(7):843–59.
3. Ionescu C, Corbu CG, Tanase C, Jonescu-Cuypers C, Nicula C, Dascalescu D, Cristea M, Voinea LM. Inflammatory biomarkers profile as microenvironmental expression in keratoconus. Dis Markers. 2016;2016:1243819.
4. McMonnies CW. Inflammation and keratoconus. Optom Vis Sci. 2015;92(2):e35–41.
5. Balasubramanian SA, Pye DC, Willcox MD. Effects of eye rubbing on the levels of protease, protease activity and cytokines in tears: relevance in keratoconus. Clin Exp Optom. 2013;96(2):214–8.
6. Romero-Jimenez M, Santodomingo-Rubido J, Wolffsohn JS. Keratoconus: a review. Cont Lens Anterior Eye. 2010;33(4):157–66. quiz 205
7. Poh R, Tan JA, Deva JP, Poo D, Yong Y, Arjunan S. Paraoxonase 1 status in keratoconus: a preliminary study of activity and polymorphism. West Indian Med J. 2012;61(6):569–73.
8. Gordon-Shaag A, Millodot M, Shneor E, Liu Y. The genetic and environmental factors for keratoconus. Biomed Res Int. 2015;2015:795738.
9. Shehadeh MM, Diakonis VF, Jalil SA, Younis R, Qadoumi J, Al-Labadi L. Prevalence of keratoconus among a Palestinian tertiary student population. Open Ophthalmol J. 2015;9:172–6.
10. Abu-Amero KK, Al-Muammar AM, Kondkar AA (2014) Genetics of keratoconus: where do we stand? J Ophthalmol, 2014:641708.
11. Abu Ameerh MA, Bussieres N, Hamad GI, Al Bdour MD. Topographic characteristics of keratoconus among a sample of Jordanian patients. Int J Ophthalmol. 2014;7(4):714–9.
12. Abu Ameerh MA, Al Refai RM, Al Bdour MD. Keratoconus patients at Jordan University hospital: a descriptive study. Clin Ophthalmol. 2012;6:1895–9.
13. Gokhale NS. Epidemiology of keratoconus. Indian J Ophthalmol. 2013;61(8):382–3.
14. Vazirani J, Basu S. Keratoconus: current perspectives. Clin Ophthalmol. 2013;7:2019–30.
15. Mohd-Ali B, Abdu M, Yaw CY, Mohidin N. Clinical characteristics of keratoconus patients in Malaysia: a review from a cornea specialist Centre. J Opt. 2012;5(1):38–42.
16. Assiri AA, Yousuf BI, Quantock AJ, Murphy PJ. Incidence and severity of keratoconus in Asir province, Saudi Arabia. Br J Ophthalmol. 2005;89(11):1403–6.
17. Ljubic A. Keratoconus and its prevalence in Macedonia. Maced J Med Sci. 2009;2(1):58–62.
18. Valdez-García JE, Sepúlveda R, Salazar-Martínez JJ, Lozano-Ramírez JF. Prevalence of keratoconus in an adolescent population. Revista Mexicana de Oftalmología. 2014;88(3):95–8.
19. Wagner H, Barr JT, Zadnik K. Collaborative Longitudinal Evaluation of Keratoconus Study Group (2007) Collaborative longitudinal evaluation of keratoconus (CLEK) study: methods and findings to date. Cont Lens Anterior Eye. 30(4):223–32.
20. Gordon-Shaag A, Millodot M, Shneor E. The epidemiology and etiology of keratoconus. Int J Keratoconus Corn Ectatic Dis. 2012;1:7–15.

11

Treating Diabetic Macular Oedema (DMO): real world UK clinical outcomes for the 0.19mg Fluocinolone Acetonide intravitreal implant (Iluvien™) at 2 years

William Fusi-Rubiano[1,2], Chandoshi Mukherjee[1,2], Mark Lane[1,2], Marie D. Tsaloumas[1], Nicholas Glover[1], Andrej Kidess[1], Alastair K. Denniston[1,3*], Helen E. Palmer[1], Avinash Manna[1] and Rupal Morjaria[1,2]

Abstract

Background: To compare visual function and structural improvements in pseudophakic eyes with diabetic macular oedema (DMO) treated with the 0.19mg Fluocinolone Acetonide (FAc) intravitreal implant (Iluvien™) in a 'real world' setting.

Methods: A single centre retrospective evaluation of patients with DMO unresponsive to conventional treatment treated with the FAc implant according to UK guidelines. Primary efficacy endpoint was best corrected visual acuity (BCVA); secondary endpoints included optical coherence tomography evaluations of the macula (a) central retinal and (b) peak macular thickness collected at annual time points. Primary safety endpoint was new rise in IOP >27mmHg or glaucoma surgery. Patients with <1 year follow-up were excluded.

Results: Twenty-nine eyes were included, with mean(SD) follow up of 792(270) days. Improvement in BCVA and reduction in macular oedema was noted at all timepoints. Mean improvement in BCVA from baseline was 6 ETDRS letters at year 1(n=29), 6.5L at year 2(n=22) and 11L at year 3(n=6). Mean central retinal thickness at baseline was 451 microns, 337 microns at year 1, 342 microns at year 2 and 314 microns at year 3. Two eyes required IOP-lowering drops post implant. Supplementary treatment for persistence or recurrence of DMO was necessary in 18 eyes over the total study period of 3 years with mean time to supplementary treatment being 12 months.

Conclusions: Our evaluation of the 0.19mg FAc implant delivered in a real-world setting, provides additional evidence that it is effective and safe in the treatment of patients with DMO, and can provide sustained benefit for patients with previously refractory disease.

Keywords: Diabetic Macular Oedema, Iluvien, Diabetic Retinopathy, Fluocinolone Acetonide implant

* Correspondence: A.Denniston@bham.ac.uk
[1]Ophthalmology Department, Queen Elizabeth Hospital Birmingham, University Hospitals Birmingham NHSFT, Mindelsohn Way, Birmingham B15 2TH, United Kingdom
[3]Academic Unit of Ophthalmology, Institute of Inflammation & Ageing, University of Birmingham, Edgbaston, Birmingham B15 2TT, United Kingdom
Full list of author information is available at the end of the article

Background

Worldwide 422 million people have diabetes [1]. A third of these people have diabetic retinopathy (DR) and of these a further third have vision threatening DR including diabetic macular oedema (DMO) [2]. In developed countries, DMO is a leading cause of blindness in the working population [3]. DMO occurs due to impairment of the blood retinal barrier and increased vascular permeability caused by anatomical and biochemical changes including pericyte loss, endothelial cell dysfunction and increased pro-inflammatory changes [4]. Vascular endothelial growth factor has a major role in these mechanisms, however the role of anti-oxidants, inflammatory agents and angiogenesis has also been shown [5–7].

For many years laser treatment was the mainstay treatment for DMO, at times supplemented by short acting corticosteroid injections (peri/intra-ocular triamcinolone). In more recent years the role of laser has been largely replaced by the use of anti-vascular endothelial growth factor (VEGF) agents (notably bevacizumab, ranibizumab and aflibercept) [8]. A significant proportion of patients with DMO are however unresponsive to anti-VEGF agents. Gonzalez et al found that 39.7% patients treated with anti-VEGF had minimal response of <5 letter gain in best corrected visual acuity (BCVA) after 3 months [9]. This 'minimal response' at 3 months was associated with worse long-term BCVA (52 weeks and 156 weeks), which may provide a simple method of identifying sub-optimal DMO responders.

Fluocinolone acetonide [FAc] 0.19mg was approved by NICE in 2013 as a treatment option for pseudophakic patients with chronic DMO that are refractory to other therapies, such as laser and anti-VEGF [10]. The main source of evidence for its efficacy was the Fluocinolone Acetonide in Diabetic Macular Edema (FAME) A and B randomized clinical trials which showed clinical effectiveness of 36 months duration [11, 12]. Although 'real-world' data is now emerging, it is still largely limited to the first two years after implantation [8]. The aim of this study was to evaluate the longer-term clinical effectiveness and safety of the FAc implant in patients with DMO treated in the context of a single tertiary centre in the UK.

Methods

This is a single centre retrospective evaluation of the use of the 0.19mg FAc implant (Iluvien™) in patients with DMO unresponsive to conventional treatment. This evaluation was approved by and registered with the relevant NHS trust (University Hospitals Birmingham NHS Foundation Trust). Patients were assessed for treatment with the FAc implant as guided by NICE (UK) Technology Appraisal (TA301) which restricts its use to refractory DMO in pseudophakic patients. Refractory DMO

was determined by clinician and assessed as an inadequate response to conventional therapy (laser and/or anti-VEGF) either no reduction in central retinal thickness or minimal reduction from treatment and a persistence in macula oedema of >250um. Post-FAc implantation, patients continued to be seen regularly to evaluate efficacy and safety, and to monitor associated retinopathy and other ocular disease. For the purposes of this evaluation, the inclusion criteria was all patients at our centre who had been treated with the FAc implant for refractory DMO and for whom there was a minimum of one year follow-up. Data was extracted anonymously from the electronic medical record (Medisoft) in March 2017. The primary efficacy endpoint was best corrected visual acuity (BCVA). Absolute BCVA was evaluated in LogMAR but for presentation of change in BCVA this was converted to number of letters to enable direct comparison to the FAME study [13]. Secondary efficacy endpoints included spectral domain optical coherence tomography (SD-OCT) evaluation of the central retinal thickness and peak macular thickness as per the Heyex™ software from Heidelberg Engineering (Heidelberg, Germany), proportion of cases requiring 'top-up' treatment, and time from baseline for 'top-up' treatment.

The primary safety endpoint was new rise in IOP over 27mmHg or glaucoma surgery. Evaluation was carried out at annual time-points up to 3 years. Patients with less than 1 year follow-up or who had received treatment for other pathology (e.g. for uveitis) were excluded.

Statistical Analysis

BCVA, mean central retinal thickness and mean peak macular thickness were evaluated against baseline for each time-point using student's unpaired t test for parametric data and Mann-Whitney test for non-parametric data. P-values were calculated with a value of less than 0.05 taken to indicate statistical significance. Statistical analysis was performed using SPSS version 20.

Results

Demographics

Overall 37 eyes (33 patients) were treated with the FAc implant between January 2014 and March 2016. Four eyes (4 patients) were excluded due to being treated for non-DMO diagnosis and a further 4 eyes (2 patients) were excluded due to having less than 1 year follow-up.

Of the 29 eyes (27 patients) included, mean age of the patients was 69.1 (range, 44-90) with an equal distribution of gender (13 females, 14 males) and laterality of eye treated (Right eye 17, left eye 12). Mean baseline BCVA was 0.77 and 97% were pseudophakic (28 of 29 eyes). Three eyes (2 patients) received the FAc implant after laser treatment alone due to unsuitability for use of anti-VEGF post recent stroke/heart disease. Three patients (3 eyes) had had previous vitrectomy. Twenty of 29 eyes had a duration of DMO more than 3 years prior to implant. Full data outcomes were available for 29 eyes at year 1, 20 at year 2 and 6 at year 3. Mean (SD) duration of DMO prior to treatment was 2.6 (0.77) years; in the subset for which 3 year data is available the duration of DMO was more than 3 years in all cases with mean (SD) duration 3.2 (0.31) years.

All patients had received either laser and/or anti-VEGF prior to treatment with the FAc implant (Table 1). Twenty six eyes had at least 1 prior laser therapy, 17 eyes had at least 1 prior ranibizumab injection, 19 eyes had at least 1 prior bevacizumab injection and 6 eyes at least 1 prior treatment with triamcinolone. 10 eyes had treatment with both ranibizumab and bevacizumab. All 3 eyes unsuitable for anti-VEGF had prior treatment with triamcinolone injection. Minimum time to FAc implant from prior treatment was 8 weeks.

Efficacy endpoints: Best corrected visual acuity

Mean (SD) BCVA at baseline was 0.77 (0.37) for all 29 eyes. BCVA improved at all time points with mean (SD) letter gain of 6 (15) at 1 year (p<0.05), 6.5 (15) at 2 years (p=0.90) and 11 (7) at 3 years (p<0.05) after implantation (Fig. 1). Of the 6 patients with at least 3 years follow-up, three eyes (3 patients) had an improvement of 15 letters or more at 3 years from baseline.

Efficacy endpoints: Retinal thickness

Mean central retinal thickness at baseline was 451 microns, and mean peak retinal thickness was 488 microns. There was a reduction in both central and peak retinal thickness at all time-points relative to baseline (Fig. 1). The mean (SD) reduction in central retinal and peak thickness was 114 (177) (p<0.001) and 124 (160) (p<0.00001) micrometers respectively at year 1, 103 (207) (p<0.005) and 104 (114) (p<0.001) micrometers at year 2, and 65 (162) (p<0.05) and 99 (90) (p<0.05) micrometers at year 3. Of the patients with at least 3 years follow-up, 50% of eyes (50% of patients) were clinically dry at 3 years from baseline (p<0.05). Case examples demonstrating OCT appearances pre- and post-FAc implant are provided in Fig. 2.

Table 1 Prior therapies, number treated and mean number of treatments for all eyes

Prior therapy	Number of eyes treated	Mean number of treatments	Range
Focal/grid macula laser	10	1.15	1-3
Ranibizumab	17	3.94	1-8
Bevacizumab	18	4.32	1-13
Triamcinolone	16	2.31	1-6

Of the 33 eyes with a clinical diagnosis of DMO treated with the FAc implant (ie including the four eyes excluded from the primary follow-up on the basis of less than one year's follow-up), 9 eyes (27%) showed no significant improvement in macular oedema with no reduction or minimal reduction in peak or central thickness at any timepoint.

Safety endpoints

There were 2 eyes (2 patients) with raised intraocular pressure (IOP) >27mmHg post injection one found at 1 month follow up and one at 6 months follow up. Both were controlled with drops alone. These cases had established raised intraocular pressure (IOP) prior to treatment with the FAc implant: one had a previous diagnosis of ocular hypertension (OHT) and one had a previous diagnosis of primary open angle glaucoma (POAG) for which they were under glaucoma specialist follow up and had been controlled with drops alone. No other ocular or systemic side effects were identified for any patient.

Persistent or recurrence of DMO requiring supplementary treatment

Supplementary treatment for either persistence of DMO (treatment failure) or recurrence of DMO (premature loss of effect) was necessary in 18 eyes. Supplementary treatment was with one or more of laser (n=4), intravitreal triamcinolone (n=3) or anti-VEGF agent (aflibercept n=11; bevacizumab n=4; ranibizumab n=3). No patients had retreatment with the FAc implant. 10 of 29 (34.5%) eyes had required supplementary treatment by 1 year, 12 of 20 (60%) eyes by 2 years and 5 of 6 (83.3%) eyes by 3 years. Mean number of extra treatments needed per eye/year was 2 at year 1, 1.85 at year 2 and 1.66 at year 3. Mean time until supplementary treatment was 12 months (range 2-22 months), with a mean of 2.6 retreatments (range 1 to 9) during the follow-up period. For the subset with 3 year follow-up, 5 out of 6 eyes needed supplementary treatment with anti-VEGF or laser. Mean time to supplementary treatment was 12.8 months in this cohort (range 10-16 months) with mean number of retreatments needed from this point being 5. In the supplementary treatment group (n=18), mean BCVA at baseline was 0.71 (64.5 L) with a mean change in BCVA was -0.18 (9 L gain (p=0.026)) at 1 year, -0.09 (4.5 L gain (p=0.26)) at 2 years, and -0.22 (11 L gain (p=0.047)) at 3 years.

In the group who did not require supplementary treatment (n=11) during the follow-up period mean BCVA at baseline was 0.82 (59 L), with a mean change in BCVA of -0.05 (2.5 L gain (p=0.28)) at 1 year, -0.14 (7 L gain (p=0.18)) at 2 years, and -0.3 (15 L gain) at 3 years (Fig. 3).

FAc implant in vitrectomised eyes

Three eyes had had previous vitrectomy prior to FAc implant, with one year data being available for 3 eyes, and

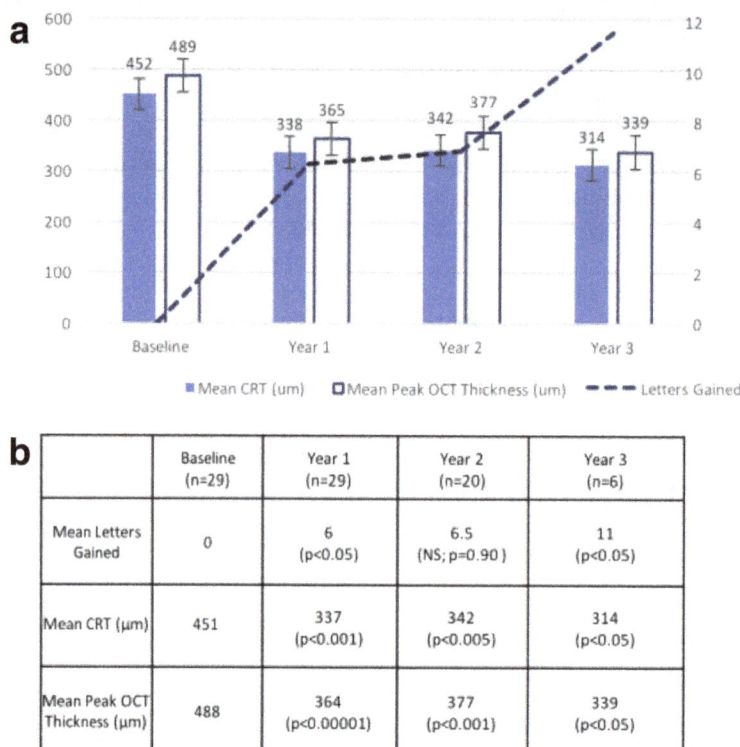

Fig. 1 Improvement in BCVA and reduction in retinal thickness at 1, 2 and 3 years after treatment with FAc implant. Graph (**a**) showing mean values for ETDRS letters gained, mean (SD) central retinal thickness (CRT) and peak macular thickness as measured by SD-OCT. Significance at each time-point was tested against baseline (**b**)

two year data for 1 eye. Mean (SD) BCVA at baseline was 0.83 (0.06), with a mean change of -0.13 (0.11) (6.5 letter gain (p=0.18)) at 1 year, and -0.13 (0.06) (6.5 letter gain (p=0.06)) at 2 years. Mean (SD) CRT was 326 (70) micrometers at baseline, with a mean change of -55.7 micrometers (116) (p=0.31) at 1 year, and -87.7 (62) (p=0.14) at 2 years. Mean peak macula thickness was 412 (77.2) micrometers thickness at baseline, with a mean change of -63.7 micrometers (81) (p=0.31) at 1 year and -84 (62) (p=0.14) at 2 years. Of the three eyes in this group, one required supplementary treatment at 22 months.

Discussion

Our study provides some of the first 'real world' data through to 3 years follow-up for the effect and safety of the 0.19 mg FAc implant in patients with DMO. Three year data for the FAc implant has hitherto been based almost exclusively on the pivotal FAME study, which demonstrated a 15 letter gain or more at 36 months in over a quarter of patients treated with low dose FAc implant and a reduction of 100 micrometers or more in CRT [11]. The effect on visual acuity was noted to be more significant in those with chronic DMO for more than 3 years compared to the cohort with a more recent diagnosis [11]. Our findings are in line with results of the FAME study, with 50% eyes in our series gaining 15

letters or more and being 'dry' on OCT analysis at three years (3 of 6 eligible eyes with three year follow-up data). All three of these eyes had had a duration of DMO more than 3 years. Worse outcomes would be expected in our cohort compared to patients being treated today as patients may have FAc offered at an earlier stage in DMO, whereas many patients in our cohort had a duration of DMO of at least 3 years prior to treatment with FAc implant. A longer duration of DMO and associated disruption to the retinal architecture is known to affect visual outcomes [14].

Other 'real world' data of the use of the FAc implant is now emerging. El-Ghrably et al have shown the additional value of treatment with the FAc implant, in patients initially treated with anti-VEGF as BCVA and CRT improved and was maintained at 12 months [15]. In our study the effects were maintained at 36 months in those who responded to the FAc implant. We further evaluated the need for supplementary treatment over the 3-year period which has not yet been reported in real-world studies. Thirty four percent of eyes had required supplementary treatment by 1 year, 60% by 2 years and 83.3% of eyes by 3 years however overall treatments needed was less than or equal to 2 at each year. None of our patients needed retreatment with the FAc implant at 3 years. This significantly lowers the retreatment burden

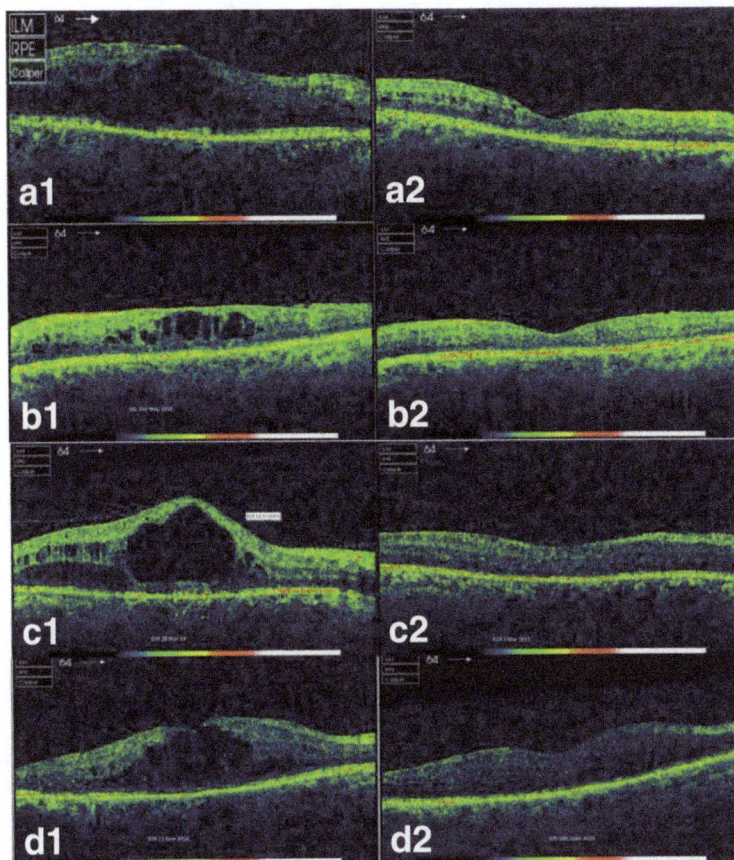

Fig. 2 SD-OCT images pre- and post-FAc implant in patients with chronic DMO. **a**. Right eye of 42 year old male with type 1 diabetes and a 4 year history of DMO treated with previous anti-VEGF, triamcinolone and grid laser. DMO (**a**1) resolved by 8 months (**a**2) **b**. Left vitrectomised eye of a patient with 5 year history of DMO. Treated with anti-VEGF, triamcinolone and grid laser. DMO (**b**1) resolved by 5 months (**b**2). **c**. Right eye of 45 year old male chronic non attender with type 1 diabetes and a 1.2 year history of DMO treated with anti-VEGF. DMO (**c**1) resolved by 3 months (**c**2). **d**. Left vitrectomised eye of 53 year old female with type 1 diabetes and 1 year history of DMO treated with anti-VEGF. DMO (**d**1) resolved by 5 months (**d**2)

when compared to a recent, large, comparative study of aflibercept, bevacizumab, or ranibizumab which reported that a mean of 9-10 injections were required to control DMO over 12 months [16]. Reduction of injection burden is an important benefit of the FAc implant, as high frequency of intravitreal injections has been shown to affect quality of life and to increase anxiety and work absences in patients with DMO [17]. Most patients want fewer injections and appointments, to achieve the same visual results [17]. Fewer supplementary treatments not only improves the quality of life of these patients, but also contributes to the cost efficacy of the FAc implant.

One question regarding the FAc implant is whether vitrectomised eyes may respond differently. In line with the study by Meireles et al [18] , we found the FAc implant to be effective in vitrectomised eyes. Of the three eyes in our series that had had previous vitrectomies, only one eye needed further treatment during the

follow-up, and this was at 1.8 years, compared to the mean supplementary treatment time of 1 year.

The major concerns with the FAc implant are cataract and glaucoma. Cataract occurred in 82-89% of phakic patients by 3 years after implantation of the FAc implant [11] which has led to the NICE (UK) guidelines which restrict its usage to pseudophakic patients with DMO. In our study 97% of eyes were pseudophakic as per the NICE recommendations. Modern cataract surgery is however extremely successful and safe, and thus it may be argued that phakic status should not be a complete bar to treatment if the FAc implant was shown to be otherwise safe and effective. A recent cost analysis has shown that single treatment with the FAc implant is more cost effective than multiple injections of ranibizumab even after allowing for the additional cost of cataract surgery [19]. Although less common than cataract, the greater concern is elevated intraocular pressure (IOP). In FAME, three year data noted an adverse event

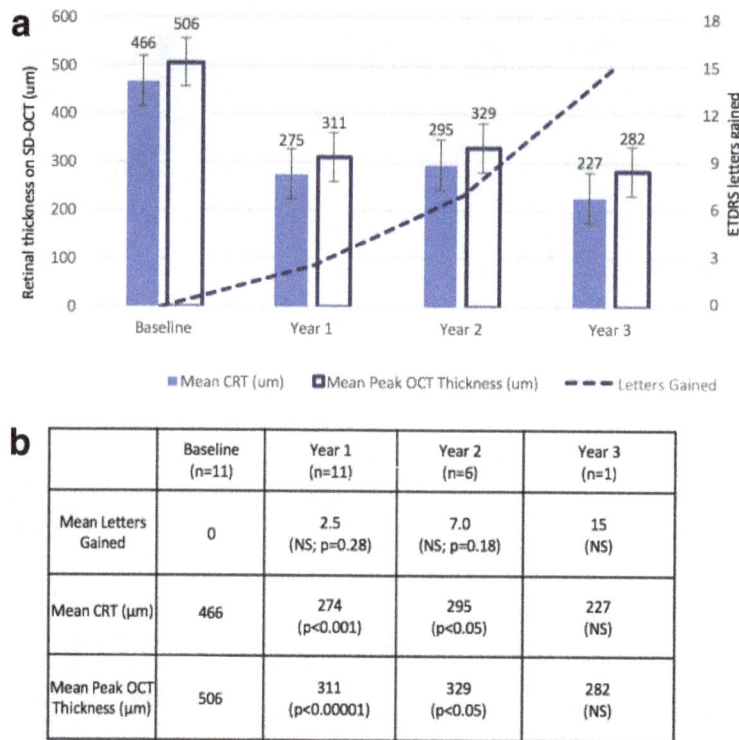

Fig. 3 (Supplementary) Improvement in BCVA and reduction in retinal thickness at 1, 2 and 3 years after treatment with FAc implant in those patients who did not require supplementary treatment. Graph (**a**) showing mean values for ETDRS letters gained, mean (SD) central retinal thickness (CRT) and peak macular thickness as measured by SD-OCT. Significance at each time-point was tested against baseline (**b**)

of elevated IOP of 37% in the standard FAc group (vs 12% in the sham group) and incisional glaucoma surgery being required in 4.8% (vs 0.5% of the sham group). It is interesting to note that our reported adverse events were significantly lower than reported in FAME, although this may in part be due to the relatively smaller number of eyes achieving the three year time-point. In our study only 2 out of 33 eyes were reported to have raised IOP and both of these had a prior history of raised IOP. These patients were successfully treated with drops and did not need surgery. Although Alfaqwi et al have previously reported that there is no additional risk with the FAc implant in patients with well controlled OHT at 12 months [20], further studies are required to evaluate the effect on IOP long-term in patients with OHT and/or POAG.

The primary limitation of our study is its retrospective design and limited numbers, although all data was collected prospectively and recorded on our electronic medical record and imaging database. Use of an electronic medical record platform is also a limitation as limited data is routinely recorded via this platform and therefore limits analysis of crucial factors such as HbA1c and type of diabetes. Use of EMR is however widespread now and is an important method of continuous medical record and source for clinical information in various

studies. An additional limitation is that there is variable follow-up, with a diminishing number of patients across the later time-points reflecting the ongoing recruitment to treatment with the FAc implant; this seemed preferable to either limiting the analysis to only that subset which had achieved three years follow-up, or to prematurely censor the follow-up period. Finally we recognize that this is a relatively small study, reflecting its single site nature. The results of the study are however in line with the FAME trials and does provide 'real world' support to those results.

Conclusions

In summary our study is the first to report 'real world' clinical outcomes of the therapeutic effects and risk profile of the FAc implant in pseudophakic patients with chronic DMO through to 36 months in UK. There was an improvement in mean VA at all time-points with a mean overall improvement in vision of 8.5 letters at 3 years ($p<0.05$), associated with a mean reduction in CRT and peak macula thickness. Although three year data was only available for a subset of our patients, 50% of these patients had a 15 letter or more improvement at this time-point, broadly comparable to the 34% with a similar benefit in the FAME study [10]. It should be noted however that almost two-thirds of the eyes in our series required further treatment within three years. The FAc implant appears to provide clinical benefit in pseudophakic patients with chronic DMO that are insufficiently responsive to first line therapies, with a significant proportion of patients benefitting for up to 3 years as shown in the FAME trials [11, 12]. The FAc implant has the added benefit of less frequent visits and fewer injections. It should be considered in all pseudophakic patients with refractive DMO, or considered after laser alone in patients where anti-VEGF is contraindicated. Our outcomes support the findings of the FAME trial that the FAc implant can be safely used in such patients and significantly improve BCVA and reduce macula oedema whilst reducing the overall cost and burden of treatment in this sight-threatening disease.

Abbreviations
BCVA: Best Corrected Visual Acuity; CRT: Central Retinal Thickness; DMO: Diabetic Macular Oedema; DR: Diabetic Retinopathy; FAc: Fluocinolone Acetonide; IOP: Intraocular Pressure; OHT: Ocular Hypertension; POAG: Primary Open Angle Glaucoma; SD: Standard Deviation; VEGF: Vascular Endothelial Growth Factor

Acknowledgements
Not applicable

Funding
Not applicable

Authors' contributions
WFR: literature review, data collection, analysis and contributor to the writing of the manuscript. CM: literature review, data collection, analysis and contributor to the writing of the manuscript. ML: literature review, data collection, analysis and contributor to the writing of the manuscript. MDT: contributor to the writing of the manuscript. NG: contributor to the writing of the manuscript. AK: contributor to the writing of the manuscript. AKD: contributor to the writing of the manuscript. HEP: contributor to the writing of the manuscript. AM: literature review, contributor to the writing of the manuscript. RM: literature review, data collection, analysis and contributor to the writing of the manuscript. All authors have read and approved the final manuscript.

Competing interests
WF-R and RM have received sponsorship from Alimera Sciences Ltd to attend Euretina 2017. HEP has received sponsorship from Alimera Sciences Ltd to attend Euretina 2016. All written material is the authors' own material.

Author details
[1]Ophthalmology Department, Queen Elizabeth Hospital Birmingham, University Hospitals Birmingham NHSFT, Mindelsohn Way, Birmingham B15 2TH, United Kingdom. [2]Sandwell & West Birmingham NHS Trust, Dudley Road, Birmingham B18 7QH, United Kingdom. [3]Academic Unit of Ophthalmology, Institute of Inflammation & Ageing, University of Birmingham, Edgbaston, Birmingham B15 2TT, United Kingdom.

References
1. Mathers CD, Loncar D. Projections of global mortality and burden of disease from 2002 to 2030. PLoS Med. 2006;3(11):e442.
2. Lee R, Wong TY, Sabanayagam C. Epidemiology of diabetic retinopathy, diabetic macula edema and related vision loss. Eye Vis (lond). 2015;2:17.
3. Romero-Aroca P. Managing diabetic macular edema: The leading cause of diabetes blindness. World Journal of Diabetes. 2011;2(6):98–104.
4. Amoaku WM, Saker S, Stewart EA. A review of therapies for diabetic macular oedema and rationale for combination therapy. Eye. 2015;29(9):1115.
5. Klaassen I, Van Noorden CJ, Schlingemann RO. Molecular basis of the inner blood–retinal barrier and its breakdown in diabetic macular edema and other pathological conditions. Prog Retin Eye Res. 2013;34:19–48.
6. Ehrlich R, Harris A, Ciulla TA, Kheradiya N, Winston DM, Wirostko B. Diabetic macular oedema: physical, physiological and molecular factors contribute to this pathological process. Acta Ophthalmol. 2010;88:279–91.
7. Joussen AM, Poulaki V, Le ML, Koizumi K, Esser C, Janicki H, et al. A central role for inflammation in the pathogenesis of diabetic retinopathy. FASEB J. 2004;18:1450–2.
8. Bailey C, Chakravarthy U, Lotery A, Menon G, Talks J, Medisoft AG. Real-world experience with 0.2 µg/day fluocinolone acetonide intravitreal implant (ILUVIEN) in the United Kingdom. Eye. 2017; https://doi.org/10.1038/eye.2017.125.
9. Gonzalez VH, Campbell J, Holekamp NM, Kiss S, Loewenstein A, Augustin AJ, et al. Early and Long-Term Responses to Anti–Vascular Endothelial Growth Factor Therapy in Diabetic Macular Edema: Analysis of Protocol I Data. American Journal of Ophthalmology. 2016;172:72–9.
10. National Institute for Health and Care Excellence. Fluocinolone acetonide intravitreal implant for treating chronic diabetic macular oedema after an inadequate response to prior therapy. London: NICE; 2014.
11. Campochiaro PA, Brown DM, Pearson A, Chen S, Boyer D, Ruiz-Moreno J, et al. Sustained delivery fluocinolone acetonide vitreous inserts provide benefit for at least 3 years in patients with diabetic macular edema. Ophthalmology. 2012;119(10):2125–32.
12. Campochiaro PA, Brown DM, Pearson A, Ciulla T, Boyer D, Holz FG, et al. Long-term benefit of sustained-delivery fluocinolone acetonide vitreous inserts for diabetic macular edema. Ophthalmology. 2011;118(4):626–35.
13. Gregori NZ, Feuer W, Rosenfeld PJ. Novel method for analyzing snellen visual acuity measurements. Retina. 2010;30(7):1046–50.
14. Gardner TW, Larsen M, Girach A, Zhi X. Diabetic macular oedema and visual loss: relationship to location, severity and duration. Acta ophthalmologica. 2009;87(7):709–13.
15. El-Ghrably I, Steel DH, Habib M, Vaideanu-Collins D, Manvikar S, Hillier RJ. Diabetic macular edema outcomes in eyes treated with fluocinolone acetonide 0.2 µg/d intravitreal implant: real-world UK experience. European journal of ophthalmology. 2017;27(3):357.
16. Diabetic Retinopathy Clinical Research Network. Aflibercept, bevacizumab, or ranibizumab for diabetic macular edema. N Engl J Med. 2015;372:1193–203.
17. Sivaprasad S, Oyetunde S. Impact of injection therapy on retinal patients with diabetic macular edema or retinal vein occlusion. Clinical ophthalmology. 2016;10:939.
18. Meireles A, Goldsmith C, El-Ghrably I, Erginay A, Habib M, Pessoa B, et al. Efficacy of 0.2 µg/day fluocinolone acetonide implant (ILUVIEN) in eyes with diabetic macular edema and prior vitrectomy. Eye. 2017;31(5):684.
19. Quhill F, Beiderbeck A. Cost advantage of fluocinolone acetonide implant (ILUVIEN®) versus ranibizumab in the treatment of chronic diabetic macular oedema. Glob Reg Health Technol Assess. 2017;3(2):00.
20. Alfaqawi F, Lip PL, Elsherbiny S, Chavan R, Mitra A, Mushtaq B. Report of 12-months efficacy and safety of intravitreal fluocinolone acetonide implant for the treatment of chronic diabetic macular oedema: a real-world result in the United Kingdom. Eye. 2017;31(4):650.

12

Epidemiology of uveitis (2013–2015) and changes in the patterns of uveitis (2004–2015) in the central Tokyo area

Shintaro Shirahama[1]* (ID), Toshikatsu Kaburaki[1], Hisae Nakahara[1], Rie Tanaka[1], Mitsuko Takamoto[2], Yujiro Fujino[3], Hidetoshi Kawashima[4] and Makoto Aihara[1]

Abstract

Background: The distribution of uveitis varies with genetic, ethnic, geographic, environmental, and lifestyle factors. Epidemiological information about the patterns of uveitis is useful when an ophthalmologist considers the diagnosis of uveitis. Therefore, it is important to identify the causes of uveitis over the years in different regions. The purposes of this study were to characterize the uveitis patients who first arrived at the University of Tokyo Hospital in 2013–2015, and to analyze the changes in the patterns of uveitis from 2004 to 2012 to 2013–2015.

Methods: We retrospectively identified 750 newly arrived patients with uveitis who visited the Uveitis Clinic in the University of Tokyo Hospital between January 2013 and December 2015, using clinical records. We extracted data on patient age, sex, diagnosis, anatomic location of inflammation, laboratory test results of blood and urine, and chest X-ray and fluorescein fundus angiography findings for each patient. In addition, we compared these data with those from 2004 to 2012 to analyze the changes in the patterns of uveitis.

Results: A definite diagnosis was established in 445 patients (59.3%). The most common diagnoses were herpetic iridocyclitis (7.5%), sarcoidosis (6.1%), Behçet's disease (4.4%), Vogt–Koyanagi–Harada disease (4.1%), and intraocular lymphoma (4.1%). The most frequent unclassified type of uveitis was suspected sarcoidosis (22.3%). Analysis of the changes in the patterns of uveitis in the central Tokyo area from 2004 to 2012 to 2013–2015 revealed notable increasing trends of herpetic iridocyclitis and intraocular lymphoma, and increasing trends of bacterial endophthalmitis, fungal endophthalmitis, and juvenile chronic iridocyclitis. In contrast, the frequency of sarcoidosis, Behçet's disease, and Vogt–Koyanagi–Harada disease decreased.

Conclusions: The patterns of uveitis changed considerably from 2004 to 2012 to 2013–2015. Continuous investigations about the epidemiology of uveitis are needed to diagnose uveitis more accurately.

Keywords: Diagnosis, Epidemiology, Japan, Trend, Uveitis

* Correspondence: aphorodite.magic@gmail.com
[1]Department of Ophthalmology, University of Tokyo Graduate School of Medicine, 7-3-1 Hongo, Bunkyo-ku, Tokyo 113-8655, Japan
Full list of author information is available at the end of the article

Background

Uveitis is a leading cause of visual blindness in developed countries [1]. Many studies have reported the patterns of uveitis in different countries and ethnicities [2–7]. The distribution of the types and etiologies of uveitis is influenced by genetic, ethnic, geographic, environmental, and lifestyle factors [8]. As a result, the patterns of uveitis vary greatly according to the population and the time of research. For example, one report from Taiwan presented data demonstrating that the incidences of herpetic anterior uveitis, acute retinal necrosis, and cytomegalovirus (CMV) retinitis have increased, while those of toxoplasmosis and tuberculosis have decreased [9], compared with findings of a previous study [10]. Therefore, it is important to analyze the epidemiology of this disease in various regions over time.

In recent years, highly advanced diagnostic methods for uveitis, including optical coherent tomography and polymerase chain reaction (PCR) analysis for infectious agents using aqueous samples, have been developed. Consequently, the number of definite diagnoses has been gradually increasing [2]. However, a definite diagnosis can still not be reached in approximately 30–40% of patients newly diagnosed with uveitis [2, 4, 5, 11].

Region-specific information about the patterns of uveitis is helpful when the clinicians consider the diagnosis for newly arrived patients. There are many reports on this topic from both Japan and other countries [3–7, 12]. Previously, we have reported the patterns of newly arrived patients with uveitis at the University of Tokyo Hospital between 2004 and 2012 [2, 11]. In this institution, retrospective analysis of newly arrived patients with uveitis have been conducted over the past 50 years [2]. Therefore, we consider that the data from our hospital are representative of the changing patterns of uveitis in Japan.

In the current study, we investigated the records of patients who visited the University of Tokyo Hospital during 2013–2015 and compared the results to those of our previous studies (2004–2012) [2, 11].

Methods

We retrospectively investigated the clinical records of 750 newly arrived patients with uveitis (363 men, 387 women) who first visited the Uveitis Clinic of the University of Tokyo Hospital (a tertiary referral center located in central Tokyo) between January 2013 and December 2015. Patients with uveitis who had first visited before 2012 due to uveitis were excluded from the study. Conversely, patients who had first visited our clinic before 2012 for other reasons and then presented with uveitis during the study period were included in this study.

We collected clinicodemographic data, including age, sex, diagnosis, anatomic location of inflammation, laboratory test results of blood and urine, and chest X-ray and fluorescein fundus angiography findings from the patients' clinical records. The ethics committee of the University of Tokyo Hospital allowed us to collect clinical data for this retrospective study.

We adopted the uveitis classification method used in a nationwide investigation of uveitis conducted in 2009 in Japan [13]. The anatomic diagnosis was evaluated according to the classification of the Standardization of Uveitis (SUN) Working Group, as anterior uveitis, intermediate uveitis, posterior uveitis, or panuveitis [14].

All patients with uveitis underwent blood tests (peripheral blood count, erythrocyte sedimentation rate, serum angiotensin-converting enzyme, glucose, rheumatoid factor, immunoglobulin [Ig] A, IgG, IgM, antinuclear antibody (double-stranded deoxyribonucleic acid [DNA] antibody and single-stranded DNA antibody), calcium, blood urea nitrogen, creatinine, creatine kinase, rapid plasma regain, *Treponema pallidum* latex agglutination, anti-human T-cell lymphotropic virus type I [HTLV-1] antibody, C-reactive protein, globulin fraction, IgM and IgG of toxoplasma, herpes simplex virus [HSV], varicella zoster virus [VZV], and CMV), urine tests, chest X-ray examination, and the Mantoux reaction test at the initial presentation. Additionally, PCR tests, β-D-glucan, HLA, interferon gamma release assays, diagnostic vitrectomy, and fluorescein angiography were performed when specific uveitis diseases were suspected; those examinations might be useful for judging the diagnosis. Quantitative PCR using aqueous humor and blood cultures was conducted when infectious uveitis was suspected; serum β-D-glucan testing (for suspected fungal endophthalmitis) and human leukocyte antigen (HLA) typing (for suspected acute anterior uveitis or Behçet's disease) were also performed. Interferon-gamma release assays were conducted when the Mantoux reaction test was strongly positive. Moreover, vitreous fluid examinations were conducted when intraocular lymphoma was suspected. If inflammation was suspected in retina and/or optic disc, fluorescein angiography was performed if the patient consented to the procedure. Information obtained from fluorescein angiography was used to determine the anatomical location of uveitis and the presence or absence of retinal vasculitis and/or chorioretinitis for consideration in differential diagnosis of uveitis.

Behçet's disease was diagnosed based on criteria established by the Behçet's Disease Research Committee of Japan [15]. For sarcoidosis, we used the criteria established by the Japanese Society of Sarcoidosis and Other Granulomatous Disorders [16, 17]. For Vogt–Koyanagi–Harada disease (VKH), we adopted previously reported criteria [18]. For herpetic iritis [19], patients with active skin lesions associated with ophthalmic herpes zoster (i.e., the vesicular rash involving the periocular skin, such as the eyelids, medial canthal area, or the tip of the nose, known as Hutchinson's sign) were clinically diagnosed and classified as VZV iritis. Patients without a skin lesion were subjected to PCR assays for HSV, VZV, and CMV DNA using anterior chamber fluid. The presence of > 100 copies/mL of viral DNA were judged as a positive finding. Patients with negative PCR results for HSV, VZV, and CMV DNA, and good response to anti-herpetic treatment were classified as herpetic iridocyclitis (clinical diagnosis), while those who did not undergo PCR assays were classified as suspected herpetic iritis. The diagnoses of bacterial and fungal endophthalmitis were based on matching of ocular symptoms suggesting bacterial or fungal etiology, the results of laboratory tests (blood culture, serum β-D-glucan), detection of bacterial or fungal DNA in aqueous humor samples by broad-range PCR [20, 21], and a response to antibiotics or antifungal drugs. As for intraocular lymphoma, we diagnosed this disease if at least two of the following four criteria were met: cytology >class 3, interleukin (IL)-10/IL-6 ratio > 1 or IL-10 > 50 pg/mL in the intraocular fluid [22], κ/λ ratio on fluorescence-activated cell sorting analysis, and positive PCR results for immunoglobulin heavy chain (IgH) gene rearrangement [23]. Regarding acute anterior uveitis (AAU), patients with unique symptoms of ankylosing spondylitis, ulcerative colitis, or psoriasis were diagnosed as having systemic disease-associated uveitis. Those with HLA-B27 were diagnosed as AAU, while those without HLA-B27 or with unknown HLA typing were diagnosed as unclassified uveitis. We diagnosed ocular tuberculosis based on a combination of ocular symptoms indicating tuberculous etiology, laboratory tests, and response to anti-tuberculosis therapy. Consequently, we used the diagnostic criteria for presumed ocular tuberculosis [24]. The diagnostic criteria for diabetic iritis in this study were (1) acute severe iridocyclitis in patients with poor glycemic control (HbA1c ≥ 8.0%) and (2) other investigations for systemic disease associated

with uveitis were negative [25]. For HTLV-1 [26], acute zonal occult outer retinopathy (AZOOR) [27], and rubella virus-associated uveitis [28], we adopted the criteria described in previous reports [26–28]. Juvenile chronic iridocyclitis was diagnosed by the typical ocular findings and clinical courses, as described in a previous report [29].

Statistical analyses were performed using the χ-squared test in SPSS for Windows, version 14.0 (SPSS Inc., Chicago, IL, USA). We compared the frequency of each disease between 2013 and 2015 with those between 2004 and 2012. A p value < 0.05 was considered statistically significant.

Results

Figure 1 shows the age distribution of the patients with uveitis that visited our institution between 2013 and 2015. The mean age was 56.4 ± 18.5 years (men: 56.9 ± 18.9 years, women: 56.1 ± 18.9 years). The most common age category was 60–69 years for both men and women. Among a total of 750 newly arrived patients with uveitis, 445 patients (59.3%) received a definite diagnosis. Table 1 presents the distribution of patients who were given a definite diagnosis. The three most common diagnoses were herpetic iridocyclitis (HSV, VZV, and CMV) in 56 patients (7.5%), sarcoidosis in 46 (6.1%), and Behçet's disease in 31 (4.4%).

Patients with herpetic iridocyclitis were divided into five groups by diagnostic method. Of these, CMV DNA positivity was the most common diagnostic method ($n = 34$, 60.7%), followed by skin lesions of herpes zoster ophthalmicus ($n = 12$, 21.4%), VZV DNA positivity ($n = 5$, 8.9%), HSV DNA positivity ($n = 3$, 5.4%), and clinical diagnosis only ($n = 2$, 3.6%) (Table 2).

Table 3 shows the distributions of patients with uveitis according to three age groups (< 20 years, 20–59 years, and ≥ 60 years). In these patients, juvenile chronic iridocyclitis, Behçet's disease, and herpetic iridocyclitis were

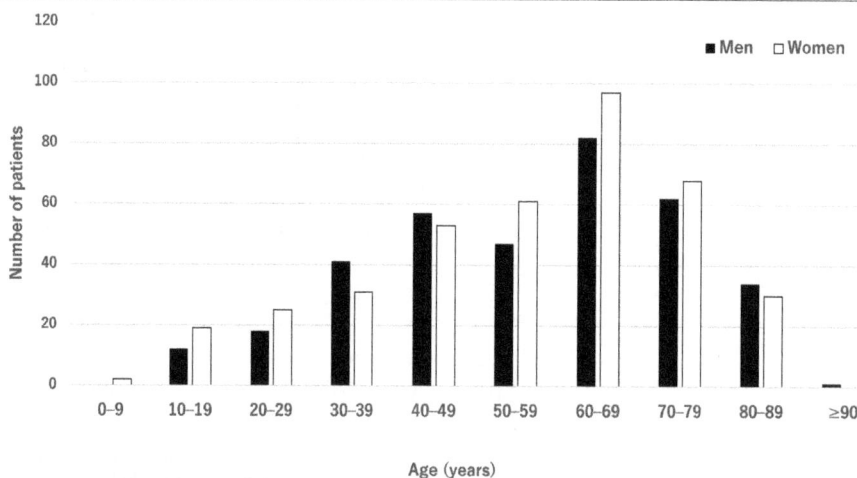

Fig. 1 Distribution of 750 patients with uveitis from 2013 to 2015 by age and sex Uveitis was more frequent in the age group of 60–69 years among both men and women

Table 1 Distribution of uveitis among new patients (2013–2015)

Patient diagnosis	No. of patients		Sex	
	No.	%	Male	Female
Herpetic iridocyclitis	56	7.5	43	13
Sarcoidosis	46	6.1	13	33
Behçet's disease	33	4.4	17	16
Vogt–Koyanagi–Harada disease	31	4.1	12	19
Intraocular lymphoma	31	4.1	21	10
Posner–Schlossman syndrome	25	3.3	15	10
Bacterial endophthalmitis	23	3.1	9	14
Fuchs heterochromic iridocyclitis	20	2.7	11	9
Juvenile chronic iridocyclitis	17	2.3	4	13
Fungal endophthalmitis	16	2.1	11	5
Acute anterior uveitis	14	1.9	8	6
Acute retinal necrosis	13	1.7	5	8
HTLV-1-associated uveitis	13	1.7	5	8
Cytomegalovirus retinitis	10	1.3	6	4
Tuberculosis	9	1.2	6	3
AZOOR	8	1.1	3	5
MEWDS	8	1.1	3	5
Psoriatic uveitis	7	0.9	4	3
Neuroretinitis	6	0.8	3	3
Lens induced uveitis	6	0.8	2	4
Toxoplasma	6	0.8	5	1
IBD	5	0.7	4	1
APMPPE	4	0.5	1	3
Diabetic iridocyclitis	4	0.5	4	0
Systemic lupus erythematosus	4	0.5	0	4
Syphilis	3	0.4	2	1
Rubella	3	0.4	2	1
Ankylosing spondylitis	2	0.3	2	0
Immune reconstitution syndrome	2	0.3	0	2
JIA	2	0.3	0	2
Multifocal choroiditis	2	0.3	1	1
RA	2	0.3	0	2
Sympathetic ophthalmia	2	0.3	1	1
Geographic chorioretinopathy	2	0.3	1	1
Multiple sclerosis	2	0.3	0	2
Sclerouveitis due to scleroderma	2	0.3	0	2
CAR	1	0.1	0	1
PIC	1	0.1	1	0
UAIM	1	0.1	0	1
Iridocyclitis due to nivolumab	1	0.1	0	1
Cat scratch disease	1	0.1	0	1

Table 1 Distribution of uveitis among new patients (2013–2015) *(Continued)*

Patient diagnosis	No. of patients		Sex	
	No.	%	Male	Female
Polymyalgia rheumatica	1	0.1	0	1
Unclassified uveitis	305	38.4	138	167
Total	750		363	387

HTLV-1 human T lymphotropic virus type-1, *AZOOR* acute zonal occult outer retinopathy, *MEWDS* multiple evanescent white dot syndrome, *IBD* inflammatory bowel disease, *APMPPE* acute posterior multifocal placoid pigment epitheliopathy, *JIA* juvenile idiopathic arthritis, *RA* rheumatoid arthritis, *CAR* cancer-associated retinopathy, *PIC* punctate inner choroidopathy, *UAIM* unilateral acute idiopathic maculopathy

the most common diagnoses, respectively. Definite diagnoses were not made for the remaining 305 patients (39.1%). Among these patients, suspected sarcoidosis was the most frequent diagnosis ($n = 167$, 22.3%), which accounted for 54.8% of all suspected diagnoses.

Table 4 shows the distribution of uveitis categorized by anatomical location (anterior uveitis, intermediate uveitis, posterior uveitis, and panuveitis). In this study, 289 out of 750 patients (38.5%) had anterior uveitis, 12 (1.6%) had intermediate uveitis, 94 (12.5%) had posterior uveitis, and 355 (47.3%) had panuveitis. The distribution of uveitis according to anatomical site did not differ from that in our previous studies [2].

Table 5 shows the shifting numbers and distributions of the uveitis cases diagnosed at the University of Tokyo Hospital over 12 years. Compared with our previous studies since 2004 [2, 11], the present analysis showed that the incidences of herpetic iridocyclitis, intraocular lymphoma, bacterial endophthalmitis, fungal endophthalmitis, and juvenile chronic iridocyclitis have been increasing. Additionally, sarcoidosis, Behçet's disease, and VKH disease have been decreasing in recent years. However, the increases or decreases of these disease frequencies were not statistically significant ($p > 0.05$ for all).

Table 6 reports the distribution of the age of patients at the first visit in this study (2013–2015) and previous studies (2004–2006, 2007–2009, and 2010–2012). The average ages of new patients were 52.0, 51.6, 53.6, and

Table 2 Diagnostic methods for herpetic iritis

Diagnostic method	No. of patients (%)
Clinical diagnosis only	2 (3.6)
Skin lesions of herpes zoster ophthalmicus and granulomatous iridocyclitis	12 (21.4)
Herpes simplex virus detection with PCR using aqueous humor	3 (5.4)
Varicella zoster virus detection with PCR using aqueous humor	5 (8.9)
Cytomegalovirus detection with PCR using aqueous humor	34 (60.7)

PCR polymerase chain reaction

Table 3 Frequency of new patients with uveitis (2013–2015) by age

< 20 years (n = 31)	No. of patients (%)	20–59 years (n = 358)	No. of patients (%)	≥60 years (n = 409)	No. of patients (%)
Juvenile chronic iridocyclitis	11 (35.5)	Behçet's disease	24 (7.1)	Herpetic iridocyclitis	37 (9.7)
Fuchs heterochronic iridocyclitis	3 (9.7)	Herpetic iridocyclitis	19 (5.7)	Sarcoidosis	27 (7.0)
Bechet disease	3 (9.7)	Sarcoidosis	19 (5.7)	Intraocular lymphoma	27 (7.0)
Posner-Schlossman syndrome	2 (6.5)	Vogt-Koyanagi-Harada disease	16 (4.8)	Bacterial endophthalmitis	20 (5.2)
HTLV-1-associated uveitis	1 (3.2)	Posner-Schlossman syndrome	13 (3.9)	Vogt-Koyanagi-Harada disease	14 (3.7)
JIA	1 (3.2)	Acute anterior uveitis	12 (3.6)	Fungal endophthalmitis	12 (3.1)
Cat scratch disease	1 (3.2)	Fuchs heterochromic iridocyclitis	10 (3.0)	HTLV-1-associated uveitis	11 (2.9)
Cytomegalovirus retinitis	1 (3.2)	MEWDS	8 (2.4)	Posner-Schlossman syndrome	10 (2.6)
Vogt-Koyanagi-Harada disease	1 (3.2)	AZOOR	7 (2.1)	Cytomegalovirus retinitis	8 (2.1)
Toxoplasma	1 (3.2)	Juvenile chronic iridocyclitis	6 (1.8)	Fuchs heterochromic iridocyclitis	7 (1.8)
Unknown	6 (19.4)	Acute retinal necrosis	6 (1.8)	Acute retinal necrosis	7 (1.8)
		Tuberculosis	6 (1.8)	Lens induced uveitis	6 (1.6)
		IBD	5 (1.5)	Behçet's disease	6 (1.6)
		Systemic lupus erythematosus	4 (1.2)	Diabetic iridocyclitis	4 (1.0)
		Psoriatic uveitis	4 (1.2)	Psoriatic uveitis	3 (0.8)
		Intraocular lymphoma	4 (1.2)	Tuberculosis	3 (0.8)
		Neuroretinitis	4 (1.2)	Syphilis	3 (0.8)
		Fungal endophthalmitis	4 (1.2)	APMPPE	3 (0.8)
		Toxoplasma	3 (0.9)	Toxoplasma	2 (0.5)
		Bacterial endophthalmitis	3 (0.9)	Acute anterior uveitis	2 (0.5)
		Rubella virus-associated uveitis	3 (0.9)	Sympathetic ophthalmia	2 (0.5)
		Multiple sclerosis	2 (0.6)	Neuroretinitis	2 (0.5)
		Ankylosing spondylitis	2 (0.6)	AZOOR	1 (0.3)
		Multifocal choroiditis and panuveitis	2 (0.6)	CAR	1 (0.3)
		APMPPE	1 (0.3)	Immune reconstitution syndrome	1 (0.3)
		Cytomegalovirus retinitis	1 (0.3)	Polymyalgia rheumatica	1 (0.3)
		Immune reconstitution syndrome	1 (0.3)	RA	1 (0.3)
		HTLV-1-associated uveitis	1 (0.3)	Sclerouveitis due to scleroderma	1 (0.3)
		JIA	1 (0.3)	Geographic chorioretinopathy	1 (0.3)
		PIC	1 (0.3)	Unknown	160 (41.8)
		RA	1 (0.3)		
		UAIM	1 (0.3)		
		Iridocyclitis due to nivolumab	1 (0.3)		
		Sclerouveitis due to scleroderma	1 (0.3)		
		Geographic chorioretinopathy	1 (0.3)		
		Unknown	139 (41.4)		
Total	31	Total	336	Total	383

HTLV-1 human T lymphotropic virus type-1, *AZOOR* acute zonal occult outer retinopathy, *MEWDS* multiple evanescent white dot syndrome, *IBD* inflammatory bowel disease, *APMPPE* acute posterior multifocal placoid pigment epitheliopathy, *JIA* juvenile idiopathic arthritis, *RA* rheumatoid arthritis, *CAR* cancer-associated retinopathy, *PIC* punctate inner choroidopathy, *UAIM* unilateral acute idiopathic maculopathy

Table 4 Shifts in the distribution of anatomic localization of uveitis (2004–2015) [2, 11]

Period	2004–2006[a]	2007–2009[a]	2010–2012[b]	2013–2015
New patients (n)	426	535	695	750
Anterior uveitis	48.8%	48.0%	50.1%	38.5%
Intermediate uveitis	–	–	1.6%	1.6%
Posterior uveitis	9.6%	15.7%	13.4%	12.5%
Panuveitis	41.5%	36.3%	35.0%	47.3%

[a]The classification of the International Ocular Inflammation Society (IOIS) was adopted. Intermediate uveitis is included in the definition of posterior uveitis [27]
[b]The classification of the Standardization of Uveitis Nomenclature (SUN) [14] was adopted

56.4 years, respectively, indicating that the average age has been gradually increasing.

Discussion

In this study, the most frequent uveitis categories in patients aged < 20, 20–59, and ≥ 60 years were juvenile chronic iridocyclitis, Behçet's disease, and herpetic iridocyclitis, respectively. A previous study conducted in our hospital (2010–2012) showed that the most frequent types of uveitis in the same age groups were juvenile chronic iridocyclitis, Behçet's disease, and sarcoidosis, respectively [11]. In comparison with the findings of the previous study, an increase in the incidence of herpetic iridocyclitis in patients aged ≥60 years was observed. A possible reason for this new finding might be the progression of aging in Japan [30]. In fact, the incidence of

Table 5 Shifts in the number and distribution (%) of diagnosed uveitis cases (2004–2015) [2, 11]

Diagnosis	2004–2006	2007–2009	2010–2012	2013–2015
Herpetic iridocyclitis	20 (4.7)	28 (5.2)	38 (5.5)	56 (7.5)
Sarcoidosis	37 (8.7)	44 (8.2)	56 (8.1)	46 (6.1)
Behçet's disease	21 (4.9)	26 (4.9)	32 (4.6)	33 (4.4)
Vogt–Koyanagi–Harada disease	27 (6.3)	37 (6.9)	28 (4.0)	31 (4.1)
Intraocular lymphoma	4 (0.9)	13 (2.4)	21 (3.0)	31 (4.1)
Posner–Schlossman syndrome	19 (4.5)	20 (3.7)	25 (3.6)	25 (3.3)
Bacterial endophthalmitis	2 (0.5)	10 (1.9)	13 (1.9)	23 (3.1)
Fuchs heterochromic iridocyclitis	9 (2.1)	10 (1.9)	11 (1.6)	20 (2.7)
Juvenile chronic iridocyclitis	3 (0.7)	7 (1.3)	11 (1.6)	17 (2.3)
Others	90 (21.1)	100 (18.7)	138 (20.0)	163 (21.7)
Unclassified uveitis	147 (34.5)	173 (32.3)	264 (38.0)	305 (40.7)
Total	426	535	695	750

The data are presented as no. of patients (%)

Table 6 Shifts in the numbers of new patients with uveitis according to age (2004–2015) [2, 11]

Age (years)	2004–2006	2007–2009	2010–2012	2013–2015
< 20	11 (2.6)	26 (4.9)	29 (4.2)	31 (3.9)
20–59	251 (58.9)	308 (57.6)	354 (50.9)	336 (44.8)
≥60	164 (38.5)	201 (37.6)	312 (44.9)	383 (51.1)
Total	426	535	695	750

The data are presented as no. of patients (%)

infections, such as herpes zoster, in the elderly has been shown to be increasing in other countries as well [31].

Compared with the previous studies from our hospital [2, 11], the ratios of herpetic iridocyclitis (7.5%), intraocular lymphoma (4.1%), bacterial endophthalmitis (3.1%), fungal endophthalmitis (2.1%), and juvenile chronic iridocyclitis (2.3%) were increased in this study.

We speculated that the increase of herpetic iridocyclitis patients may be attributed to the recurring use of PCR assays for HSV, VZV, and CMV DNA using anterior chamber fluid. The increase in intraocular lymphoma may be due to two reasons. First, that we passively conducted diagnostic vitrectomy for patients suspected of having intraocular lymphoma. Second, that there has been an increase in the number of patients with primary central nervous system lymphoma [32]. The increases of patients with bacterial and fungal endophthalmitis were considered to be due to advances in the relevant diagnostic methods. Broad-range real-time PCR for bacterial DNA [19] and fungus DNA [20] were employed using both anterior chamber fluid and vitreous fluid. Moreover, the increase of juvenile chronic iridocyclitis might be related to the increasing number of patients aged < 20 years old in our hospital. In Japan, juvenile chronic iridocyclitis was not commonly associated with juvenile idiopathic arthritis [33]. The number of patients with juvenile chronic iridocyclitis without juvenile idiopathic arthritis in this study was also larger than the number of patients with both juvenile chronic iridocyclitis and juvenile idiopathic arthritis.

Notably, the ratios of scleritis, sarcoidosis, Behçet's disease, and VKH have been gradually decreasing over the past years in our institution. We cannot find adequate reasons for the decreasing frequencies of these diseases.

Another interesting finding of this study is the trend for increasing age of newly arrived patients with uveitis. Compared to the data from 2004 to 2006, the average age of the patients with uveitis in the current study (2013–2015) was 4.6 years higher. A possible reason for the older age of patients with uveitis might be the rapid aging of the Japanese population [30]. Thus, it can be expected that the frequencies of herpetic iridocyclitis and intraocular lymphoma will be further increasing in the future in Japan. Indeed, the average age of patients with herpetic iridocyclitis or intraocular lymphoma in the current study was 62.5 ± 14.8 years and 72.0 ± 12.0 years, respectively. Further studies should be continued to clarify the trends of the patterns of uveitis.

The limitations of this study include its retrospective design, that it was conducted in a tertiary referral center, and that the study period was only 3 years. However, 750 patients were included in this study, and we believe that the current study's findings could reflect the current trends of uveitis in Japan.

Conclusions

The recent patterns of uveitis in the central Tokyo area revealed increasing trends of herpetic iridocyclitis and intraocular lymphoma. Because the patterns of uveitis are continuously changing, ongoing investigations of the predominant types of uveitis are needed.

Abbreviations

AAU: Acute anterior uveitis; AZOOR: Acute zonal occult outer retinopathy; CMV: Cytomegalovirus; DNA: Deoxyribonucleic acid; HLA: Human leukocyte antigen; HSV: Herpes simplex virus; HTVV-1: Anti-human T-cell lymphotropic virus type I; Ig: Immunoglobulin; IgH: Immunoglobulin heavy chain; IL: Interleukin; PCR: Polymerase chain reaction; VKH: Vogt–Koyanagi–Harada disease; VZV: Varicella zoster virus

Funding

This study was supported in part by a Grant-in-Aid for Science Research for Behçet's Disease from the Ministry of Health, Labour and Welfare of Japan (No. 50056096).

Authors' contributions

SS was involved in study design, data collection, analysis of the results, and drafting of the manuscript. TK participated in study design, data collection, and reviewing and editing of the manuscript. HN, RT, and MT made substantial contributions to the acquisition of data. YF, HK, and MA were involved in critically revising the manuscript for important intellectual content. All authors read and approved the final manuscript.

Competing interests

The authors declare that they have no competing interests.

Author details

[1]Department of Ophthalmology, University of Tokyo Graduate School of Medicine, 7-3-1 Hongo, Bunkyo-ku, Tokyo 113-8655, Japan. [2]Department of Ophthalmology, Saitama Red Cross Hospital, 1-5 Shintoshin, Chuo-ku, Saitama-shi, Saitama 330-8553, Japan. [3]Department of Ophthalmology, Tokyo Shinjuku Medical Center, 5-1 Tsukudo-cho, Shinjuku-ku, Tokyo 162-8543, Japan. [4]Department of Ophthalmology, Jichi Medical University, 3311-1 Yakushiji, Shimotsuke-City, Tochigi, Japan.

References

1. Durrani OM, Tehrani NN, Marr JE, Moradi P, Stavrou P, Murray PI. Degree, duration, and causes of visual loss in uveitis. Br J Ophthalmol. 2004;88:1159–62.
2. Nakahara H, Kaburaki T, Takamoto M, Okinaga K, Matsuda J, Konno Y, et al. Statistical analyses of endogeneous uveitis patients (2007-2009) in Central Tokyo area and comparison with previous studies (1963-2006). Ocul Immunol Inflamm. 2015;23:291–6.
3. Merrill PT, Kim J, Cox TA, Betorr CC, McCallum RM, Jaffe GJ. Uveitis in the southeastern United States. Curr Eye Res. 1997;16:865–74.
4. Goto H, Mochizuki M, Yamaki K, Kotake S, Usui M, Ohno S. Epidemiological survey of intraocular inflammation in Japan. Jpn J Ophthalmol. 2007;51:41–4.
5. Keino H, Nakashima C, Watanabe T, Taki W, Hayakawa R, Sugitani A, et al. Frequency and clinical features of intraocular inflammation in Tokyo. Clin Exp Ophthalmol. 2009;37:595–601.
6. Al-Shakarchi FI. Pattern of uveitis at a referral center in Iraq. Middle East Afr J Ophthalmol. 2014;21:291–5.
7. Llorenç V, Mesquida M, Sainz de la Maza M, Keller J, Molins B, Espinosa G, et al. Epidemiology of uveitis in a western urban multiethnic population. Acta Ophthalmol. 2015;93:561–7.
8. Baarsma GS. The epidemiology and genetics of endogenous uveitis: a review. Curr Eye Res. 1992;11:1–9.
9. Chen SC, Chuang CT, Chu MY, Sheu SJ. Patterns and etiologies of uveitis at a tertiary referral center in Taiwan. Ocul Immunol Inflamm. 2017;25(sup1):S31–8.
10. Chou LC, Sheu SJ, Hong MC, Hsiao YC, Wu TT, Chuang CT, et al. Endogenous uveitis: experiences in Kaohsiung Veterans General Hospital. J Chin Med Assoc. 2003;66:46–50.
11. Nakahara H, Kaburaki T, Tanaka R, Takamoto M, Ohtomo K, Karakawa A, et al. Frequency of uveitis in the central Tokyo area (2010–2012). Ocul Immunol Inflamm. 2017;25(sup1):S8–S14.
12. Al Dhibi HA, Al Shamsi HA, Al-Mahmood AM, Al Taweel HM, Al Shamrani MA, Arevalo JF, et al. Patterns of uveitis in a tertiary care referral institute in Saudi Arabia. Ocul Immunol Inflamm. 2017;25:388–95.
13. Ohguro N, Sonoda KH, Takeuchi M, Matsumura M, Mochizuki M. The 2009 prospective multi-center epidemiologic survey of uveitis in Japan. Jpn J Ophthalmol. 2012;56:432–5.
14. Jabs DA, Nussenblatt RB, Rosenbaum JT, Standardization of Uveitis Nomenclature (SUN) Working Group. Standardization of uveitis nomenclature for reporting clinical data Results of the First International Workshop. Am J Ophthalmol. 2005;140:509–16.
15. Suzuki Kurokawa M, Suzuki N. Behçet's disease. Clin Exp Med. 2004;4:10–20.
16. The Japanese Society of Sarcoidosis and Other Granulomatous Disorders. Diagnostic standard and guidelines for sarcoidosis-2006. Nippon Sarcoidosis Gakkai Zasshi. 2007;27:89–102.
17. Kawaguchi T, Hanada A, Horie S, Sugamoto Y, Sugita S, Mochizuki M. Evaluation of characteristic ocular signs and systemic investigations in ocular sarcoidosis patients. Jpn J Ophthalmol. 2007;51:121–6.
18. Read RW, Holland GN, Rao NA, Tabbara KF, Ohno S, Arellanes-Garcia L, et al. Revised diagnostic criteria for Vogt-Koyanagi-Harada disease: report of an international committee on nomenclature. Am J Ophthalmol. 2001;131:647–52.
19. Namba K, Goto H, Kaburaki T, Kitaichi N, Mizuki N, Asukata Y, et al. A major review: current aspects of ocular Behçet's disease in Japan. Ocul Immunol Inflamm. 2015;23(Suppl 1):S1–23.
20. Ogawa M, Sugita S, Shimizu N, Watanabe K, Nakagawa I, Mochizuki M. Broad-range real-time PCR assay for detection of bacterial DNA in ocular samples from infectious endophthalmitis. Jpn J Ophthalmol. 2012;56:529–35.
21. Ogawa M, Sugita S, Watanabe K, Shimizu N, Mochizuki M. Novel diagnosis of fungal endophthalmitis by broad-range real-time PCR detection of fungal 28S ribosomal DNA. Graefes Arch Clin Exp Ophthalmol. 2012;250:1877–83.
22. Cassoux N, Giron A, Bodaghi B, Tran TH, Baudet S, Davy F, et al. IL-10 measurement in aqueous humor for screening patients with suspicion of primary intraocular lymphoma. Invest Ophthalmol Vis Sci. 2007;48:3253–9.
23. Kaburaki T, Taoka K, Matsuda J, Yamashita H, Matsuda I, Tsuji H, et al. Combined intravitreal methotrexate and immunochemotherapy followed by reduced-dose whole-brain radiotherapy for newly diagnosed B-cell primary intraocular lymphoma. Br J Haematol. 2017; https://doi.org/10.1111/bjh.14848.
24. Cimino L, Herbort CP, Aldigeri R, Salvarani C, Boiardi L. Tuberculous uveitis, a resurgent and underdiagnosed disease. Int Ophthalmol. 2009;29:67 74.
25. Oswal KS, Sivaraj RR, Murray PI, Stavrou P. Clinical course and visual outcome in patients with diabetes mellitus and uveitis. BMC Res Notes. 2013;6:167.
26. Mochizuki M, Tajima K, Watanabe T, Yamaguchi K. Human T lymphotropic virus type 1 uveitis. Br J Ophthalmol. 1994;78:149–54.
27. Francis PJ, Marinescu A, Fitzke FW, Bird AC, Holder GE. Acute zonal occult outer retinopathy: towards a set of diagnostic criteria. Br J Ophthalmol. 2005;89:70–3.

28. Quentin CD, Reiber H. Fuchs heterochromic cyclitis: rubella virus antibodies and genome in aqueous humor. Am J Ophthalmol. 2004;138:46–54.
29. Ohno S, Char DH, Kimura SJ, O'Connor GR. HLA antigens and antinuclear antibody titres in juvenile chronic iridocyclitis. Br J Ophthalmol. 1977;61:59–61.
30. Nishi N, Yoshizawa T, Okuda N. Effects of rapid aging and lower participation rate among younger adults on the short-term trend of physical activity in the National Health and nutrition survey, Japan. Geriatr Gerontol Int. 2017;17:1677–82.
31. Rimland D, Moanna A. Increasing incidence of herpes zoster among Veterans. Clin Infect Dis. 2010;50:1000–5.
32. Citterio G, Reni M, Gatta G, Ferreri AJM. Primary central nervous system lymphoma. Crit Rev Oncol Hematol. 2017;113:97–110.
33. Keino H, Watanabe T, Taki W, Nakayama M, Nakamura T, Yan K, et al. Clinical features of uveitis in children and adolescents at a tertiary referral Centre in Tokyo. Br J Ophthalmol. 2017;101:406–10.

13

Identification of H_2O_2 induced oxidative stress associated microRNAs in HLE-B3 cells and their clinical relevance to the progression of age-related nuclear cataract

Song Wang[1], Chenjun Guo[1], Mengsi Yu[2], Xiaona Ning[1], Bo Yan[3], Jing Zhao[3], Angang Yang[3] and Hong Yan[1,4*]

Abstract

Background: This study is aimed to screen out the microRNAs (miRNAs) associated with H_2O_2 induced oxidative stress in human lens epithelial B3 (HLE-B3) cell lines and investigate their relations with the progression of age-related nuclear cataract.

Methods: H_2O_2 was used to induce oxidative stress in HLE-B3 cells. A genome-wide expression profiling of miRNAs in HLE-B3 cells was performed to select the differentially expressed miRNAs before and after H_2O_2 treatment. The selected miRNAs were validated by RT-PCR and fluorescence in situ hybridization (FISH). Clinical specimens were divided into three groups according to the Lens Opacities Classification System III (LOCSIII) and the expression levels of the selected miRNAs were tested by RT-PCR in the three groups. Bioinformatics analyses were applied to predict the target genes of the miRNA hits and construct the miRNA regulatory network. The expression level of MAPK14 was analyzed by Western blot.

Results: The H_2O_2 induced oxidative stress model of HLE-B3 cells was established. Nineteen upregulated and 30 downregulated miRNAs were identified as differentially expressed miRNAs. Seven of the total 49 were validated in the cell model. RT-PCR of the clinical samples showed that the expression levels of miR-34a-5p, miR-630 and miR-335-3p were closely related with the severity of nuclear opacity. The images taken from FISH confirmed the results of RT-PCR. There were 172 target genes of the three miRNAs clustered in the category of response to stress. The regulatory network demonstrated that 23 target genes were co-regulated by multiple miRNAs. MAPK14 was the target gene of three miRNAs and the result were verified by Western blot.

Conclusion: Up-regulation of miR-34a-5p and miR-630 and down-regulation of miR-335-3p are related with the progression of age-related nuclear cataract and the underlying mechanism awaits further functional research to reveal.

Keywords: Age-related nuclear cataract, Oxidative stress, microRNA, Bioinformatics analysis

* Correspondence: zeratulws@126.com
[1]Department of Ophthalmology, Tangdu Hospital, Fourth Military Medical University, 1 Xinsi Road, Xi'an, Shaanxi 710038, People's Republic of China
[4]Chongqing Key Laboratory of Ophthalmology and Chongqing Eye Institute, The First Affiliated Hospital of Chongqing Medical University, 1 Youyi Road, Chongqing 400016, People's Republic of China
Full list of author information is available at the end of the article

Background

Human lenses are transparent in young people, but changes occur as the body ages. These changes include the development of a hard, compact nucleus, local opacity, and, finally, the development of a pathological cataract [1]. By far, many factors such as diabetes mellitus, ultraviolet, systemic drugs and congenital diseases are known to be related to cataract formation. Among these factors, oxidative stress with the generation of reactive oxygen species (ROS) is thought to be a major predisposing factor in age-related cataracts [2]. Substantial data suggest that, with increasing age, the lens nucleus becomes more susceptible to oxidation and less able to repair oxidative damage [3, 4].

MicroRNAs (miRNAs) are evolutionarily well-conserved, small non-coding transcripts. It plays an important role in the post-transcriptional regulation of target mRNA via mRNA degradation or translational repression through binding with 3′-untranslated regions (UTRs) of target genes [5–7]. Accumulating evidences demonstrated that miRNAs play a critical role in multiple pathological processes of mammalian lens [8–10]. A clinical research revealed that the expression profile of miRNAs in cataractous lenses is different from transparent lenses [1]. And further mechanistic study showed that miR-26, miR-30a and miR-211 involved in the formation of cataract through targeting certain mRNAs [11–13]. However, there has no record of a systemic screening for oxidative stress associated miRNAs in human lens epithelial cells (HLECs).

In the present study, we used hydrogen peroxide to induce oxidative damage in human lens epithelium B3 (HLE-B3) cells and monitored the status of cell viability and apoptosis. Subsequently, the miRNA transcriptome profiles of control and oxidized cells were determined by microarray and the differentially expressed miRNAs were validated by RT-PCR. The central epithelium of cataractous human lenses was divided into three groups according to the Lens Opacities Classification System III (LOCSIII) [14] and the expression levels of the distinct miRNAs were verified in these specimens. Finally, bioinformatics analysis was used to find novel targets of cataractogenesis.

Methods

Cell culture and treatment

HLE-B3 cells purchased from the American Type Culture Collection (ATCC, Manassas, VA, USA) were grown as a monolayer in DMEM supplemented with 20% heat-inactivated fetal bovine serum (FBS) at 37 °C in a humidified atmosphere of 5% CO_2 and 21% O_2. Twenty-four h before the day of the experiment, cells were switched to hypoxic conditions (1% O_2 to mock physiological environment [15]). At 85–90% confluence,

the cells were treated with the indicated concentration of H_2O_2 for 24 h.

Tissue extraction and grouping

Forty five lens epithelium samples, collected from 45 patients (patient age range was 57–86 years, free of other ocular diseases), were obtained by intact continuous curvilinear capsulorhexis. Cataract type and severity were graded in accordance with the LOCSIII. All LOCSIII scorings among subjects were carried out and consisted up to at least three ophthalmologists.

The research population was divided into three groups according to the grading of nuclear opacity ($0 < N \le 2$, $2 < N \le 4$, $4 < N \le 6$). There were no statistically significant differences between each group with respect to age or sex of the patient ($P > 0.05$, Independent Sample t-test). This study was performed according to the tenets of the Declaration of Helsinki for Research Involving Human Tissue. Verbal consent was obtained from each patient following an explanation of the surgery procedure and the purpose of this research. The Moral and Ethical Committee of the Fourth Military Medical University approved the verbal consent.

Cell viability

The MTT assay was used to monitor the viability of HLE-B3 cells. Cells were plated at a density of 5×10^3 cells/well in 96-well microplates. After incubation, cells were treated with different concentrations of H_2O_2 for a different duration time. Then cells were incubated with 20 μl of MTT solution (0.5 mg/ml) for 4 h at 37 °C. The incubation was stopped by removing the culture medium and 200 μl DMSO was added to solubilize formazan. The absorbance was measured at 490 nm by a microplate reader (Bio-Rad, West Berkeley, CA).

Detection of cell apoptosis by flow cytometry

Cells were incubated in a six-well plate at a density of 5×10^5 cells per well. After treatment, the cells were washed twice with PBS and harvested by trypsin digestion. Cells were collected and centrifuged at 500 rpm for 5 min, the supernatant was discarded, and 5 μl of Annexin V-FITC and 10 μl of propidium iodide (PI) were added to the cell pellet followed by 15 min incubation in the dark at room temperature. Samples were analyzed by flow cytometry within 60 min of processing.

Hoechst staining

Cells were stained with 10 μg/ml Hoechst 33,258 in the dark at room temperature for 5 mins, after which the cells were washed twice with PBS. The nuclear morphology of stained cells was examined using a fluorescence microscope with an excitation of 350 nm and emission of 460 nm. Nonspecific fluorescence values were subtracted from the experimental fluorescence values. At least 100 cells in three different fields were counted, and the data are presented as the percentage of viable cells out of the total number of cells.

RNA isolation and real-time PCR

Total RNA from cells and tissues were isolated using TRIzol Reagent (Invitrogen, Carlsbad, CA, USA) according to manufacturer's instructions. RNA content was measured using a Nanodrop-2000 (Thermo Fisher Scientific, Waltham, MA, USA). First strand cDNA was synthesized from the total RNA of the HLE-B3 cells and tissue samples using the miScript Reverse Transcription Kit (Qiagen, Germany) in accordance with the manufacturer's recommended protocol. The quantitative real-time PCR (qRT-PCR) was conducted using the SYBR Green dye (TaKaRa, Japan). Real-time PCR was performed in triplicate on CFX96 Real Time PCR Detection System (Bio-Rad, West Berkeley, CA). The $2^{-\Delta\Delta CT}$ method was used to determine the relative gene expression, and mature miRNA were normalized to U6-snRNA.

Microarray analysis

For microRNA expression analysis, total RNA, including microRNA, was isolated from treated and control groups of HLE-B3 cells according to the manufacturer's instructions and analyzed using Affymetrix GeneChip miRNA 2.0 arrays (Affymetrix, Santa Clara, CA, USA) containing 4560 probe sets for human small RNAs. All of the steps of the procedure were performed according to the standardized protocol for Affymetrix miRNA 2.0 arrays. The intensity values for microRNA transcripts were calculated using Affymetrix GeneChip Command Console 3.2. The quality control for the microarray was performed with the Affymetrix miRNA QC Tool.

Western blot analysis

Cells were harvested, rinsed in PBS, and lysed in RIPA buffer containing 5% PMSF for 1 h on ice. After the mixture was centrifuged at 12,000×g for 10 min at 4 °C, insoluble materials were removed. Identical amount (50 μg of protein) of cell lysates were boiled for 5 min, size fractionated by SDS-PAGE, and electrophoretically transfected on to PVDF membranes. After being incubated with blocking solution including 5% powered milk in TBST buffer (10 mM Tris–HCl, 150 mM NaCl, and 0.1% Tween-20) for 1 h at room temperature, the membranes were immunoblotted with primary antibodies (Cell Signaling Technology, USA. Catalogue 9211, 9212). Primary antibodies were identified using HRP-conjugated secondary antibody at a 1:10,000 dilution and visualized by the ECL detection system.

Fluorescence in situ hybridization (FISH)

Specific probes of miR-34a-5p, miR-630 and miR-335-3p were used in FISH and the sequences are 5'-ACAAC-CAGCTAAGACACTGCCA-3' for miR-34a-5p, 5'-ACCT TCCCTGGTACTGAATACT-3' for miR-630 and 5'-GGT CAGGAGCAATAATGAAAAA-3' for miR-335-3p. In brief, HLEB-B3 cells were treated with H_2O_2 for 24 h. 5' cy3-labelled probes were specific to the miRNAs. Nuclei were stained by 4,6-diamidino-2-phenylindole (DAPI). All the procedures were conducted according to the manufactory's instruction (Genepharma, Shanghai, China). All images were observed using fluorescent microscopy (Nikon, Eclipse CI, Tokyo, Japan).

Bioinformatics analysis of the differentially expressed microRNAs

Target genes of the distinct miRNAs were determined by the union of miRNA target predictions from TargetScan 7.1 [7] (http://www.targetscan.org) and miRanda [16] (http://www.microrna.org). The picked genes were further analyzed according to the PANTHER classification system [17] (http://www.pantherdb.org). Finally, visualization of the miRNA-mRNA regulatory network was achieved by Cytoscape [18].

Statistical analysis

Statistical analyses and data imaging were performed using GraphPad Prism version 5.00 (GraphPad Inc., La Jolla, CA, USA). Quantitative data was presented as means±SD from at least three separate experiments. Two-tailed Student's t-test was used to evaluate experiments with two experimental groups. The results were considered statistically significant when $^*P < 0.05$; $^{**}P < 0.01$; $^{***}P < 0.001$.

Results
H_2O_2 treatment decreased the viability of HLE-B3 cells

In the current study, we used H_2O_2 to generate excessive ROS, which can permeate cellular membranes and enter into the cells to cause oxidative damage. The viability of HLE-B3 cells exposed to various concentrations of H_2O_2 after 24 h incubation was investigated by MTT assay. Generally, the toxicity of H_2O_2 increased in a dose-dependent manner as shown in Fig. 1a. From 0 μM to 75 μM, cell viability decreased gently. However, from 75 μM to 100 μM, cell viability dropped drastically from $76.22 \pm 2.64\%$ to $33.76 \pm 2.20\%$. Meanwhile we found that, at the concentration of 75 μM, H_2O_2 decreased the viability of HLE-B3 cells in a time-dependent manner (Fig. 1a). Therefore, in order to achieve the balance between oxidative damage and cell survival, the treatment of 75 μM H_2O_2 for 24 h was chosen to induce oxidative stress on HLE-B3 cells for further research.

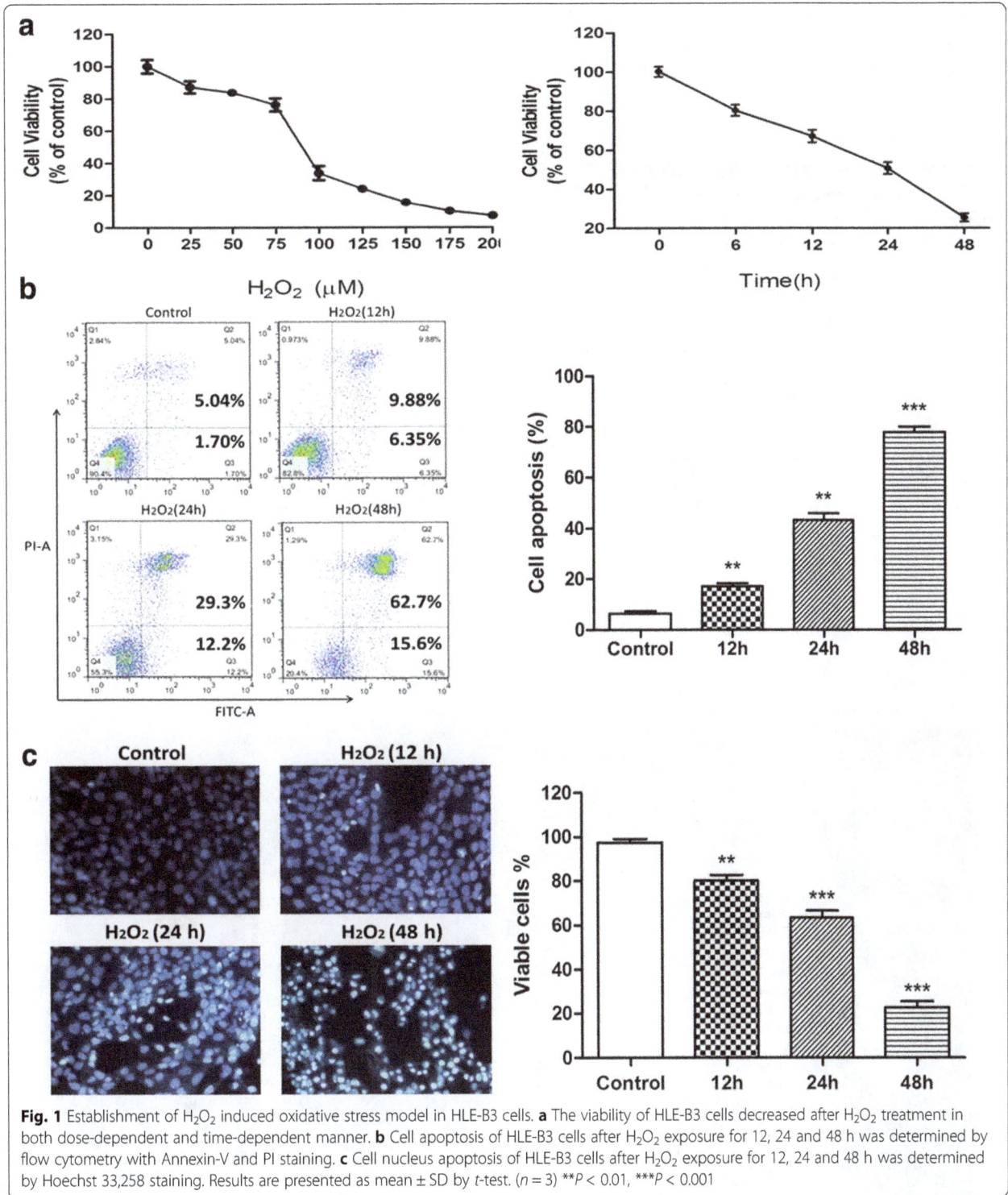

Fig. 1 Establishment of H_2O_2 induced oxidative stress model in HLE-B3 cells. **a** The viability of HLE-B3 cells decreased after H_2O_2 treatment in both dose-dependent and time-dependent manner. **b** Cell apoptosis of HLE-B3 cells after H_2O_2 exposure for 12, 24 and 48 h was determined by flow cytometry with Annexin-V and PI staining. **c** Cell nucleus apoptosis of HLE-B3 cells after H_2O_2 exposure for 12, 24 and 48 h was determined by Hoechst 33,258 staining. Results are presented as mean ± SD by t-test. ($n = 3$) **$P < 0.01$, ***$P < 0.001$

H_2O_2 treatment induced apoptosis in HLE-B3 cells

Flow cytometry was used to quantify the rate of apoptosis using double staining of Annexin V-FITC and PI. As the results shown in Fig. 1b, HLE-B3 cells treated with 75 µM H_2O_2 showed significant apoptosis, besides, the apoptosis rate increased in a time-dependent manner. To validate the flow cytometric data for H_2O_2-induced apoptotic cell death, Hoechst 33,258 staining was used to detect apoptotic cell nucleus. Normal nuclear morphology (round blue nuclei) was observed in the H_2O_2-free control group (Fig. 1c). However, chromatin condensation and strong fluorescent spots were observed in HLE-B3 cells treated with 75 μM H_2O_2. The percentage of Hoechst-positive cells correlated closely with the percentage of Annexin V-positive cells in Fig. 1b.

Microarray screening for microRNAs associated with H_2O_2 induced oxidative stress in HLE-B3 cells

Microarray analysis was used to characterize the H_2O_2 induced miRNAs. Microarray data revealed that after H_2O_2 treatment, 19 miRNAs were upregulated 2-fold relative to the control group; 30 miRNAs were downregulated 2-fold (Fig. 2a). Ultimately, according to the miRNAs' fold change and expression level, five up-regulated miRNAs (miR-630, miR-222-5p, miR-210-3p, miR-34a-5p and miR-34b-5p) and two down-regulated miRNAs (miR-335-3p and miR-15b-3p) were chosen for microarray validation by RT-PCR (Table 1). The result of the PCR analysis confirmed the differentially expressed miRNAs selected by microarray (Fig. 2b).

Table 1 Fold change of the seven selected miRNAs and their forward primer sequences used for RT-PCR

miRNA Name	Fold Change	Forward Primer for RT-PCR
miR-630	4.14	GCGAGTATTCTGTACCAGGGAAGGT
miR-222-5p	3.84	CGCTCAGTAGCCAGTGTAGATCCT
miR-210-3p	3.23	CTGTGCGTGTGACAGCGG
miR-34a-5p	2.59	CTGGCAGTGTCTTAGCTGGTTGT
miR-34b-5p	2.44	GCGTAGGCAGTGTCATTAGCTGATTG
miR-335-3p	0.45	CGGCGTTTTTCATTATTGCTCCTGACC
miR-15b-3p	0.33	CGGGCGAATCATTATTTGCTGCTCTA

The association between the oxidation-induced miRNAs and nuclear opacity

To identify the connections between the grading of nuclear opacity and expression levels of miRNAs, Pearson correlation coefficient was introduced (Fig. 3). For miR-34a-5p, miR-630 and miR-335-3p, close relations ($R = 0.691, 0.617, -0.594$) between LOCSIII grading and their expression levels were found and they were

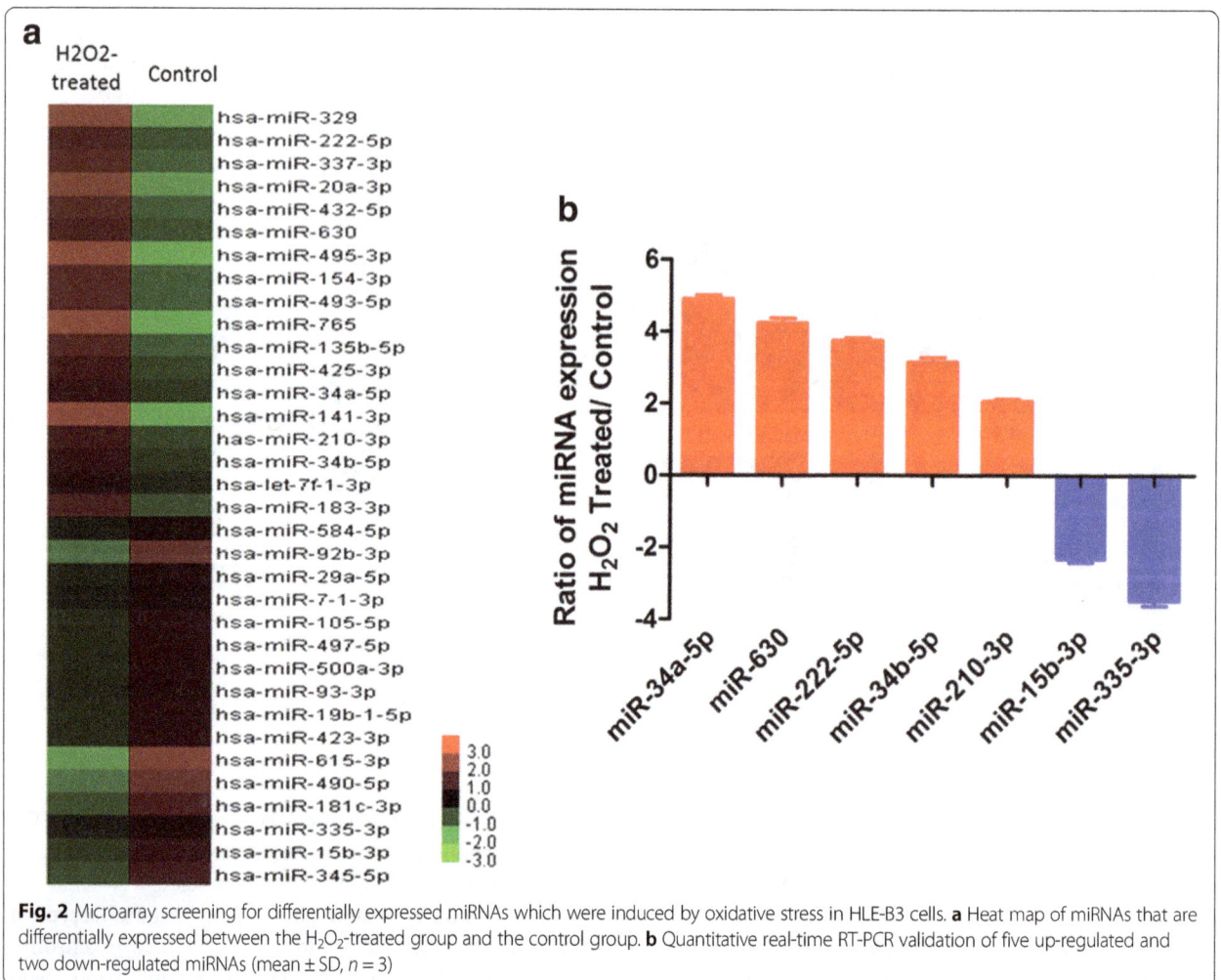

Fig. 2 Microarray screening for differentially expressed miRNAs which were induced by oxidative stress in HLE-B3 cells. **a** Heat map of miRNAs that are differentially expressed between the H_2O_2-treated group and the control group. **b** Quantitative real-time RT-PCR validation of five up-regulated and two down-regulated miRNAs (mean ± SD, $n = 3$)

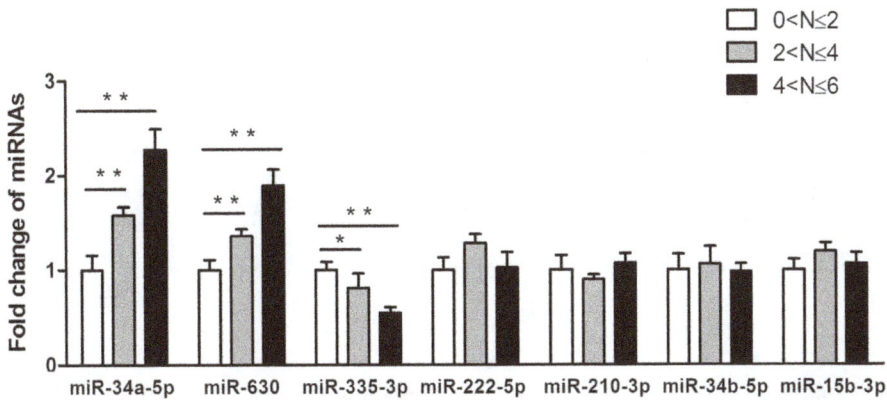

Fig. 3 Relevance of expression levels of the seven miRNAs to the severity of lens nuclear opacity. Forty five samples were divided into three groups according to their grading of nuclear opacity. Each group contained 15 samples. The expression level of each miRNA in $0 < N \leq 2$ group was defined as 1. Up-regulation of miR-34a-5p and miR-630 are closely related to a higher severity score of nuclear cataract, while down-regulation of miR-335-3p is associated with the increase of nuclear opacity (mean ± SD, $n = 3$). *$P < 0.05$, **$P < 0.01$

statistically significant ($P < 0.001$). However, for miR-222-5p, miR-210-3p, miR-34b-5p and miR-15b-3p, the relations were moderate ($R = 0.436, 0.428, 0.398, 0.489$) and statistically insignificant ($P > 0.05$).

Then we compared the expression levels of miR-34a-5p, miR-630 and miR-335-3p in each subgroup (Fig. 3). In miR-34a-5p and miR-630, higher scores of nuclear opacity associated with greater levels of both miRNAs ($0 < N \leq 2$ as control, $P < 0.01$). Meanwhile, in miR-335-3p, higher grading correlated with lower levels of miR-335-3p ($0 < N \leq 2$ as control, $P < 0.05$).

Validation of the levels of miR-34a-5p, miR-630 and miR-335-3p by FISH

After evaluating the PCR results of HLE-B3 cells and clinical samples, we chose miR-34a-5p, miR-630 and miR-335-3p as the key miRNAs in our research. In order to further validate the PCR tests, FISH was applied and images were taken to estimate the difference visually. As

Fig. 4 showed that, after 24 h of H_2O_2 treatment, the expression levels of miR-630 and miR-34a-5p were elevated while miR-335-3p was down-regulated. The results were in accordance with the microarray and PCR tests.

Identification of target genes and analysis of the miRNA/ target gene network

According to Targetscan and miRanda, there were 1532, 1323 and 1275 genes predicted to be the target genes of miR-34a-5p, miR-630 and miR-335-3p. Predictions from the algorithms were submitted to the PANTHER classification system. First, genes were distributed to different biological processes. Then we picked the process of response to stress, which is a subcategory of response to stimulus, as our target process. The picked genes from the algorithms were further analyzed according to the PANTHER classification system, in which 68, 50 and 54 genes were clustered in the response to stress process (Fig. 5a-c). The network of miRNA/targets was

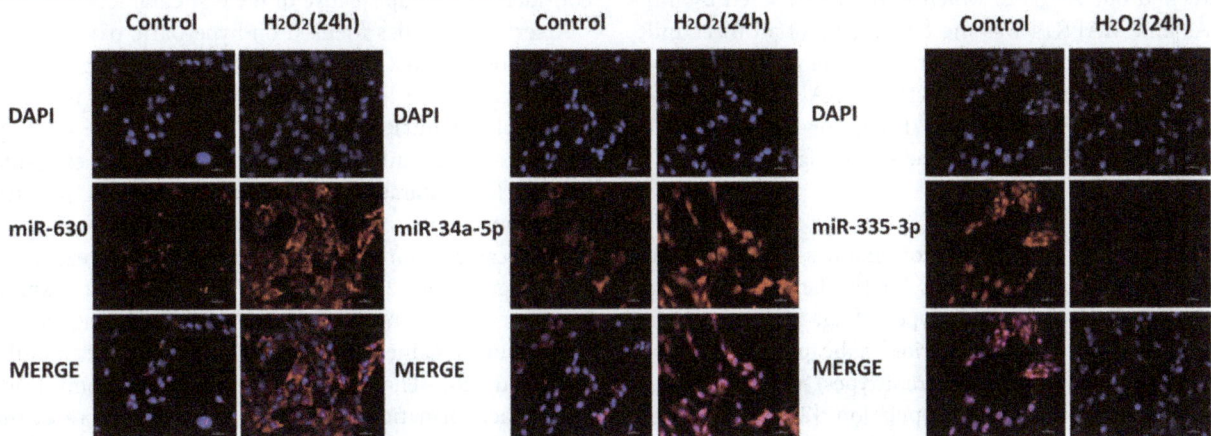

Fig. 4 The expression of three key miRNAs in HLE-B3 cells were assessed by FISH. (400×, scale bar is 25 μm)

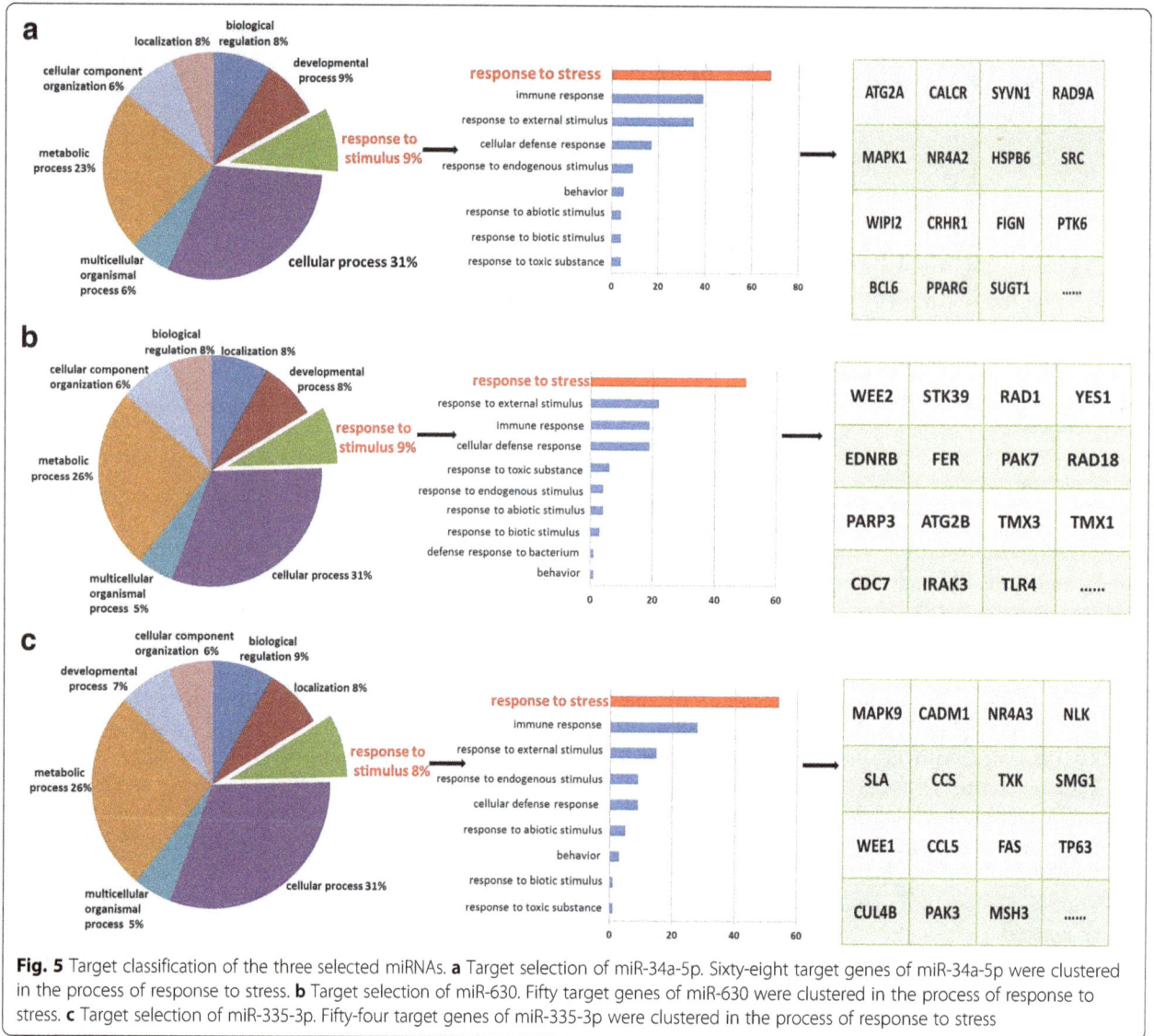

Fig. 5 Target classification of the three selected miRNAs. **a** Target selection of miR-34a-5p. Sixty-eight target genes of miR-34a-5p were clustered in the process of response to stress. **b** Target selection of miR-630. Fifty target genes of miR-630 were clustered in the process of response to stress. **c** Target selection of miR-335-3p. Fifty-four target genes of miR-335-3p were clustered in the process of response to stress

constructed using Cytoscape (Fig. 6). Furthermore, we screened out 23 genes which were co-regulated by miR-NAs and MAPK14 was the target gene of all three miR-NAs (Tables 2 and 3). Western blot analysis showed that the level of phospho-MAPK14 (p-MAPK14) increased when cells were exposed to H_2O_2 for 24 h while the level of MAPK14 remained the same (Fig. 7).

Discussion

Cataract is the leading cause of blindness worldwide and age-related cataract accounts for the largest percentage [19]. There are three main types of age-related cataract: nuclear, cortical or posterior subcapsular cataracts (PSC). Among the three different types, nuclear cataracts predominate in Chinese population [20]. Researchers and ophthalmologists found out multiple risk factors of nuclear cataracts, including malnutrition, smoking,

larger lens and family history. Notably, oxidative stress is considered the major cause of nuclear cataracts [2].

A series of studies focused on hyperbaric oxygen therapy discovered that the treatment, whether long-term or short-term, could lead to a myopic shift, then incipient or full-blown nuclear cataracts [21–23]. These findings provide a direct link between excessive oxygen exposure and nuclear cataract. Further evidence is that patients undergoing vitrectomy had significantly higher rates of nuclear cataract formation (60–95%) within 2 years after the surgery [24–27]. Research revealed that oxygen levels near the lens increased markedly during vitrectomy and remained significantly elevated for months afterward [28]. The hypothesis is that vitrectomy leads to cataract formation by increasing the exposure of the lens to oxygen and Lou's research explained in detail about the mechanism of protein aggregation and

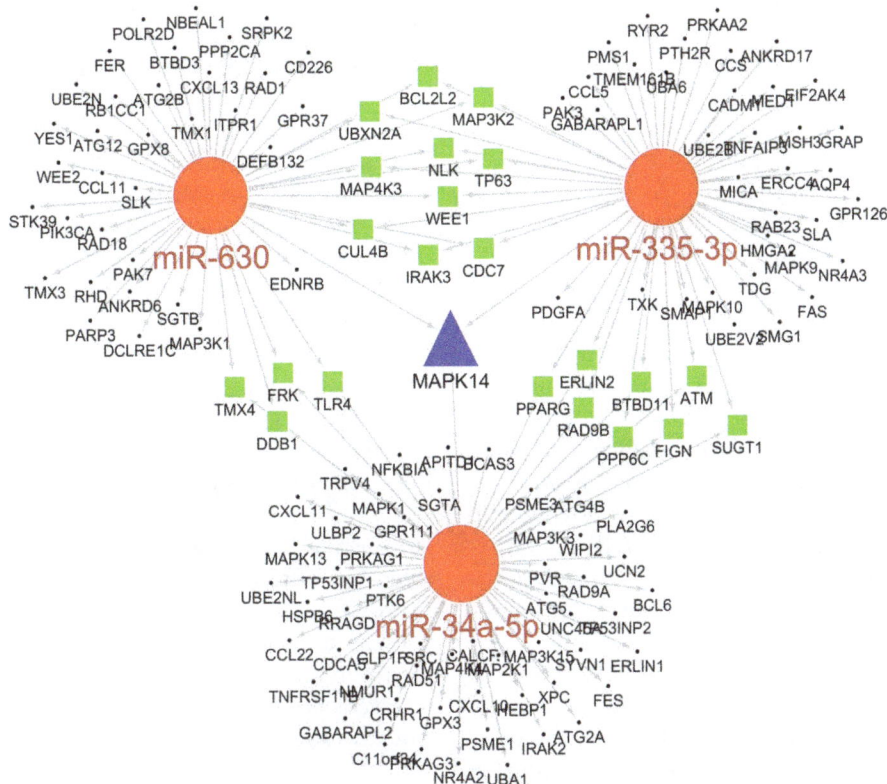

Fig. 6 Network of the miRNAs and their target genes in the process of response to stress. Red circles, miRNAs; black dots, target genes regulated by one miRNA; green squares, target genes regulated by two miRNAs; blue triangle, target gene regulated by three miRNAs

cataract formation caused by oxidation overload [29]. In the present study, in order to simulate the physiological environment of lens, which is in a natural state of hypoxia [30], we switched the HLE-B3 cells into the 1% O_2 incubator 24 h before the H_2O_2 treatment.

The miRNAs have recently emerged as a prominent class of gene regulators. Although miRNAs have been identified as key regulators of multiple pathways involved in cataract formation and development, there is no systemic screening for oxidative stress and cell apoptosis associated miRNAs in HLECs. In the current study, after the induction of cell apoptosis by H_2O_2, the authors used microarray to identify the crucial miRNAs.

Among the seven selected miRNAs, which were validated in HLE-B3 cells by RT-PCR, three of them were proven to be correlated with age-related nuclear cataract and they are miR-34a-5p, miR-630 and miR-335-3p.

MiR-34a-5p is one of the most explored miRNAs in oxidative stress and cell senescence [31]. Bai et al. found that miR-34a-5p suppressed mitochondrial anti-oxidative enzymes with a concomitant increase in intracellular ROS level [32]. Ito et al. found that miR-34a increased with age in endothelial cells in senescent human umbilical cord vein endothelial cells and in the hearts and spleens of older mice [31]. The regulation of miR-34a-5p/SIRT 1 pathway was investigated in multiple disease and aging

Table 2 Target genes clustered in response to stress by PANTHER classification system

MiRNA	Clustered target genes
miR-34a-5p	ATG2A, CALCR, SYVN1, RAD9A, TP53INP2, MAPK14, MAPK1, NR4A2, BTBD11, HSPB6, NMUR1, WIPI2, CRHR1, MAP3K15, FIGN, PTK6, TRPV4, BCL6, RRAGD, ATG4B, MAP2K1, TNFRSF11B, PPARG, CCL22, GABARAPL2, ERLIN2, PVR, SUGT1, SRC, GPR111, NFKBIA, MAPK13, XPC, GLP1R, FRK, C11orf34, TLR4, TP53INP1, SGTA, ERLIN1, UBA1, TMX4, UCN2, UNC45A, APITD1, CDCA5, HEBP1, ATM, PSME1, CXCL11, ATG5, MAP3K3, RAD9B, PSME3, DDB1, ULBP2, FES, BCAS3, PRKAG1, PRKAG3, PLA2G6, PPP6C, RAD51, IRAK2, UBE2NL, MAP4K4, GPX3,CXCL10
miR-630	WEE2, MAP3K2, MAP4K3, STK39, DEFB132, MAPK14, ANKRD6, RAD1, ATG12, SGTB, MAP3K1, YES1, RB1CC1, BCL2L2, EDNRB, WEE1, FER, PAK7, DCLRE1C,UBXN2A, RAD18, PARP3, SLK, ATG2B, TMX3, BTBD3, TMX1, GPR37, CDC7, PPP2CA, IRAK3, TP63, RHD, FRK, CXCL13, POLR2D, GPX8, ITPR1, TLR4, SLK, UBE2N, SRPK2, CUL4B, TMX4, NBEAL1, CD226, CCL11, PIK3CA, DDB1, NLK
miR-335-3p	MAPK9, CADM1, MAP3K2, PRKAA2, MAP4K3, NR4A3, GRAP, MAPK14, EIF2AK4, BTBD11, NLK, ANKRD17, SLA, CCS, UBE2B, FIGN, PPP6C, TXK, ERCC4, PDGFA, GPR126, BCL2L2, SMG1, WEE1, CCL5, UBXN2A, PPARG, FAS, ERLIN2, RYR2, CDC7, SUGT1, MED1, AQP4, TDG, PTH2R, IRAK3, PMS1, UBA6, MICA, TP63, HMGA2, TNFAIP3, CUL4B, SMAP1, PAK3, GABARAPL1, UBE2V2, ATM, MSH3, MAPK10, RAD9B, TMEM161B,RAB23

Table 3 Genes targeted by at least two miRNAs in the cluster of response to stress

Co-regulated miRNAs	Target genes
miR-34a-5p/miR-630	DDB1, TMX4, FRK, TLR4
miR-34a-5p/miR-335-3p	PPARG, ERLIN2, RAD9B, BTBD11, PPP6C, ATM, FIGN, SUGT1
miR-630/miR-335-3p	UBXN2A, BCL2L2, MAP3K2, MAP4K3, NLK, TP63, WEE1, CUL4B, IRAK3, CDC7
miR-34a-5p/miR-630/ miR-335-3p	MAPK14

models for its effect on aging and oxidative damage [33–35]. In the present research, our data demonstrated that the expression level of miR-34a-5p in the oxidized HLE-B3 cells is 2.59 fold higher compared to the control group. In the clinical specimens, the miRNA's abundance increases as the LOCSIII grading climbs. Among the seven selected miRNAs, it is ranked NO.1 in not only the Pearson correlation coefficient but also the ratio of fold change. Our findings are in accordance with Chien's research [36].

Mir-630 has been studied in oncology. Researchers focused on the regulatory effect of miR-630 on epithelial-to-mesenchymal transition (EMT). Through targeting FoxM1 [37] and Slug [38], overexpression of miR-630 is capable of suppressing EMT in various carcinomas. However, there is no report concerning about the correlation of miR-630 with cataract. In our study, the level of miR-630 in HLECs elevated drastically at the presence of H_2O_2 (4.14 fold) and this trend remained the same in the cataractous human lenses. Further mechanistic study is needed to confirm the involvement of miR-630 in cataractogenesis, but we can speculate that miR-630 may play an important role in the formation of PSC and posterior capsular opacification (PCO) for its influence in EMT.

Opinions about the role of miR-335-3p in tumor progression are controversial. Some believed that miR-335-3p is an oncogene for its effect on induction of multidrug resistance [39] and cancer-associated fibroblasts [40], while others viewed miR-335-3p as a tumor suppressor [41, 42]. This difference could be explained by the diversity of miRNA's function. Although the function of miR-335-3p in cataract formation is unclear, the results of our experiment, for the first time, offered evidence that down-regulation of miR-335-3p may be the cause or effect of age-related nuclear cataract.

According to the results of bioinformatics analysis, there were 23 genes co-regulated by the three miRNAs in the process of response to stress. Most of all, we found that MAPK14 was the target gene of all three miRNAs and the Western blot analysis indicated that oxidative stress could induce the phosphorylation and activation of MAPK14. Since it was co-regulated by three miRNAs, the specific mechanism needs further research. Mitogen-activated protein kinase 14 (MAPK14) is a member of the MAP kinase family, which is activated by various environmental stresses and proinflammatory cytokines [43, 44]. Although there is no report considering the connection between MAPK14 and cataract, our finding suggests the possibility of MAPK14's involvement in cataract formation via its response to oxidative stress.

Conclusions

In conclusion, our research is the first to conduct a microarray screening for oxidative stress and cell apoptosis associated miRNAs in HLECs. The selected miRNAs were further validated by clinical samples from age-related nuclear cataract patients, which suggest that miR-34a-5p, miR-630 and miR-335-3p might be potential regulators of cataract formation. Among them, miR-630 and miR-335-3p are first reported in the field of cataract research. Further mechanism research is needed to identify these miRNAs' target genes and functions and these miRNAs may serve as molecular targets for the diagnosis and treatment of age-related cataract.

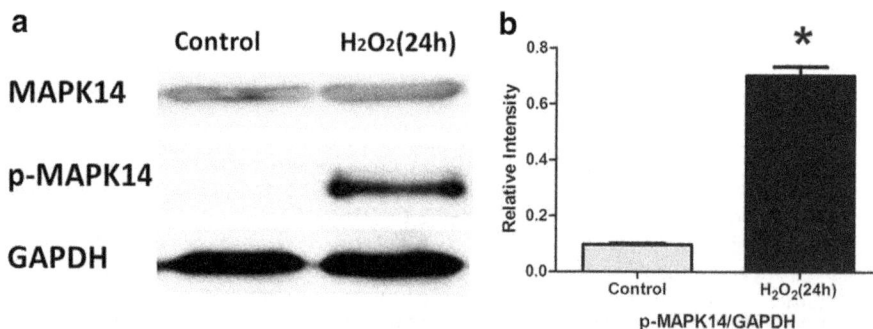

Fig. 7 Western blot analysis of MAPK14 and p-MAPK14 in H_2O_2 treated HLE-B3 cells. **a** The expression level of MAPK14 remained the same after 24 h H_2O_2 treatment while p-MAPK14 increased significantly. **b** Quantitative analysis of the relative intensity of protein levels in HLE-B3 cells. ($n = 3$, *$P < 0.05$)

Abbreviations

EMT: Epithelial-to-mesenchymal transition; FISH: Fluorescence in situ hybridization; HLEs: Human lens epithelial cells; LOCSIII: Lens Opacities Classification System III; MAP K14: Mitogen-activated protein kinase 14; miRNA: MicroRNA.; PCO: Posterior capsular opacification.; PI: Propidium iodide.; PSC: Posterior subcapsular cataracts.; qRT-PCR: Quantitative real-time PCR.; ROS: Reactive oxygen species.; UTRs: Untranslated regions.

Acknowledgements

The author thanks Dr. Xiao Zhang for his generous help in bioinformatics analysis.

Funding

This work was supported by the National Natural Science Foundation of China (Grant No. 81370997).

Authors' contributions

HY, AGY, JZ and SW designed the experiments; BY, MSY and SW performed the experiments; SW analyzed the data; HY performed capsulorrhexis during cataract surgery; CJG and XNN collected clinical samples for this study; SW wrote the paper. All authors read and approved the final manuscript.

Competing interests

The authors declare that they have no competing interests.

Author details

[1]Department of Ophthalmology, Tangdu Hospital, Fourth Military Medical University, 1 Xinsi Road, Xi'an, Shaanxi 710038, People's Republic of China. [2]Department of Dermatology, Xijing Hospital, Fourth Military Medical University, 169 West Changle Road, Xi'an, Shaanxi 710032, People's Republic of China. [3]The State Key Laboratory of Cancer Biology, Department of Biochemistry and Molecular Biology, Fourth Military Medical University, 169 West Changle Road, Xi'an, Shaanxi 710032, People's Republic of China. [4]Chongqing Key Laboratory of Ophthalmology and Chongqing Eye Institute, The First Affiliated Hospital of Chongqing Medical University, 1 Youyi Road, Chongqing 400016, People's Republic of China.

References

1. Wu C, Lin H, Wang Q, Chen W, Luo H, Chen W, Zhang H. Discrepant expression of microRNAs in transparent and cataractous human lenses. Invest Ophthalmol Vis Sci. 2012;53(7):3906–12.
2. Truscott RJ. Age-related nuclear cataract-oxidation is the key. Exp Eye Res. 2005;80(5):709–25.
3. Giblin FJ. Glutathione: a vital lens antioxidant. J Ocul Pharmacol Ther. 2000; 16(2):121–35.
4. Beebe DC, Holekamp NM, Shui YB. Oxidative damage and the prevention of age-related cataracts. Ophthalmic Res. 2010;44(3):155–65.
5. Yang M, Li Y, Padgett RW. MicroRNAs: small regulators with a big impact. Cytokine Growth Factor Rev. 2005;16(4):387–93.
6. Zeng Y, Yi R, Cullen BR. MicroRNAs and small interfering RNAs can inhibit mRNA expression by similar mechanisms. Proc Natl Acad Sci U S A. 2003; 100(17):9779–84.
7. Bartel DP. MicroRNAs: target recognition and regulatory functions. Cell. 2009;136(2):215–33.
8. Ryan DG, Oliveira-Fernandes M, Lavker RM. MicroRNAs of the mammalian eye display distinct and overlapping tissue specificity. Mol Vis. 2006;12:1175–84.
9. Karali M, Peluso I, Gennarino VA, Bilio M, Verde R, Lago G, Dolle P. Banfi S: miRNeye: a microRNA expression atlas of the mouse eye. BMC Genomics. 2010;11:715.
10. Makarev E, Spence JR, Del Rio-Tsonis K, Tsonis PA. Identification of microRNAs and other small RNAs from the adult newt eye. Mol Vis. 2006;12:1386–91.
11. Chen X, Xiao W, Chen W, Liu X, Wu M, Bo Q, Luo Y, Ye S, Cao Y, Liu Y. MicroRNA-26a and -26b inhibit lens fibrosis and cataract by negatively regulating Jagged-1/notch signaling pathway. Cell Death Differ. 2017;24(8):1431–42.
12. Zhang L, Wang Y, Li W, Tsonis PA, Li Z, Xie L, Huang Y. MicroRNA-30a regulation of epithelial-mesenchymal transition in diabetic cataracts through targeting SNAI1. Sci Rep. 2017;7(1):1117.
13. Zeng K, Feng QG, Lin BT, Ma DH, Liu CM. Effects of microRNA-211 on proliferation and apoptosis of lens epithelial cells by targeting SIRT1 gene in diabetic cataract mice. Biosci Rep. 2017;37(4).
14. Chylack LT Jr, Wolfe JK, Singer DM, Leske MC, Bullimore MA, Bailey IL, Friend J, McCarthy D, Wu SY. The Lens opacities classification system III. The longitudinal study of cataract study group. Arch Ophthalmol. 1993;111(6):831–6.
15. Neelam S, Brooks MM, Cammarata PR. Lenticular cytoprotection. Part 1: the role of hypoxia inducible factors-1alpha and -2alpha and vascular endothelial growth factor in lens epithelial cell survival in hypoxia. Mol Vis. 2013;19:1–15.
16. Betel D, Koppal A, Agius P, Sander C, Leslie C. Comprehensive modeling of microRNA targets predicts functional non-conserved and non-canonical sites. Genome Biol. 2010;11(8):R90.
17. Mi H, Muruganujan A, Casagrande JT, Thomas PD. Large-scale gene function analysis with the PANTHER classification system. Nat Protoc. 2013;8(8):1551–66.
18. Shannon P, Markiel A, Ozier O, Baliga NS, Wang JT, Ramage D, Amin N, Schwikowski B, Ideker T. Cytoscape: a software environment for integrated models of biomolecular interaction networks. Genome Res. 2003;13(11):2498–504.
19. West S. Epidemiology of cataract: accomplishments over 25 years and future directions. Ophthalmic Epidemiol. 2007;14(4):173–8.
20. Sasaki H, Jonasson F, Shui YB, Kojima M, Ono M, Katoh N, Cheng HM, Takahashi N, Sasaki K. High prevalence of nuclear cataract in the population of tropical and subtropical areas. Dev Ophthalmol. 2002;35:60–9.
21. Palmquist BM, Philipson B, Barr PO. Nuclear cataract and myopia during hyperbaric oxygen therapy. Br J Ophthalmol. 1984;68(2):113–7.
22. Evanger K, Haugen OH, Irgens A, Aanderud L, Thorsen E. Ocular refractive changes in patients receiving hyperbaric oxygen administered by oronasal mask or hood. Acta Ophthalmol Scand. 2004;82(4):449–53.
23. Fledelius HC, Jansen EC, Thorn J. Refractive change during hyperbaric oxygen therapy. A clinical trial including ultrasound oculometry. Acta Ophthalmol Scand. 2002;80(2):188–90.
24. Cherfan GM, Michels RG, de Bustros S, Enger C, Glaser BM. Nuclear sclerotic cataract after vitrectomy for idiopathic epiretinal membranes causing macular pucker. Am J Ophthalmol. 1991;111(4):434–8.
25. de Bustros S, Thompson JT, Michels RG, Enger C, Rice TA, Glaser BM. Nuclear sclerosis after vitrectomy for idiopathic epiretinal membranes. Am J Ophthalmol. 1988;105(2):160–4.
26. Thompson JT, Glaser BM, Sjaarda RN, Murphy RP. Progression of nuclear sclerosis and long-term visual results of vitrectomy with transforming growth factor beta-2 for macular holes. Am J Ophthalmol. 1995;119(1):48–54.
27. Van Effenterre G, Ameline B, Campinchi F, Quesnot S, Le Mer Y. Haut J: [is vitrectomy cataractogenic? Study of changes of the crystalline lens after surgery of retinal detachment]. J Fr Ophtalmol. 1992;15(8–9):449–54.
28. Holekamp NM, Shui YB, Beebe DC. Vitrectomy surgery increases oxygen exposure to the lens: a possible mechanism for nuclear cataract formation. Am J Ophthalmol. 2005;139(2):302–10.
29. Lou MF. Redox regulation in the lens. Prog Retin Eye Res. 2003;22(5):657–82.
30. McNulty R, Wang H, Mathias RT, Ortwerth BJ, Truscott RJ, Bassnett S. Regulation of tissue oxygen levels in the mammalian lens. J Physiol. 2004; 559(Pt 3):883–98.
31. Ito T, Yagi S, Yamakuchi M. MicroRNA-34a regulation of endothelial senescence. Biochem Biophys Res Commun. 2010;398(4):735–40.
32. Bai XY, Ma Y, Ding R, Fu B, Shi S. Chen XM: miR-335 and miR-34a promote renal senescence by suppressing mitochondrial antioxidative enzymes. J Am Soc Nephrol. 2011;22(7):1252–61.
33. Guo Y, Li P, Gao L, Zhang J, Yang Z, Bledsoe G, Chang E, Chao L, Chao J. Kallistatin reduces vascular senescence and aging by regulating microRNA-34a-SIRT1 pathway. Aging Cell. 2017;16(4):837–46.
34. Zhang H, Zhao Z, Pang X, Yang J, Yu H, Zhang Y, Zhou H, Zhao J. MiR-34a/sirtuin-1/foxo3a is involved in genistein protecting against ox-LDL-induced oxidative damage in HUVECs. Toxicol Lett. 2017;277:115–22.
35. Xia C, Shui L, Lou G, Ye B, Zhu W, Wang J, Wu S, Xu X, Mao L, Xu W, et al. 0404 inhibits hepatocellular carcinoma through a p53/miR-34a/SIRT1 positive feedback loop. Sci Rep. 2017;7(1):4396.

36. Chien KH, Chen SJ, Liu JH, Chang HM, Woung LC, Liang CM, Chen JT, Lin TJ,
     Chiou SH, Peng CH. Correlation between microRNA-34a levels and lens
     opacity severity in age-related cataracts. Eye (Lond). 2013;27(7):883–8.
37. Feng J, Wang X, Zhu W, Chen S, Feng C. MicroRNA-630 suppresses
     epithelial-to-mesenchymal transition by regulating FoxM1 in gastric Cancer
     cells. Biochemistry (Mosc). 2017;82(6):707–14.
38. Sun Y, Cai J, Yu S, Chen S, Li F, Fan C. MiR-630 inhibits endothelial-mesenchymal
     transition by targeting slug in traumatic heterotopic ossification. Sci Rep. 2016;6:
     22729.
39. Tang R, Lei Y, Hu B, Yang J, Fang S, Wang Q, Li M, Guo L. WW domain
     binding protein 5 induces multidrug resistance of small cell lung cancer
     under the regulation of miR-335 through the hippo pathway. Br J Cancer.
     2016;115(2):243–51.
40. Kabir TD, Leigh RJ, Tasena H, Mellone M, Coletta RD, Parkinson EK, Prime SS,
     Thomas GJ, Paterson IC, Zhou D, et al. A miR-335/COX-2/PTEN axis regulates
     the secretory phenotype of senescent cancer-associated fibroblasts. Aging
     (Albany NY). 2016;8(8):1608–35.
41. Yu Y, Gao R, Kaul Z, Li L, Kato Y, Zhang Z, Groden J, Kaul SC, Wadhwa R. Loss-of-
     function screening to identify miRNAs involved in senescence: tumor suppressor
     activity of miRNA-335 and its new target CARF. Sci Rep. 2016;6:30185.
42. Liu ZF, Liang ZQ, Li L, Zhou YB, Wang ZB, Gu WF, Tu LY, Zhao J. MiR-335
     functions as a tumor suppressor and regulates survivin expression in
     osteosarcoma. Eur Rev Med Pharmacol Sci. 2016;20(7):1251–7.
43. Sathish Kumar P, Viswanathan MBG, Venkatesan M, Balakrishna K. Bauerenol,
     a triterpenoid from Indian Suregada angustifolia: induces reactive oxygen
     species-mediated P38MAPK activation and apoptosis in human
     hepatocellular carcinoma (HepG2) cells. Tumour Biol. 2017;39(4):
     1010428317698387.
44. Dragoni S, Hudson N, Kenny BA, Burgoyne T. Endothelial MAPKs direct
     ICAM-1 signaling to divergent inflammatory functions. J Immunol. 2017;
     198(10):4074–85.

Prevalence and risk factors of retinopathy of prematurity in Iran

Milad Azami[1], Zahra Jaafari[2], Shoboo Rahmati[2], Afsar Dastjani Farahani[3] and Gholamreza Badfar[4*]

Abstract

Background: Retinopathy of prematurity (ROP) refers to the developmental disorder of the retina in premature infants and is one of the most serious and most dangerous complications in premature infants. The prevalence of ROP in Iran is different in various parts of Iran and its prevalence is reported to be 1–70% in different regions. This study aims to determine the prevalence and risk factors of ROP in Iran.

Methods: This review article was conducted based on the preferred reporting items for systematic review and meta-analysis (PRISMA) protocols. To find literature about ROP in Iran, a comprehensive search was done using MeSH keywords in several online databases such as PubMed, Ovid, Science Direct, EMBASE, Web of Science, CINAHL, EBSCO, Magiran, Iranmedex, SID, Medlib, IranDoc, as well as the Google Scholar search engine until May 2017. Comprehensive Meta-analysis Software (CMA) Version 2 was used for data analysis.

Results: According to 42 studies including 18,000 premature infants, the prevalence of ROP was reported to be 23.5% (95% CI: 20.4–26.8) in Iran. The prevalence of ROP stages 1, 2, 3, 4 and 5 was 7.9% (95% CI: 5.3–11.5), 9.7% (95% CI: 6.1–15.3), 2.8% (95% CI: 1.6–4.9), 2.9% (95% CI: 1.9–4.5) and 3.6% (95% CI: 2.4–5.2), respectively. The prevalence of ROP in Iranian girls and boys premature infants was 18.3% (95% CI: 12.8–25.4) and 18.9% (95% CI: 11.9–28.5), respectively. The lowest prevalence of ROP was in the West of Iran (12.3% [95% CI: 7.6–19.1]), while the highest prevalence was associated with the Center of Iran (24.9% [95% CI: 21.8–28.4]). The prevalence of ROP is increasing according to the year of study, and this relationship is not significant ($p = 0.181$). The significant risk factors for ROP were small gestational age ($p < 0.001$), low birth weight ($p < 0.001$), septicemia ($p = 0.021$), respiratory distress syndrome ($p = 0.036$), intraventricular hemorrhage ($p = 0.005$), continuous positive pressure ventilation ($p = 0.023$), saturation above 50% ($p = 0.023$), apnea ($p = 0.002$), frequency and duration of blood transfusion, oxygen therapy and phototherapy ($p < 0.05$), whereas pre-eclampsia decreased the prevalence of ROP ($p = 0.014$).

Conclusion: Considering the high prevalence of ROP in Iran, screening and close supervision by experienced ophthalmologists to diagnose and treat the common complications of pre-maturity and prevent visual impairment or blindness is necessary.

Keywords: Meta-analysis, Retinopathy of prematurity, Iran, Prevalence, Risk factor

* Correspondence: Gh_badfar@yahoo.com
[4]Department of Pediatrics, Behbahan Faculty of Medical Sciences, Behbahan, Iran
Full list of author information is available at the end of the article

Background

Retinopathy of prematurity (ROP) refers to the developmental disorder of the retina in premature infants and is one of the most serious and most dangerous complications in premature infants.

Embryonic retinal arteries start to grow in the third month of pregnancy and their development ends at birth. Therefore, the stages of evolution of the eye are defective in premature infants, and the growth of the vessels is either stopped or unusual, and ultimately, the vessels become very fragile, which can lead to visual impairment in severe cases [1].

Despite considerable progress made in the treatment of ROP, it is still a common cause of reduced vision in children in developed countries, and its prevalence is increasing [2–4]. This is a preventable disease and responds to treatments appropriately if diagnosed at early stages, but in case of delayed diagnosis and treatment, it may lead to blindness [5].

The first incidences of ROP were reported in the 1940s and 1950s, mainly as a result of the use of supplemental oxygen without supervision (first epidemic). Although the survival of premature infants improved in the following decades, and despite improved monitoring methods for oxygen supplements, ROP emerged with an increasing incidence (second epidemic) [6]. Over the past decade, the increasing incidence of ROP blindness has been recorded in low-income countries. Studies show that ROP is the leading cause of blindness in China, Southeast Asia, South America, Latin America, and Eastern Europe, especially in urban centers of newly industrialized countries, and this is referred to as the "third epidemic" [7].

ROP is a multifactorial disease and the most important risk factors are preterm delivery, especially before the 32nd week of gestation and birth weight less than 1500 g. Apnea, intraventricular hemorrhage, various maternal factors (diabetes, preeclampsia, mother's smoking), respiratory disorders, infection, vitamin E deficiency, heart disease, increased blood carbon dioxide, increased oxygen (O_2) consumption, decreased PH, decreased blood O2, bradycardia, transfusion, amount of received oxygen and duration of ventilation are other risk factors for ROP [8–10].

The prevalence of ROP in different regions of Iran is different and its prevalence is reported to be 1–70% in different regions [11–14]. Considering the abovementioned issues and the importance of the subject, as well as the diversity of reports in Iranian studies, it is necessary to carry out more extensive and precise studies. Meta-analysis is a method that collects and analyzes multiple research data with a common purpose to provide a reliable estimate of the impact of some interventions or observations in medicine [15, 16]. Obviously, the sample size in meta-analysis becomes larger by collecting data from several studies and therefore the range of changes and probabilities will be reduced; therefore, the significance of statistical results increases [16, 17]. This study aims to determine the incidence and risk factors for ROP in Iran.

Methods

Study protocol

This review article was conducted based on the preferred reporting items for systematic review and meta-analysis (PRISMA) protocols [16]. The study was conducted in five stages: design and search strategy, a collection of articles and their systematic review, evaluation of inclusion and exclusion criteria, qualitative evaluation and statistical analysis of data. To avoid bias in the study, each of the above steps was carried out by two researchers independently. In case of differences in the results obtained by the two researchers, a third researcher intervened to reach an agreement.

Search strategy

To find literature about ROP in Iran, a comprehensive search was done using the terms (Retinopathy of Prematurity [MeSH]) AND ("Incidence" [MeSH] OR "Epidemiology" [MeSH]), OR ("Prevalence" [MeSH]) AND ("Iran" [MeSH]) in 7 international databases including PubMed, Ovid, Science Direct, EMBASE, Web of Science, CINAHL, EBSCO, and 5 national databases including Magiran, Iranmedex, SID, Medlib, IranDoc, as well as Google Scholar search engine until May 2017. References to all relevant articles were reviewed. Due to the inability of Iranian databases to search using Boolean operators (AND, OR and NOT), searches on these databases were only performed using the keywords.

Inclusion and exclusion criteria

Articles with the following characteristics were chosen for meta-analysis: 1. Original research papers published either in Persian or English; 2. Medical dissertations; 3. Review of the prevalence or risk factors for ROP. The exclusion criteria were: 1. Non-random sample for estimating the prevalence; 2. Being irrelevant to the topic; 3. Congress papers; 4. Sample size other than premature infants; 5. Non-Iranian studies; 6. Review articles, case reports, editorials; 7. Duplicate studies and 8. Low-quality studies.

ROP detection criteria

ROP was diagnosed by an expert through examination of retinas of infants using indirect ophthalmoscope.

Selection of studies

First, all related articles (articles with affiliations containing Iranian authors) were collected and a list of titles was prepared at the end of the search and removal of duplicates. After blinding the specifications of the articles by on researcher (Milad Azami), including the name of the journal and the name of the author, the full text of the articles was presented to the researchers. Each article was studied by two researchers independently (Gholamreza Badfar, Afsar Dastjani Farahani). If the article was rejected, the reason for this rejection was mentioned. In case of disagreement between the two authors, the article was judged by the team of researchers.

Quality of studies
Using the standard modified Newcastle Ottawa Scale (NOS) checklist [18], which included 8 sections. Thus, the minimum and maximum score available on this checklist were 0 and 8, respectively. Accordingly, the studies were divided into three categories: 1. low quality with a score less than 5; 2. moderate quality with a score of 5–6; and 3. high quality with a score of 7–8. Finally, the moderate to high quality studies were selected for the meta-analysis stage.

Data extraction
The raw data of the prepared articles were extracted using a premade checklist. The checklist includes the name of the authors, published year the year of study, the location of the study, the study design, quality score, sample size, the prevalence of ROP, the ROP detection criteria, the prevalence of ROP based on gender (ROP) and ROP risk factors.

Statistical analysis
In each study, the prevalence of ROP was considered as the probability of binomial distribution. To evaluate the heterogeneity of the studies, Cochran's Q test and I^2 index were used [19]. There are three categories for the I^2 index: heterogeneity lower than 25%, heterogeneity between 25% and 75% and heterogeneity more than 75%. Considering the heterogeneity of the studies, a random effects model was used to combine ROP prevalence. For ROP risk factors, the fixed effects model and the random effects model were used, respectively in the case of low heterogeneity and high heterogeneity in the meta-analysis [20, 21]. Sensitivity analysis was performed to identify the influence of a single study on the combined result incidence or any risk factors (with ≥ 7 studies). In order to identify the cause of heterogeneity of ROP prevalence, sub-groups analysis of ROP were carried out based on geographical region, province and quality of studies, while the meta-regression model (method of moments) was carried out based on the year of studies [22]. Egger and Begg's tests were used to identify publications bias. Data analysis was performed using Comprehensive Meta-Analysis Software Version 2 and the significance level in the tests was considered to be lower than 0.05.

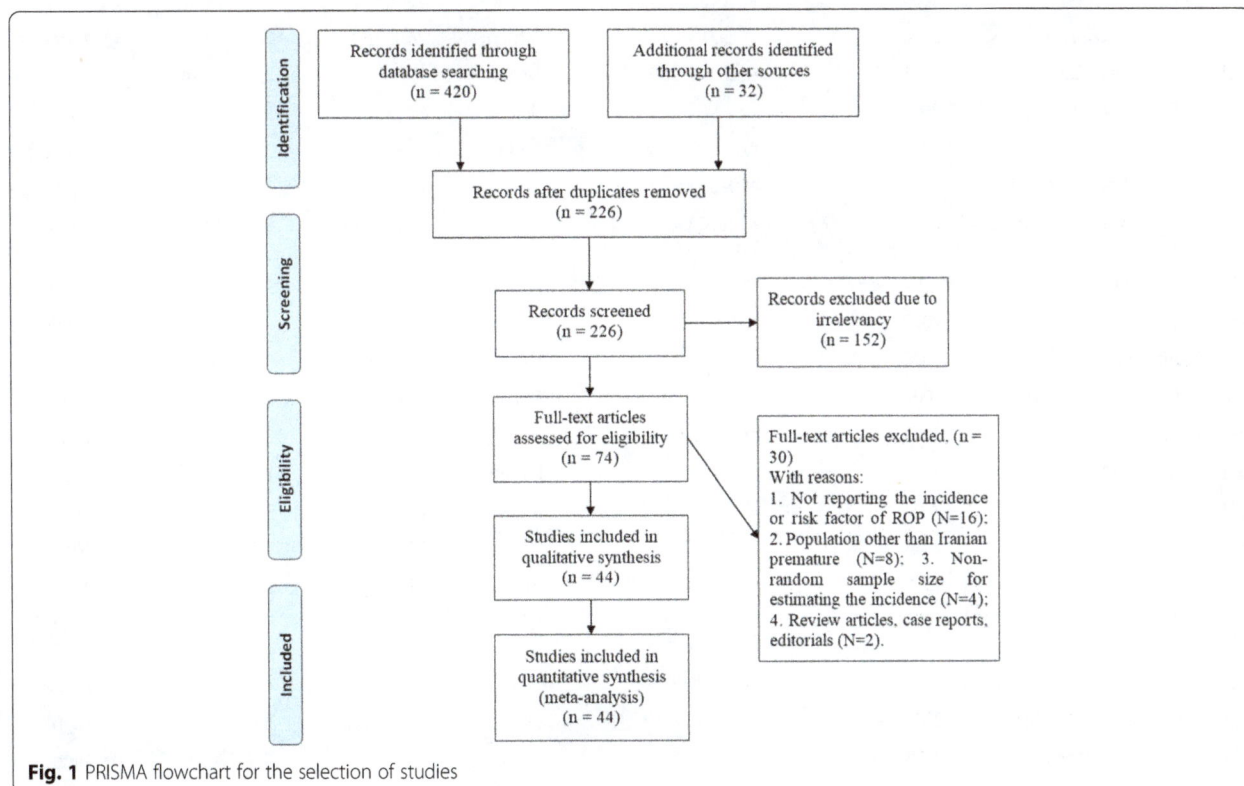

Fig. 1 PRISMA flowchart for the selection of studies

Table 1 Summary of demographic characteristics in studies into a meta-analysis

Ref.	First author, Published Year	Year of study	GA[a] (week)	BW[b] (gr)	Place	Sample size			Prevalence (%)	Quality
						All	Non-ROP[c]	ROP		
[11]	Naderian Gh, 2011	2009	< 34	And ≤ 1800	Isfahan	100	71	29	29	Moderate
[11]	Naderian Gh(1), 2011	2009	< 34	And ≤ 1800	Isfahan	100	58	42	42	Moderate
[12, 13]	Mostafa Gharebagh M, 2012	2008	< 34	–	Tabriz	71	41	30		High
[14]	Nakhshab M, 2016	2014	< 30 or < 34[d]	–	Sari	146	122	24	16.44	High
[52]	Naderian G, 2009	2002	25–34	And 600–1800	Isfahan	796	662	134	16.8	Moderate
[53]	Hosseini H, 2009	2006	< 34	–	Shiraz	1024	1004	20	1.95	High
[54]	Karkhaneh R, 2005	2000	≤ 37	And ≤ 2500	Tehran	185	162	23	12.4	High
[55]	Naderian G, 2010	2003	–	–	Isfahan	604	498	106	17.5	High
[56]	Mansouri M, 2007	2004	≤ 32	And ≤ 1500	Tehran	147	103	44	29.9	High
[57]	Nakshab M, 2003	2001	–	≤ 2500	Sari	68	60	8	11.7	High
[58]	Daraie G, 2016	2008	< 37	Or < 2000	Semnan	270	267	3	1.1	Moderate
[59]	Fayazi A, 2009	2005	< 32	Or < 1500 or 1500–2500*	Tabriz	399	370	29	7.26	Moderate
[60]	Sadeghi K, 2008	2006	< 36	And < 2000	Tabriz	150	124	26	17.3	Moderate
[61]	Ebrahimiadib N, 2016	2011	< 37	Or < 3000	Tehran	1896	1326	570	30.06	Moderate
[62]	Ghaseminejad A, 2011	2006	≤ 36	And ≤ 2500	Kerman	83	59	24	29	High
[63]	Khatami F, 2008	2000	< 34	Or < 2000	Mashhad	50	36	14	28	Moderate
[64]	Sabzehei MK, 2013	2007	–	< 1500	Tehran	414	343	71	17.14	Moderate
[65]	Saeidi R, 2009	2005	≤ 32	Or < 1500	Mashhad	47	43	4	8.5	Moderate
[66]	Azin Far B, 2005	2001	< 29	And < 1500	Babol	100	56	44	44	High
[67]	Karkhanehyousefi N, 2009	2009	–	–	Babol	100	61	39	39	Moderate
[68]	Ebrahimzadeh A, 2009	2003	–	–	Tehran	1343	874	469	34.9	High
[69]	Mirzaee SA, 2010	2008	–	< 2000	Tehran	74	50	24	324	Moderate
[70]	Mousavi Z, 2009	2001	24–36	And 600–2900	Tehran	797	540	257	32.24	Moderate
[71]	Fouladinejad M, 2009	2004	≤ 34	–	Gorgan	89	84	5	5.6	High
[72]	Mousavi S, 2008	2001	24–36	And 600–2800	Tehran	693	474	219	31.6	Moderate
[73]	Sadeghzadeh M, 2016	2001	–	450–3000	Zanjan	78	77	1	1.2	Moderate
[74]	Bayat-Mokhtari M, 2010	2006	–	< 1500 Or 1500–2000*	Shiraz	199	115	84	42	High
[75]	Karkhaneh R, 2001	1997	< 37	Or < 2500	Tehran	150	141	9	6	High
[76]	Babaei H, 2012	2009	–	≤ 1500	Kermanshah	84	73	11	13.1	Moderate
[77]	Abrishami M, 2013	2006	< 32	–	Mashhad	122	90	32	26.2	High
[78]	Riazi-Esfahani M, 2008	2002	≤ 37	And ≤ 2500	Tehran	165	125	40	24.24	Moderate
[79]	Alizadeh Y, 2015	2005	≤ 36	And ≤ 2500	Rasht	310	246	64	20.6	High
[80]	Mousavi SZ, 2010	2003	–	–	Tehran	605	415	190	31.4	Moderate
[81]	Mousavi Z, 2010	2003	–	–	Tehran	1053	673	380	36.1	High
[82]	Feghhi M, 2012	2006	< 32	And ≤ 2000	Ahvaz	576	393	183	32	High
[83]	Afarid M, 2012	2006	≤ 32	And ≤ 2000	Shiraz	787	494	293	37.2	Moderate
[84]	Ahmadpourkacho M, 2014	2009	< 28	And < 1500 or 1500–2000*	Babol	256	76	180	70.31	High
[85]	AhmadpourKacho M, 2014	2007	< 34	And < 2000	Babol	155	85	70	45.2	Moderate
[86]	Rasoulinejad SA, 2016	2007	< 36	And < 2500	Babol	680	374	306	45	High
[87]	Karkhaneh R, 2008	2003	< 37	–	Tehran	953	624	329	34.5	High

Table 1 Summary of demographic characteristics in studies into a meta-analysis *(Continued)*

Ref.	First author, Published Year	Year of study	GA[a] (week)	BW[b] (gr)	Place	Sample size			Prevalence (%)	Quality
						All	Non-ROP[c]	ROP		
[88]	Khalesi N, 2015	2013	–	–	Tehran	120	60	60		Moderate
[89]	Ebrahim M, 2010	2004	< 37	–	Babol	173	140	33	19.1	High
[90]	Roohipoor R, 2016	2012	≤ 37	And ≤ 3000	Tehran	1932	1362	570	3	High
[91]	Mansouri M, 2016	2013	< 34	Or < 2000	Sanandaj	47	42	5	10.6	High

[a]Gestational age; [b]Birth weight; [c]Retinopathy of prematurity; [d]With unstable condition

Results

Search results and characteristics
In the initial search, 452 studies were found to be related to the topic. Two independent researchers reviewed the title and the abstract. If the title or abstract was likely to be related to the topic, the full text was reviewed. After reviewing the full text of 74 relevant articles, 30 articles were omitted due to lacking the necessary criteria and finally 44 qualified studies entered the qualitative assessment stage (Fig. 1). Table 1 shows the characteristics of each study.

Prevalence
Reviewing 42 studies with a total sample size of 18,000 premature infants, the prevalence of ROP in Iran was estimated to be 23.5% (95% CI: 20.4–26.8). The lowest and highest prevalence was related to the studies in Semnan (2008) (1.1%) (58) and in Babol (2009) (70.3%) (84), respectively (Fig. 2).

Sensitivity analysis and cumulative analysis for ROP
The sensitivity analysis of the prevalence or risk factors of ROP and its 95% confidence interval (CI) was estimated simultaneously regardless of one study and the results showed that the incidence or risk factors of ROP were not significantly changed before and after the deletion of each study. (Fig. 3a). Cumulative analysis for incidence of ROP based on the year of publication is shown in Fig. 3b.

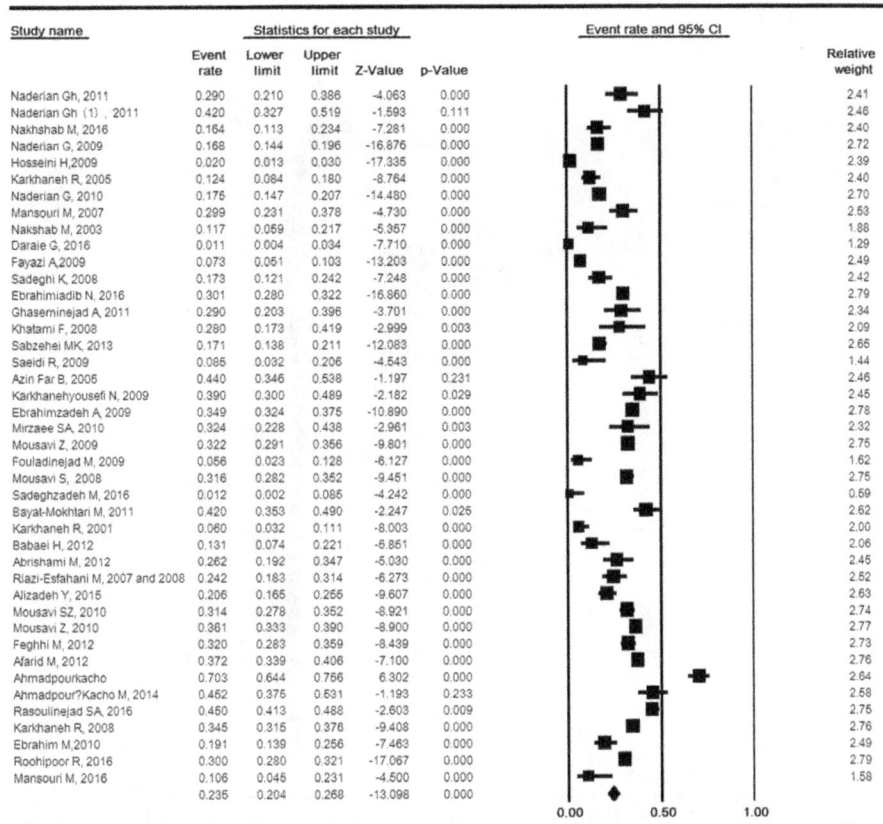

Fig. 2 The prevalence of retinopathy of prematurity in Iran. Random effects model

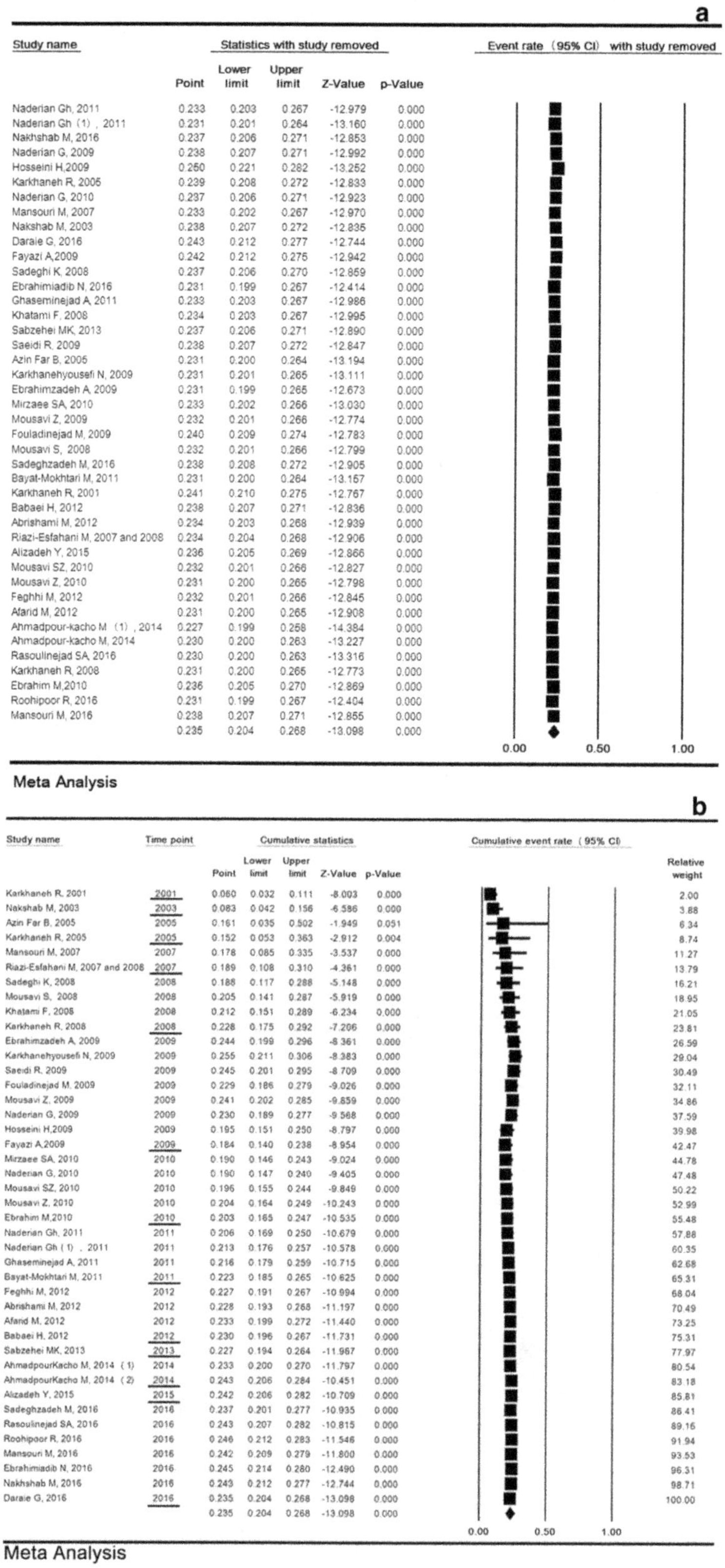

a

Study name	Statistics with study removed					Event rate (95% CI) with study removed
	Point	Lower limit	Upper limit	Z-Value	p-Value	
Naderian Gh, 2011	0.233	0.203	0.267	-12.979	0.000	
Naderian Gh (1), 2011	0.231	0.201	0.264	-13.160	0.000	
Nakhshab M, 2016	0.237	0.206	0.271	-12.853	0.000	
Naderian G, 2009	0.238	0.207	0.271	-12.992	0.000	
Hosseini H,2009	0.250	0.221	0.282	-13.252	0.000	
Karkhaneh R, 2005	0.239	0.208	0.272	-12.833	0.000	
Naderian G, 2010	0.237	0.206	0.271	-12.923	0.000	
Mansouri M, 2007	0.233	0.202	0.267	-12.970	0.000	
Nakshab M, 2003	0.238	0.207	0.272	-12.835	0.000	
Daraie G, 2016	0.243	0.212	0.277	-12.744	0.000	
Fayazi A,2009	0.242	0.212	0.275	-12.942	0.000	
Sadeghi K, 2008	0.237	0.206	0.270	-12.859	0.000	
Ebrahimiadib N, 2016	0.231	0.199	0.267	-12.414	0.000	
Ghaseminejad A, 2011	0.233	0.203	0.267	-12.986	0.000	
Khatami F, 2008	0.234	0.203	0.267	-12.995	0.000	
Sabzehei MK, 2013	0.237	0.206	0.271	-12.890	0.000	
Saeidi R, 2009	0.238	0.207	0.272	-12.847	0.000	
Azin Far B, 2005	0.231	0.200	0.264	-13.194	0.000	
Karkhanehyousefi N, 2009	0.231	0.201	0.265	-13.111	0.000	
Ebrahimzadeh A, 2009	0.231	0.199	0.265	-12.673	0.000	
Mirzaee SA, 2010	0.233	0.202	0.266	-13.030	0.000	
Mousavi Z, 2009	0.232	0.201	0.266	-12.774	0.000	
Fouladinejad M, 2009	0.240	0.209	0.274	-12.783	0.000	
Mousavi S, 2008	0.232	0.201	0.266	-12.799	0.000	
Sadeghzadeh M, 2016	0.238	0.208	0.272	-12.905	0.000	
Bayat-Mokhtari M, 2011	0.231	0.200	0.264	-13.157	0.000	
Karkhaneh R, 2001	0.241	0.210	0.275	-12.767	0.000	
Babaei H, 2012	0.238	0.207	0.271	-12.836	0.000	
Abrishami M, 2012	0.234	0.203	0.268	-12.939	0.000	
Riazi-Esfahani M, 2007 and 2008	0.234	0.204	0.268	-12.906	0.000	
Alizadeh Y, 2015	0.236	0.205	0.269	-12.866	0.000	
Mousavi SZ, 2010	0.232	0.201	0.266	-12.827	0.000	
Mousavi Z, 2010	0.231	0.200	0.265	-12.798	0.000	
Feghhi M, 2012	0.232	0.201	0.266	-12.845	0.000	
Afarid M, 2012	0.231	0.200	0.265	-12.908	0.000	
Ahmadpour-kacho M (1), 2014	0.227	0.199	0.258	-14.384	0.000	
Ahmadpour-kacho M, 2014	0.230	0.200	0.263	-13.227	0.000	
Rasoulinejad SA, 2016	0.230	0.200	0.263	-13.316	0.000	
Karkhaneh R, 2008	0.231	0.200	0.265	-12.773	0.000	
Ebrahim M,2010	0.236	0.205	0.270	-12.869	0.000	
Roohipoor R, 2016	0.231	0.199	0.267	-12.404	0.000	
Mansouri M, 2016	0.238	0.207	0.271	-12.855	0.000	
	0.235	0.204	0.268	-13.098	0.000	

| | | | | | | 0.00   0.50   1.00 |

Meta Analysis

b

Study name	Time point	Cumulative statistics					Cumulative event rate (95% CI)	Relative weight
		Point	Lower limit	Upper limit	Z-Value	p-Value		
Karkhaneh R, 2001	2001	0.060	0.032	0.111	-8.003	0.000		2.00
Nakshab M, 2003	2003	0.083	0.042	0.156	-6.586	0.000		3.88
Azin Far B, 2005	2005	0.161	0.035	0.502	-1.949	0.051		6.34
Karkhaneh R, 2005	2005	0.152	0.053	0.363	-2.912	0.004		8.74
Mansouri M, 2007	2007	0.178	0.085	0.335	-3.537	0.000		11.27
Riazi-Esfahani M, 2007 and 2008	2007	0.189	0.108	0.310	-4.361	0.000		13.79
Sadeghi K, 2008	2008	0.186	0.117	0.288	-5.148	0.000		16.21
Mousavi S, 2008	2008	0.205	0.141	0.287	-5.919	0.000		18.95
Khatami F, 2008	2008	0.212	0.151	0.289	-6.234	0.000		21.05
Karkhaneh R, 2008	2008	0.228	0.175	0.292	-7.206	0.000		23.81
Ebrahimzadeh A, 2009	2009	0.244	0.199	0.296	-8.361	0.000		26.59
Karkhanehyousefi N, 2009	2009	0.255	0.211	0.306	-8.383	0.000		29.04
Saeidi R, 2009	2009	0.245	0.201	0.295	-8.709	0.000		30.49
Fouladinejad M, 2009	2009	0.229	0.186	0.279	-9.026	0.000		32.11
Mousavi Z, 2009	2009	0.241	0.202	0.285	-9.859	0.000		34.86
Naderian G, 2009	2009	0.230	0.189	0.277	-9.568	0.000		37.59
Hosseini H,2009	2009	0.195	0.151	0.250	-8.797	0.000		39.98
Fayazi A,2009	2009	0.184	0.140	0.238	-8.954	0.000		42.47
Mirzaee SA, 2010	2010	0.190	0.146	0.243	-9.024	0.000		44.78
Naderian G, 2010	2010	0.190	0.147	0.240	-9.405	0.000		47.48
Mousavi SZ, 2010	2010	0.196	0.155	0.244	-9.849	0.000		50.22
Mousavi Z, 2010	2010	0.204	0.164	0.249	-10.243	0.000		52.99
Ebrahim M,2010	2010	0.203	0.165	0.247	-10.535	0.000		55.48
Naderian Gh, 2011	2011	0.206	0.169	0.250	-10.679	0.000		57.88
Naderian Gh (1), 2011	2011	0.213	0.176	0.257	-10.578	0.000		60.35
Ghaseminejad A, 2011	2011	0.216	0.179	0.259	-10.715	0.000		62.68
Bayat-Mokhtari M, 2011	2011	0.223	0.185	0.265	-10.625	0.000		65.31
Feghhi M, 2012	2012	0.227	0.191	0.267	-10.994	0.000		68.04
Abrishami M, 2012	2012	0.228	0.193	0.268	-11.197	0.000		70.49
Afarid M, 2012	2012	0.233	0.199	0.272	-11.440	0.000		73.25
Babaei H, 2012	2012	0.230	0.196	0.267	-11.731	0.000		75.31
Sabzehei MK, 2013	2013	0.227	0.194	0.264	-11.967	0.000		77.97
AhmadpourKacho M, 2014 (1)	2014	0.233	0.200	0.270	-11.797	0.000		80.54
AhmadpourKacho M, 2014 (2)	2014	0.243	0.206	0.284	-10.451	0.000		83.18
Alizadeh Y, 2015	2015	0.242	0.206	0.282	-10.709	0.000		85.81
Sadeghzadeh M, 2016	2016	0.237	0.201	0.277	-10.935	0.000		86.41
Rasoulinejad SA, 2016	2016	0.243	0.207	0.282	-10.815	0.000		89.16
Roohipoor R, 2016	2016	0.246	0.212	0.283	-11.546	0.000		91.94
Mansouri M, 2016	2016	0.242	0.209	0.279	-11.800	0.000		93.53
Ebrahimiadib N, 2016	2016	0.245	0.214	0.280	-12.490	0.000		96.31
Nakhshab M, 2016	2016	0.243	0.212	0.277	-12.744	0.000		98.71
Daraie G, 2016	2016	0.235	0.204	0.268	-13.098	0.000		100.00
		0.235	0.204	0.268	-13.098	0.000		

| | | | | | | | 0.00   0.50   1.00 | |

Meta Analysis

Fig. 3 Sensitivity analysis (**a**) and cumulative analysis based on the year of publication (**b**) for prevalence of retinopathy of prematurity in Iran. Random effects model

Subgroup analysis of ROP prevalence based on geographic region

In the reviewed studies, 2, 4, 12, 4, and 20 studies were related to the West, East, North, South, and Center of Iran, respectively. The prevalence of ROP in the five regions of Iran is shown in Table 2 and the lowest incidence of ROP was in west of Iran (12.3% [95% CI: 7.6–19.1]), while the highest prevalence was related to the center of Iran (24.9% [95% CI: 21.8–28.4]) (Table 2).

Subgroup analysis of ROP prevalence based on province

Table 2 and Fig. 4 show the prevalence of ROP based on Iran's provinces. The highest prevalence was in provinces of Mazandaran (34.8%) and Khuzestan (32%), and the lowest prevalence was in the provinces of Semnan (1.1%) and Zanjan (1.2%).

Subgroup analysis of ROP prevalence based on the quality of studies

The prevalence of ROP in moderate and high-quality studies was 23.5% (95% CI: 16.6–28.0) and 23.5% (95% CI: 19.1–28.7), respectively, and the difference was not statistically significant ($p = 0.995$) (Table 2).

The prevalence of ROP based on gender

The prevalence of ROP in girls and boys premature infants was 18.3% (95% CI: 12.8–25.4) and 18.9% (95% CI: 11.9–28.5), respectively. Their difference was not statistically significant ($P = 0.501$) (Table 2).

The prevalence of ROP based on stage

The prevalence of stages 1, 2, 3, 4 and 5 were reported in 10, eight, nine, five, and five studies, respectively. Fig. 5 shows the prevalence of ROP at different stages. The

Table 2 The prevalence of ROP based on region, gender, provinces and quality of studies

Variable		Studies (N[a])	Sample (N)	Heterogeneity		95% CI[b]	Prevalence (%)
				I[2]	P-Value		
Region	Center	20	12,355	93.65	< 0.001	21.8 to 28.4	24.9
	East	4	302	57.79	0.07	17 to 33	24.1
	North	12	2626	97.09	< 0.001	15.9 to 37.1	25
	South	4	2586	98.60	< 0.001	9.2 to 37.1	20.5
	West	2	131	0	0.67	7.6 to 19.1	12.3
	Test for subgroup differences: Q = 9.67, df(Q) = 4, P = 0.046						
Gender	Boys	11	1467	92.65	< 0.001	11.9 to 28.5	18.9
	Girls	11	1184	85.02	< 0.001	12.8 to 25.4	18.3
	Rate ratio of boys to girls: OR[c] = 1.07(0.86 to 1.33, P = 0.501)						
Provinces	Khozestan	1	576	0	–	28.3 to 35.9	32
	Mazandaran	8	1678	95.77	< 0.001	23.5 to 48.2	34.8
	Isfahan	4	1600	92.48	< 0.001	16.5 to 35	24.6
	Golestan	1	89	0	–	2.3 to 12.8	5.6
	Kerman	1	83	0	–	20.3 to 39.6	29
	Kermanshah	3	84	0	–	7.4 to 22.1	13.1
	Razavi Khorasan	3	219	67.89	0.044	12.4 to 34.2	21.3
	Guilan	1	310	0	–	16.5 to 25.5	20.9
	Kurdistan	1	47	0	–	4.5 to 23.1	10.6
	Semnan	1	270	0	–	0.4 to 3.4	1.1
	Fars	3	2010	99.09	< 0.001	4 to 50.8	17.2
	East Azarbaijan	2	549	91.32	0.001	4.6 to 25	11.3
	Tehran	14	10,407	91.32	< 0.001	25.1 to 31	28
	Zanjan	1	78	0	–	0.2 to 8.5	1.2
	Test for subgroup differences: Q = 97.59, df(Q) = 13, P < 0.001						
Quality	Medium	20	7760	63.68	< 0.001	16.6 to 28.0	23.5
	High	22	10,240	96.65	< 0.001	19.1 to 28.7	23.5
	Test for subgroup differences: Q = 0, df(Q) = 1, P = 0.995						

[a]Number
[b]Confidence interval

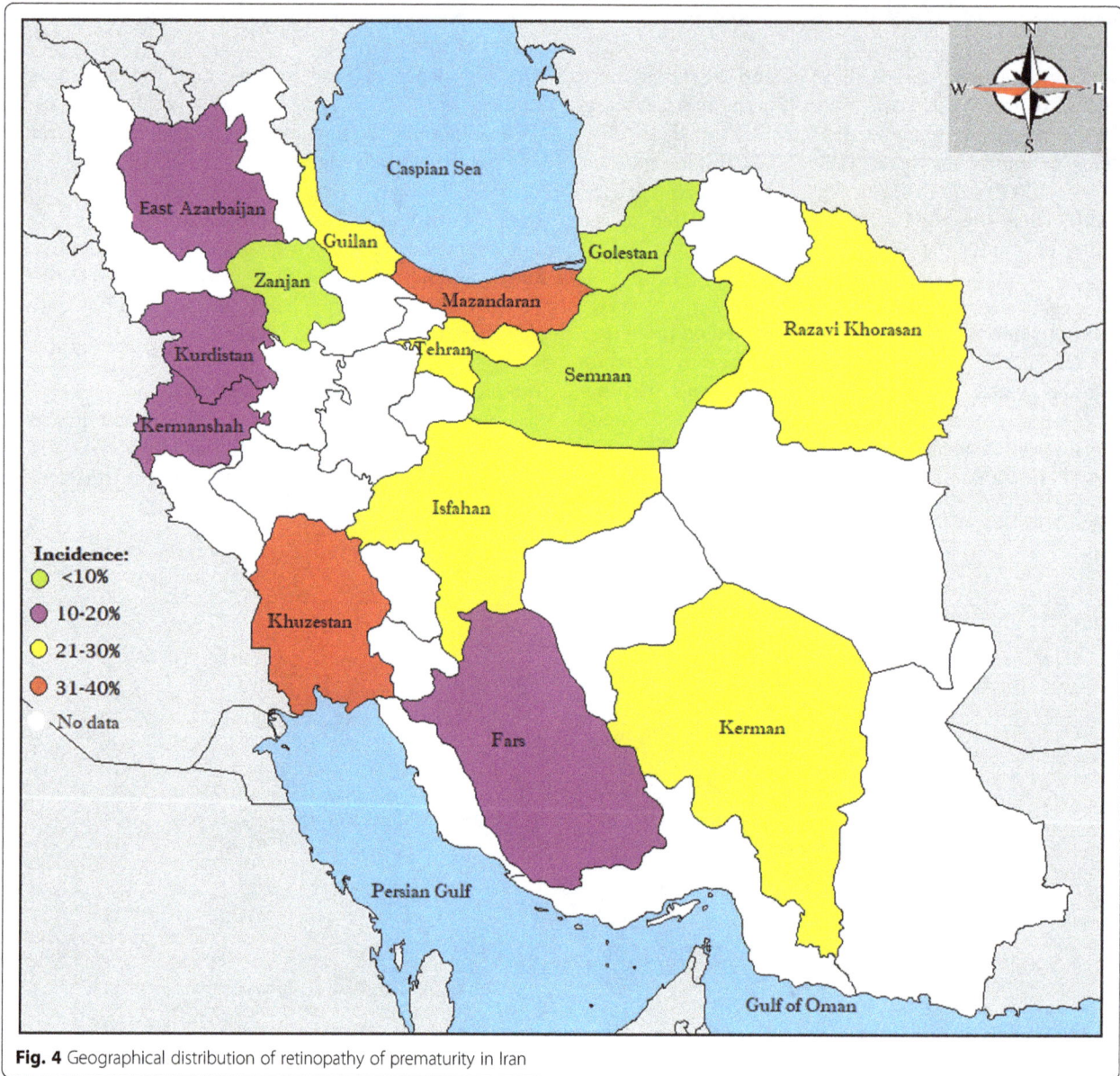

Fig. 4 Geographical distribution of retinopathy of prematurity in Iran

prevalence of stages 1, 2, 3, 4 and 5 was 7.9% (95% CI: 5.3–11.5), 9.7% (95% CI: 6.1–15.3), 2.8% (95% CI: 1.6–4.9), 2.9% (95% CI: 1.9–4.5), and 3.6% (95% CI: 2.4–5.2), respectively.

Meta-regression

Meta-regression model in Fig. 6 shows that the incidence of ROP is increasing according to the year of study, and this relationship is not statistically significant (meta-regression coefficient: 0.034, 95% CI -0.016 to 0.085, $P = 0.181$).

Publication bias

The significance level of publication bias in the reviewed studies was 0.003 and 0.002 according to Egger and Begg's tests, respectively, which is shown in Fig. 7.

ROP risk factors

The meta-analysis results of evaluating the risk factors of ROP are shown in Table 3. ROP risk factors include certain variables such as continuous positive pressure (CPAP) ($P = 0.023$), the prevalence of blood transfusion ($P = 0.001$), septicemia ($P = 0.021$), weight < 1000 g ($P < 0.001$), weight < 1500 g ($P < 0.0001$), frequency of phototherapy ($P < 0.0001$), the frequency of oxygen therapy ($P = 0.049$), apnea ($P = 00.2$), intraventricular hemorrhage (IVH) ($P = 0.005$), respiratory distress syndrome (RDS) ($P = 0.036$), gestational age (GA) ≤ 28 W(week) ($P < 0.001$), GA ≤ 32 W ($P < 0.001$), saturation over 50% ($P < 0.001$), mean GA ($P < 0.001$), mean weight ($P < 0.0001$), oxygen therapy duration ($P < 0.001$) and phototherapy

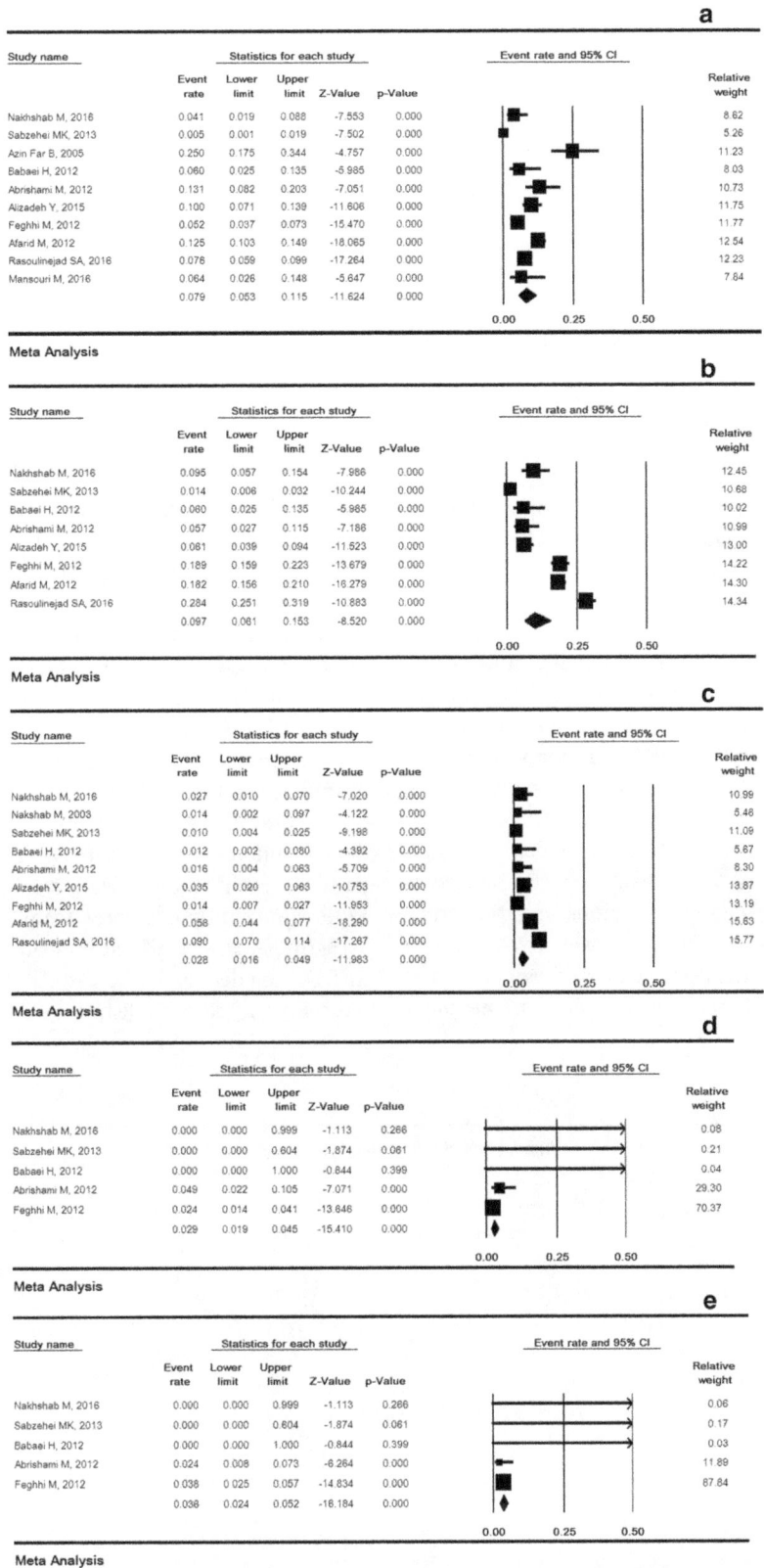

Fig. 5 The prevalence of stages I (**a**), II (**b**), III (**c**), IV (**d**), V (**e**) retinopathy of prematurity. Random effects model

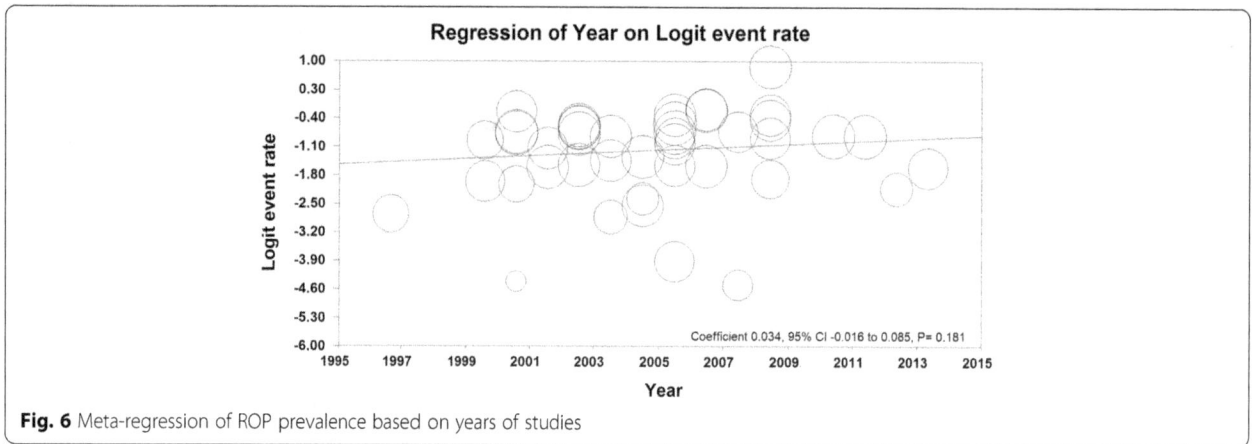

Fig. 6 Meta-regression of ROP prevalence based on years of studies

duration ($P < 0.0001$); however, preeclampsia significantly decreases the prevalence of ROP ($P = 0.014$).

Discussion

The present study is the first systematic and meta-analytic review on the prevalence and risk factors of ROP in Iran. The results of this meta-analysis showed that the prevalence of ROP in 18,000 Iranian premature infants was 23.5%, and the prevalence for stages 1, 2, 3, 4 and 5 was 7.9%, 9.7%, 2.8%, 2.9% and 3.6%, respectively. In this study, the level of heterogeneity was high for ROP studies (95.6%). The results of the subgroup analysis showed that geographic regions and the provinces could be a cause of high heterogeneity. However, this difference can be a reflection of studies conducted on different samples based on the GA or neonatal weight.

ROP is still a major cause of potentially preventable blindness around the world [23]. According to guidelines published by the American Academy of Ophthalmology, the American Academy of Children, and the American Association for Ophthalmology for Children and Strabismus for ROP screening, infants weighing less than 1500 g or GA ≤ 30 weeks, and infants weighing between 1500 and 2000 g or GA > 30 weeks with an unstable clinical course should receive dilated ophthalmoscopy examinations for ROP [24].

The prevalence of ROP in various studies is mainly due to differences in mean GA and birth weight of infants in each study. Based on GA, the prevalence of ROP significantly decreases from 77.9% in GA 24–25 to 1.1% in GA 30–31, which indicates the direct role of GA in ROP incidence. These results are completely consistent with the data published in other literature [25–31]. Moreover, in a meta-analysis study in Iran, the

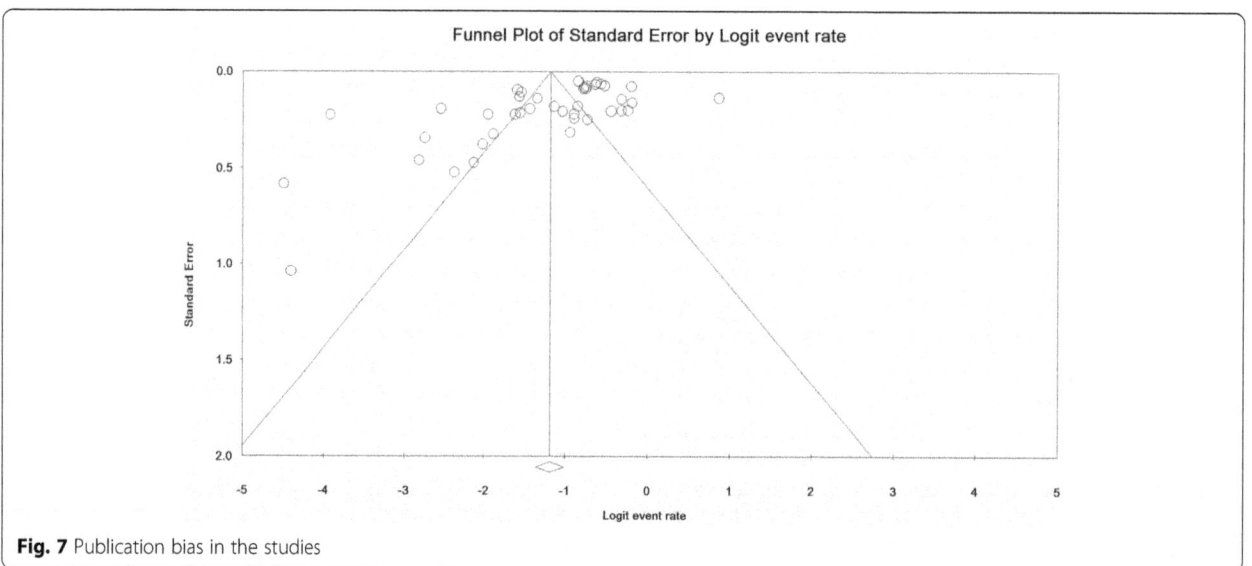

Fig. 7 Publication bias in the studies

Table 3 Risk factor for retinopathy of prematurity in Iran

Variables	Studies(N^a)	Sample (N) Case	Control	Heterogeneity I^2	P-Value	OR (95%CI^b)	P-Value	Model in Meta-analysis
Twin birth	4	804	1868	46.97	0.129	1.62 (0.94 to 2.81)	0.081	Random^c
Mechanical ventilation	6	1131	2493	73.35	0.002	1.81 (0.80 to 1.73)	0.39	Random
Continuous positive pressure ventilation	2	62	131	64.11	0.095	3.97 (1.21 to 13.01)	0.023	Random
Blood transfusion (N)	16	1820	4167	91.34	< 0.001	2.38 (1.43 to 3.94)	0.001	Random
Septicemia	11	1327	2965	80.75	< 0.001	1.96 (1.10 to 3.48)	0.021	Random
Birth weight < 1000 g	9	573	2093	59.65	0.011	4.16 (2.35 to 7.35)	< 0.001	Random
Birth weight < 1500 g	10	559	1984	43.34	0.069	3.74 (2.54 to 5.49)	< 0.001	Random
Phototherapy (N)	11	1380	3355	80.69	< 0.001	1.50 (1.00 to 2.27)	0.049	Random
Oxygen therapy (N)	14	726	3124	87.39	< 0.001	3.06 (1.29 to 7.27)	0.011	Random
Need for resuscitation	2	56	212	86.50	0.006	5.01 (0.18 to 135.71)	0.338	Random
Apnea	3	114	492	72.08	0.028	4.41 (1.70 to 11.40)	0.002	Random
Congenital heart disease	2	50	246	67.29	0.08	2.13 (0.10 to 45.62)	0.626	Random
Inter-ventricular hemorrhage	11	1223	3178	76.36	< 0.001	2.24 (1.2 to 3.95)	0.005	Random
Acidosis	3	132	296	62.62	0.069	2.56 (0.81 to 8.06)	0.106	Random
Cesarean section	4	375	830	47.88	0.124	1.08 (0.53 to 2.18)	0.82	Random
Preeclampsia	2	108	237	0	0.82	0.12 (0.02 to 0.65)	0.014	Fixed^d
Respiratory distress syndrome	11	2039	2618	80.13	< 0.001	1.64 (1.03 to 2.61)	0.036	Random
Saturation above 50%	4	118	656	30.30	0.23	8.35 (3.14 to 22.18)	< 0.001	Random
Normal Vaginal Delivery	4	375	830	46.63	0.132	1.01 (0.50 to 2.02)	0.969	Random
Multiple pregnancy	6	1199	2518	40.20	0.137	0.92 (0.73 to 1.16)	0.517	Random
Gestational age ≤ 28	6	551	1440	75.88	< 0.001	5.20 (2.31 to 11.73)	< 0.001	Random
Gestational age ≤ 32	9	689	1885	64.84	0.004	7.88 (4.62 to 13.46)	< 0.001	Random
Birth weight (gr)	7	1495	2893	97.30	< 0.001	0.98 (0.97 to 0.99)	< 0.001	Random
Gestational age (week)	7	1495	2893	84.20	< 0.001	0.67 (0.59 to 0.770)	< 0.001	Random

Variables	Studies(N^a)	Sample (N) Case	Control	Heterogeneity I^2	P-Value	Mean Difference (95% CI^b)	P-Value	
Gestational age (weeks)	18	1835	4126	94.53	< 0.001	2.08 (1.50 to 2.66)	< 0.001	Random
Birth weight (gr)	19	1782	4519	95.94	< 0.001	305.39 (236.09 to 374.69)	< 0.001	Random
Oxygen therapy (day)	11	1399	3214	96.04	< 0.001	−4.36 (−6.09 to −2.63)	< 0.001	Random
Phototherapy (days)	4	78	308	83.80	< 0.001	−2.08 (−3.81 to −0.35)	< 0.001	Random
Apgar score in the first minute	3	174	216	63.30	0.66	1.07 (0.45 to 1.68)	0.001	Random
Apgar score	3	64	272	76.34	0.015	0.43 (−0.25 to −1.13)	0.21	Random
Mechanical ventilation (days)	2	114	154	88.81	0.003	−4.53 (−9.17 to 0.10)	0.55	Random
Bilirubin (mg/di)	3	54	186	7.70	0.33	−0.27 (−1.40 to 0.86)	0.63	Random
Blood transfusion (duration)	2	98	151	0	0.98	−0.69 (−0.96 to −0.42)	< 0.001	Fixed
clinical risk index for babies	2	161	250	58.84	0.11	−0.62 (−1.40 to 0.16)	0.11	Random

^{a}Number
^{b}Confidence interval
^{c}Random effects model
^{d}Fixed effects model

prevalence of prematurity was reported to be 9.2% (95% CI: 7.6–10.7) [32]. Therefore, the high prevalence of ROP in Iran (23.5%) can be explained by the high prevalence of prematurity.

In a study by Tabarez-Carvajal et al. among 3018 premature infants, the incidence of stages 1, 2, 3, 4, and 5 was reported to be 8.34%, 8.78%, 1.9%, 0.03%, and 0.30%, respectively [33]. In another study by Abdel HA et al.,

Table 4 Risk factor for retinopathy of prematurity in other studies

Study details	GA (weeks)	BW (gr)	Risk factors
Reyes et al., 2017. Oman [46]	< 32	< 1500	low BW, low GA, duration of invasive ventilation, duration of oxygen therapy, duration of nasal CPAP, late onset clinical or proven sepsis
Shah et al., 2005 Singapore [40]	< 32	< 1500	Preeclampsia, low BW, prolonged duration of ventilation, pulmonary hemorrhage and CPAP
Yau et al., 2016, China [45]	< 32 and > 32	< 1500	low GA, low BW, preeclampsia, gestational diabetes mellitus, inotrope use, postnatal hypotension, apgar score (1 min, 5 min and 10 min), respiratory distress syndrome, bronchopulmonary dysplasia, invasive mechanical ventilation, surfactant use, oxygen supplement, patent ductus arteriosus, thrombocytopenia, blood transfusion, anemia, NSAID use, sepsis
Abdel HA et al., 2012, Egypt [34]	< 32 and > 32	< 1500 and > 1500	low GA, oxygen therapy, frequency of blood transfusions and sepsis
Chen et al., 2011, USA [41]	< 30	< 1500	low GA, Sepsis, oxygen exposure
Hadi and Hamdy, 2013, Egypt [37]	< 32	< 1250	low GA, low BW, Ventilation, blood transfusions, sepsis, Patent ductus arteriosus, IVH
Nair et al., 2001, Oman [36]	< 32	< 1500	low BW, Low GA, TPN

BW Birth weight, *GA* Gestational age, *PDA* Patent ductus arteriosus, *CPAP* Continuous positive pressure ventilation, *IVH* Intraventricular hemorrhage, *TPN* Total parenteral nutrition

the prevalence of ROP stage 1 was 10.4%, stage 2 was 5.2% and stage 3 was 3.45%, and none of the infants had ROP at stages 4 or 5 [34]. But in the present study, the prevalence of ROP stages 4 and 5 was higher.

ROP is a multi-factorial disease, and in the present study, the strongest risk factor for ROP was prematurity and low birth weight. Most studies have demonstrated that prematurity and low birth weight are the strongest predictive factors of ROP, which indicates the crucial role of factors associated with the progression of the ROP disease [35–45].

After low birth weight and prematurity, exposure to oxygen for a long period and saturation over 50% were the most important risk factors for ROP in this study, which was consistent with the results of many other studies [42–47]. Due to inadequate antioxidant defense system, premature infants are not evolved to live in an oxygen-rich ectopic environment [48, 49]. Oxidative stress is the result of various organs' exposure to free radicals of oxygen after being exposed to high concentrations of oxygen, which can lead to the progression of many pathogens such as ROP, necrotizing enterocolitis, IVH, bronchopulmonary dysplasia, and periventricular leukomalacia [50, 51].

In this study, other significant relationships with ROP were also found, including frequency and duration of blood transfusion, phototherapy, septicemia, apnea, IVH, and RDS. The comparison between the risk factors in our study and other reports is shown in Table 4.

Conclusion

Finally, it can be concluded that the present systematic review and meta-analysis summarizes the results of previous studies and provides a comprehensive view of ROP in Iran. Although the prevalence of ROP in Iran is similar to some developing countries, it is much higher than some other countries. Therefore, this fact highlights the importance of preventing and treating ROP and its following complications. To achieve a more favorable level and reduce the prevalence in the coming years, screening and close monitoring by experienced ophthalmologists are essential to diagnose and treat the common complications of prematurity and prevent visual impairment or blindness.

Abbreviations
CI: Confidence interval; GA: Gestational age; IVH: Intraventricular hemorrhage; PRISMA: Preferred Reporting Items for Systematic Reviews and Meta-Analyses Protocols; RDS: Respiratory Distress Syndrome; ROP: Retinopathy of prematurity; W: Week

Acknowledgements
We thanks Behbahan University of Medical Sciences for the financial support.

Funding
Behbahan University of Medical Sciences.

Authors' contributions
MA was involved in study concept and design, acquisition of data, search, quality evaluation of studies, drafting of the manuscript, analysis and interpretation of data, critical revision of the manuscript for important intellectual content, approval of final version, and accountable for accuracy and integrity of the work. ZJ was involved in search, interpretation of data, acquisition of data, quality evaluation of studies, drafting of the manuscript, and approval of final version. ShR was involved in search, analysis and interpretation of data, quality evaluation of studies, drafting of the manuscript, and approval of final version. GhB was involved in study concept and design, acquisition of data, quality evaluation of studies, drafting of the manuscript, critical revision of the manuscript for important intellectual content, approval of final version, administrative, technical or material

support and accountable for accuracy and integrity of the work. ADF was involved in search critical revision of the manuscript for important intellectual content, and approval of final version.

Competing interests
The authors declare that they have no competing interests.

Author details
[1]Student Research Committee, Ilam University of Medical Sciences, Ilam, Iran. [2]Student Research Committee, Ilam University of Medical Sciences, Ilam, Iran. [3]Iranian National ROP Committee, Tehran, Iran. [4]Department of Pediatrics, Behbahan Faculty of Medical Sciences, Behbahan, Iran.

References
1. Zin A, Gole GA. Retinopathy of prematurity-incidence today. Clin Perinatol. 2013;40(2):185–200.
2. Gergely K, Gerinec A. Retinopathy of prematurity–epidemics, incidence, prevalence, blindness. Bratisl Lek Listy. 2009;111(9):514–7.
3. Zin A. R etinopathyof P re maturity-I ncidence to day. 2013.
4. Kliegman RM, Behrman RE, Jenson HB,et al. Nelson textbook of pediatrics E-book: Elsevier health sciences; 2007.
5. Wilson CM, Ells AL, Fielder AR. The challenge of screening for retinopathy of prematurity. Clin Perinatol. 2013;40(2):241–59.
6. Gibson DL, Sheps SB, Schechter MT, et al. Retinopathy of prematurity: a new epidemic? Pediatrics. 1989;83:486–92.
7. Augsburger JJBN. Yanoff M, Duker JS, editors. Ophtalmology. St. Louis, MO: Mosby 2004. p. 1097–102.
8. Senthil MP, Salowi MA, Bujang MA, et al. Risk factors and prediction models for retinopathy of prematurity. Malays J Med Sci. 2015;22(5):57.
9. GEBEŞÇE A, USLU H, KELEŞ E, et al. Retinopathy of prematurity: incidence, risk factors, and evaluation of screening criteria. Turk J Med Sci. 2016;46(2): 315–20.
10. Edy Siswanto J, Sauer PJ. Retinopathy of prematurity in Indonesia: Incidence and risk factors. J Neonatal Perinatal Med. 2017;10(1):85-90. https://doi.org/10.3233/NPM-915142.
11. Naderian GIR, Mohammadizadeh M, Najafabadi FBZ, et al. The frequency of retinopathy of prematurity in premature infants referred to an ophthalmology Clinic in Isfahan. J Isfahan Med Sch. 29(128):126–30.
12. Gharebagh M, Sadeghi K, Zarghami N, Mostafidi H. Evaluation of vascular endothelial growth factor, leptin and insulin-like growth factor in precocious retinopathy. Urmia Med J. 2012;23(2):183–90.
13. Gharehbaghi MM, Peirovifar A, Sadeghi K. Plasma leptin concentrations in preterm infants with retinopathy of prematurity (ROP). Iran J Neonatol. 2012;3(1):12–6.
14. Nakhshab MAA, Dargahi S, Farhadi R, et al. The incidence rate of retinopathy of prematurity and related risk factors: a study on premature neonates hospitalized in two hospitals in sari, Iran, 2014-2015. J Kerman Univ Med Sci. 2016;23(3):296–307.
15. Badfar G, Shohani M, Nasirkandy MP, et al. Epidemiology of hepatitis B in pregnant Iranian women: a systematic review and meta-analysis. Arch Virol. 2018;163(2):319-330. https://doi.org/10.1007/s00705-017-3551-6.
16. Moher D, Liberati A, Tetzlaff J, Altman DG, PRISMA Group. Preferred reporting items for systematic reviews and meta-analyses: the PRISMA statement. PLoS Med. 2009;6(7):e1000097. https://doi.org/10.1371/journal.pmed.1000097. Epub 2009 Jul 21
17. Sayehmiri K, Tavan H, Sayehmiri F, et al. Prevalence of epilepsy in Iran: a meta-analysis and systematic review. Iran J Child Neurol. 2014;8(4):9–17.
18. Wells GA, Shea B, O'Connell D, Peterson J, Welch V, Losos M, et al. The Newcastle-Ottawa Scale (NOS) for assessing the quality of nonrandomized studies in meta-analysis. 2011. Available: www.ohri.ca/programs/clinical_epidemiology/oxford.asp. Accessed 25 Nov 2012.
19. Higgins JP, Green S. Cochrane handbook for systematic reviews of interventions, vol. 4. Hoboken: Wiley; 2011.
20. Ades A, Lu G, Higgins J. The interpretation of random-effects meta-analysis in decision models. Med Decis Mak. 2005;25(6):646–54.
21. Borenstein M, Hedges LV, Higgins J, et al. A basic introduction to fixed-effect and random-effects models for meta-analysis. Res Synth Methods. 2010;1(2):97–111.
22. Borenstein M, Hedges LV, Higgins J, Rothstein HR. Meta-Regression. Introduction to meta-analysis; 2009. p. 187–203.
23. Clemett R, Darlow R Results of screening low-birth-weight infants for retinopathy of prematurity. Curr Opin Ophthalmol. 1999;10:155–63.
24. Ophthalmology AAoPSo. Screening examination of premature infants for retinopathy of prematurity. Pediatrics. 2013;131(1):189–95.
25. Isaza G, Arora S. Incidence and severity of retinopathy of prematurity in extremely premature infants. Can J Opthalmol. 2012;47:296–300.
26. Hwang JH, Lee EH, Kim EA. Retinopathy of prematurity among very-low-birth-weight infants in Korea: incidence, treatment, and risk factors. J Korean Med Sci. 2015;30(Suppl 1):S88S94.
27. Gunn DJ, Cartwright DW, Gole GA. Incidence of retinopathy of prematurity in extremely premature infants over an 18-year period. Clin Exp Ophthalmol. 2012;40:93–9.
28. Cerman E, Balci SY, Yenice OS, et al. Screening for retinopathy of prematurity in a tertiary ophthalmology Department in Turkey: incidence, outcomes, and risk factors. Ophthalmic Surg Lasers Imaging Retina. 2014;45: 550–5.
29. Mitsiakos G, Papageorgiou A. Incidence and factors predisposing to retinopathy of prematurity in inborn infants less than 32 weeks of gestation. Hippokratia. 2016;20(2):121–6.
30. Bas AY, Koc E, Dilmen U; ROP Neonatal Study Group. Incidence and severity of retinopathy of prematurity in Turkey. Br J Ophthalmol. 2015;99(10):1311-4. https://doi.org/10.1136/bjophthalmol-2014-306286.
31. Group ETfRoPC. The incidence and course of retinopathy of prematurity: findings from the early treatment for retinopathy of prematurity study. Pediatrics 2005;116(1):15–23.
32. Vakilian K, Ranjbaran M, Khorsandi M, et al. Prevalence of preterm labor in Iran: a systematic review and meta-analysis. Int J Reprod Biomed. 2015;13(12):743–8.
33. Tabarez-Carvajal AC, Montes-Cantillo M, Unkrich KH, et al. Retinopathy of prematurity: screening and treatment in Costa Rica. Br J Ophthalmol. 2017; 101(12):1709–13. https://doi.org/10.1136/bjophthalmol-2016-310005. [Epub ahead of print]
34. Abdel HA, Mohamed GB, Othman MF. Retinopathy of prematurity: a study of incidence and risk factors in NICU of al-Minya University Hospital in Egypt. J Clin Neonatol. 2012;1(2):76–81. https://doi.org/10.4103/2249-4847.96755.
35. Bassiouny MR. Risk factors associated with retinopathy of prematurity: a study from Oman. J Trop Pediatr. 1996;42:355–8.
36. Nair PM, Ganesh A, Mitra S, et al. Retinopathy of prematurity in VLBW and extreme LBW babies. Indian J Pediatr. 2003;70:303–6.
37. Hadi AM, Hamdy IS. Correlation between risk factors during the neonatal period and appearance of retinopathy of prematurity in preterm infants in neonatal intensive care units in Alexandria, Egypt. Clin Ophthalmol. 2013;7:831–7.
38. Ratra D, Akhundova L, Das MK. Retinopathy of prematurity like retinopathy in full-term infants. Oman J Ophthalmol. 2017;10(3):167-172. https://doi.org/10.4103/ojo.OJO_141_2016.
39. Sahin A, Sahin M, Türkcü FM, et al. Incidence of retinopathy of prematurity in extremely premature infants. ISRN Pediatr. 2014;2014:134347.
40. Shah VA, Yeo CL, Ling YL, et al. Incidence, risk factors of retinopathy of prematurity among very low birth weight infants in Singapore. Ann Acad Med Singap. 2005;34:169–78.
41. Chen M, Citil A, McCabe F, et al. Infection, oxygen, and immaturity: interacting risk factors for retinopathy of prematurity. Neonatology. 2011;99:125–32.
42. Darlow BA, Hutchinson JL, Henderson-Smart DJ, et al. Prenatal risk factors for severe retinopathy of prematurity among very preterm infants of the Australian and New Zealand neonatal network. Pediatrics. 2005;115:990–6.
43. Badriah C, Amir I, Elvioza SR, et al. Prevalence and 325 risk factors of retinopathy of prematurity. Paediatr Indones. 2012;52:138–44. 327
44. Rizalya D, Rudolf T, Rohsiswatmo R. Screening for 328 retinopathy of prematurity in hospital with limited facil- 329 ities. Sari Pediatri. 2012;14:185–90.
45. Yau GS, Lee JW, Tam VT, et al. Incidence and risk factors of retinopathy of prematurity from 2 neonatal intensive care units in a Hong Kong Chinese population. Asia Pac J Ophthalmol. 2016;5(3):185–91. https://doi.org/10.1097/APO.0000000000000167.
46. Reyes ZS, Al-Mulaabed SW, Bataclan F, et al. Retinopathy of prematurity: revisiting incidence and risk factors from Oman compared to other countries. Oman J Ophthalmol. 2017;10(1):26–32.
47. Yu VY, Upadhyay A. Neonatal management of the growth-restricted infant. Semin Fetal Neonatal Med. 2004;9:403–9.
48. Weinberger B, Laskin DL, Heck DE, et al. Oxygen toxicity in premature infants. Toxicol Appl Pharmacol. 2002;181:60–7.

49. Hardy P, Beauchamp M, Sennlaub F, et al. New insights into the retinal circulation: inflammatory lipid mediators in ischemic retinopathy. Prostaglandins Leukot Essent Fatty Acids. 2005;72:301–25.

50. O'Donovan DJ, Fernandes CJ. Free radicals and diseases in premature infants. Antioxid Redox Signal. 2004;6:169–76.

51. Yoon HS. Neonatal innate immunity and toll-like receptor. Korean J Pediatr. 2010;53:985–8.

52. Naderian G, Parvaresh M, Rismanchiyan A, et al. Refractive errors after laser therapy for retinopathy of prematurity. Int J Ophthalmol. 2009;15(1):13–8.

53. Hosseini H, Farvardin M, Attarzadeh A, et al. Advanced retinopathy of prematurity at Poostchi ROP clinic, Shiraz. Bina J Ophthalmol 2009; 15(1):19–25.

54. Karkhaneh RER, Ghojehzadeh L, Kadivar M, et al. Incidence and risk factors of retinopathy of prematurity. Bina J Ophthalmol. 2005;11(1):81–90.

55. Nadeian GMH, Hadipour M, Sajjadi H. Prevalence and rsskfactor for retinopathy of prematuority in isfahan. Bina J Ophthalmol. 2010;15(3):208–13.

56. Mansouri MRKM, Karkhaneh R, Riazi Esfahani M, et al. Prevalence and risk factors of retinopathy of prematurity in very low birth weight or low gestational age infants. Bina J Ophthalmol. 2007;12(4):428–34.

57. Nakhshab MBG, Amiri A, Ashaghi M. Prevalence of preterm infant retinopathy in neonatal intensive care unit Buali Sari Hospital. J Mazandaran Univ Med Sci. 2003;13(39):63–70.

58. Daraie G, Nooripoor S, Ashrafi AM, et al. Incidence of retinopathy of prematurity and some related factors in premature infants born at amir–al–momenin hospital in Semnan. Iran Koomesh. 2016;17(2):297–303.

59. Fayazi AHM, Fayzollazade M, GHolzar A, et al. Prevalence of retinopathy in preterm infants admitted to neonatal intensive care unit of Alzahra hospital in Tabriz. J Tabriz Univ Med Sci. 2009;30(4):63–6.

60. Sadeghi KHA, Hashemi F, Haydarzade M, et al. Prevalence and risk factors of retinopathy in preterm infants. J Tabriz Univ Med Sc. 2008;30(2):73–7.

61. Ebrahimiadib N, Roohipour R, Karkhaneh R, et al. Internet-based versus conventional referral system for retinopathy of prematurity screening in Iran. Ophthalmic Epidemiol. 2016;23(5):292–7.

62. Ghaseminejad A, Niknafs P. Distribution of retinopathy of prematurity and its risk factors. Iran J Pediatr. 2011;21(2):209.

63. Khatami SF, Yousefi A, Bayat GF, et al. Retinopathy of prematurity among 1000-2000 gram birth weight newborn infants. Iran J Pediatr. 2008;18(2):137–42.

64. Sabzehei MK, Afjeh SA, Farahani AD, et al. Retinopathy of prematurity: incidence, risk factors, and outcome. Arch Iran Med. 2013;16(9):507.

65. Saeidi R, Hashemzadeh A, Ahmadi S, et al. Prevalence and predisposing factors of retinopathy of prematurity in very low-birth-weight infants discharged from NICU. Iran J Pediatr. 2009;19(1):59–63.

66. Azinfar MAM, Pasha Z, Amad M. Prevalence of premature newborns discharged from NICU and infants in Shafizadeh Ami Children's hospital [dissertation]. Babol, Iran; Babol Univ Med; 2005.

67. Karkhanehyousefi NRA, Mekaniki A. Prevalence of retinopathy in immature newborns referred to eye Clinic of Shahid Beheshti Hospital in Babol [dissertation]. Babol, Iran; Babol Univ Med; 2009.

68. Ebrahimzade MKR, Esfahani M, Kadpour M, et al. The prevalence of retinopathy in preterm infants in preterm infants referred to Farabi hospital from the beginning of the year 2002 to the beginning of 2008 and the evaluation of short-term laser therapy results [dissertation]. Tehran: Islamic Azad Univ Med; 2009.

69. Mirzaee SA, Mohagheghi P. Determine the prevalence of retinopathy (ROP) in infants admitted to the NICU department of Milad Hospital [dissertation]. Tehran: Islamic Azad Univ Med; 2010.

70. Mousavi SZ, Karkhaneh R, Riazi-Esfahani M, et al. Retinopathy of prematurity in infants with late retinal examination. J Ophthalmic Vis Res. 2009;4(1):24.

71. Foladinezhad MMM, GHarib M, SHishari F, Soltani M. Frequency, severity and some risk factors of retinopathy in premature infants of Taleghani Hospital in Gorgan. J Gorgan Univ Med Sc. 2009;11(2):51–4.

72. Mousavi SZKR, Riazi-Esfahani M, Mansouri MR, et al. Incidence, severity and risk factors for retinopathy ofPrematurity in premature infants with late retinal examination. Bina J Ophthalmol. 2008;13(4):412–7.

73. Sadeghzadeh M, Khoshnevisasl P, Parvaneh M, et al. Early and late outcome of premature newborns with history of neonatal intensive care units admission at 6 years old in Zanjan. Northwestern Iran Iran J Child Neurol. 2016;10(2):67.

74. Bayat-Mokhtari M, Pishva N, Attarzadeh A, et al. Incidence and risk factors of retinopathy of prematurity among preterm infants in shiraz/Iran. Iran J Pediatr. 2010;20(3):303.

75. Karkhaneh R, Shokravi N. Assessment of retinopathy of prematurity among 150 premature neonates in Farabi eye hospital. Acta Med Iran. 2001;39(1):35–8.

76. Babaei H, Ansari MR, Alipour AA, et al. Incidence and risk factors for retinopathy of prematurity in very low birth weight infants in Kermanshah. Iran World Appl Sci J. 2012;18(5):600–4.

77. Abrishami M, Maemori G-A, Boskabadi H, et al. Incidence and risk factors of retinopathy of prematurity in Mashhad. Northeast Iran Red Crescent Med J. 2013;15(3):229.

78. Riazi-Esfahani M, Alizadeh Y, Karkhaneh R, et al. Retinopathy of prematurity: single versus multiple-birth pregnancies. J Ophthalmic Vis Res. 2008;3(1):47.

79. Alizadeh Y, Zarkesh M, Moghadam RS, et al. Incidence and risk factors for retinopathy of prematurity in north of Iran. J Ophthalmic Vis Res. 2015;10(4):424.

80. Mousavi SZ, Karkhaneh R, Roohipoor R, et al. Screening for retinopathy of prematurity: the role of educating the parents. J Ophthalmol. 2010;22(2):13–8.

81. MousavibS Zb EM, Roohipoor R, Jabbarvand M, et al. Characteristics of advanced stages of retinopathy of prematurity. J Ophthalmol. 2010;22(2):19–24.

82. Feghhi M, Altayeb SMH, Haghi F, et al. Incidence of retinopathy of prematurity and risk factors in the south-western region of Iran. Middle East Afr J Ophthalmol. 2012;19(1):101.

83. Afarid M, Hosseini H, Abtahi B. Screening for retinopathy of prematurity in south of Iran. Middle East Afr J Ophthalmol. 2012;19(3):277.

84. Ahmadpour-kacho M, Zahed Pasha Y, Rasoulinejad SA, et al. Correlation between retinopathy of prematurity and clinical risk index for babies score. J Tehran Univ Med S. 2014;72(6):404–11.

85. Ahmadpour-Kacho M, Jashni Motlagh A, Rasoulinejad SA, et al. Correlation between hyperglycemia and retinopathy of prematurity. Pediatr Int. 2014; 56(5):726–30.

86. Rasoulinejad SA, Montazeri M. Retinopathy of prematurity in neonates and its risk factors: a seven year study in northern iran. Open Ophthalmol J. 2016;10:17.

87. Karkhaneh R, Mousavi S-Z, Riazi-Esfahani M, et al. Incidence and risk factors of retinopathy of prematurity in a tertiary eye hospital in Tehran. Br J Ophthalmol. 2008;92(11):1446–9.

88. Khalesi N, Shariat M, Fallahi M, et al. Evaluation of risk factors for retinopathy in preterm infant: a case-control study in a referral hospital in Iran. Minerva Pediatr. 2015;67(3):231–7.

89. Ebrahim M, Ahmad RS, Mohammad M. Incidence and risk factors of retinopathy of prematurity in Babol. North of Iran Ophthalmic Epidemiol. 2010;17(3):166–70.

90. Roohipoor R, Karkhaneh R, Farahani A, et al. Retinopathy of prematurity screening criteria in Iran: new screening guidelines. Arch Dis Child Fetal Neonatal Ed. 2016;101(4):F288–F93.

91. Mansouri M, Hemmatpour S, Sedighiani F, et al. Factors associated with retinopathy of prematurity in hospitalized preterm infants in Sanandaj. Iran Electronic physician. 2016;8(9):2931.

15

The increasing prevalence of myopia and high myopia among high school students

Min Chen[1,2], Aimin Wu[3], Lina Zhang[1,4], Wei Wang[1,2], Xinyi Chen[1,2], Xiaoning Yu[1,2] and Kaijun Wang[1,2*]

Abstract

Background: Myopia is the leading cause of preventable blindness in children and young adults. Multiple epidemiological studies have confirmed a high prevalence of myopia in Asian countries. However, fewer longitudinal studies have been performed to evaluate the secular changes in the prevalence of myopia, especially high myopia in China. In the present study, we investigated trends in the prevalence of myopia among high school students in Fenghua city, eastern China, from 2001 to 2015.

Methods: This was a population-based, retrospective study. Data were collected among 43,858 third-year high school students. Noncycloplegic autorefraction was used to determine refractive error, which was defined as low myopia, moderate myopia, high myopia and very high myopia according to the spherical equivalent from the worse eye of each participant. The prevalence of myopia was calculated and the annual percentage change (APC) was used to quantify the time trends. All analyses were conducted using the SPSS, Stata and Graphpad Prism software.

Results: From 2001 to 2015, the prevalence of overall myopia increased from 79.5% to 87.7% (APC =0.59%), with a significant increase of moderate myopia (38.8% to 45.7%, APC = 0.78%), high myopia (7.9% to 16.6%, APC = 5.48%) and very high myopia (0.08% to 0.92%, APC = 14.59%), while the prevalence of low myopia decreased from 32.7% to 24.4% (APC = − 1.73%). High myopia and very high myopia contributed the major part of the increasing trend of myopia prevalence (contribution rate 27.00% and 69.07%, respectively).

Conclusions: During the 15-year period, there was a remarkable increase in the prevalence of high and very high myopia among high school students, which might become a serious public health problem in China for the next few decades.

Keywords: Epidemiology, Myopia, High myopia, Prevalence, High school student

* Correspondence: ze_wkj@zju.edu.cn
[1]Eye Center, the 2nd Affiliated Hospital, Medical College of Zhejiang University, Hangzhou, China
[2]Zhejiang Provincial Key Lab of Ophthalmology, Hangzhou, China
Full list of author information is available at the end of the article

Background

Myopia is the leading cause of preventable blindness in children and young adults [1]. Recently, there has been growing evidence that the prevalence of myopia has increased rapidly in many parts of the world, especially in East and South Asia [2, 3]. For example, the prevalence of myopia were 96.5% in 19-year-old males in Seoul in 2010 [4]. In Taiwan, the prevalence of myopia in male military conscripts aged 18 to 24 years was 86.1% in 2010–2011 [5]. In China, the prevalence of myopia was 95.5% in university students in Shanghai [6], 84.6% in school children in Shandong [7]. Dramatic increases were also seen in other parts of the world [8, 9]. It has been estimated that myopia will affect nearly 5 billion people by the year 2050 and become a major public health challenge [10].

Due to its high prevalence in China, people tend to ignore the importance of myopia prevention and control, especially in high and very high myopia. High myopia-associated complications such as retinal detachment, macular lesions, peripapillary deformation and myopia choroidal neovascularization may lead to severe and irreversible visual loss [11]. Related complications of high myopia will become one of the main causes of visual impairment in the next few decades in the world [12, 13]. Jung et al. reported that the prevalence of high myopia was 21.6% in 19-year-old males in Seoul in 2010 [4]. In Singapore, the prevalence of high myopia slightly increased from 13.1% (1996–1997) to 14.7% (2009–2010) in young male subjects [14].

In the present study, we analyzed longitudinal data obtained from high school students in Fenghua city, eastern China from 2001 to 2015, to evaluate secular trends in myopia prevalence, especially in high and very high myopia, to provide guidance for the future management of myopia in China.

Methods

Study population

This retrospective study was conducted from 2001 to 2015, in Fenghua city, a county-level city located in the eastern part of Zhejiang province, China. There were seven high schools in this city. As part of the physical examination that students undertake for the National College Entrance Examination, the refractive status of all the third-year students (grade 12) were routinely collected each year. Fenghua people's hospital was in charge of the physical examination in this district. All students were registered by name, gender, age, visual activity and refractive status. The database was kept by the hospital and we retrieved the data between 2001 and 2015 for analysis, with the official permission from the hospital. Ethical approval was obtained from the Medical College of Zhejiang University and Fenghua people's hospital Ethics Review Board. The study adhered to the tenets of the Declaration of Helsinki.

Eye examination

Eye examination was conducted by two experienced ophthalmologists and two qualified optometrists from the ophthalmology department of Fenghua people's hospital. All subjects underwent a measurement of uncorrected visual acuity (UCVA) at 5 m (Standard Logarithmic Visual Acuity E chart). If UCVA was lower than 5.0, best-corrected visual acuity (BCVA) was measured with subjective refraction. A slit lamp examination was performed to exclude opacity of optical media.

Refraction error measurement

Refractive error (RE) of each subject was measured by automatic refractometer (AR-600; Nidek Ltd., Tokyo, Japan) without cycloplegia. The spherical equivalent refraction (SER) was calculated by the addition of the spherical refraction and half the cylindrical refraction. The baseline SER from the worse eye of each student was used for analysis, which was divided in to five groups: non-myopia (SER less than -0.5 D), low myopia (SER between -0.5 D and -3.0 D), moderate myopia (SER between -3.0 D and -6.0 D), high myopia (SER greater than -6.0 D), and very high myopia (SER greater than -10.0 D).

Meta-analysis

A meta-analysis was performed to evaluate myopia prevalence among young adults. A comprehensive literature search was conducted in PubMed and web of science covering publications up to December 2, 2017 by two independent authors, using the following key words ("myopia" OR "refractive error" OR "vision disorder") AND ("prevalence" OR "epidemiology" OR "incidence") AND ("young adults" OR "students"). Articles were selected based on title, abstract and full texts. The major inclusion criteria for this study were mentioning visual disorders and myopia prevalence among 16 to 39 years old young adults, and exclusion criteria were lack of reference to the prevalence of visual disorders, unrelated studies, and low quality of articles. The methodological quality evaluation of eligible studies was based on the following factors: specific diagnostic criteria, clear refraction method and matched age group. Two authors (XN Y and MC) independently review and extracted data form the eligible studies. The following information was extracted from each article: first author, publication date, region and ethnicity, gender composition, mean age, sample size, refraction method, myopia definition, prevalence of myopia and high myopia etc. Statistical analysis was conducted using Stata 12.0 software (Stata Corp., Texas, USA). A Q-statistic test was applied and $P < 0.10$

was considered to be statistically significant. Besides, I^2 value was used to evaluate the heterogeneity, with > 50% as high degree of heterogeneity [15]. When no significant heterogeneity was observed among studies, the summary was pooled by using the fixed-effects model. Otherwise, the random-effects model was applied instead [16, 17]. Egger's linear regression test [18] and Begg's funnel plot [19] were used to assess the Potential publication bias.

Statistical analysis
Median [interquartile range (IQR)] and percentage were reported in the descriptive analyses for the continuous variables and the categorical variables, respectively. Myopia prevalence was calculated for fifteen 1-year time intervals from 2001 to 2015. Chi-squared test was used to compare the differences in myopia prevalence between males and females. The annual percentage change (APC) for myopia prevalence was used to quantify the time trends [20, 21]. A regression line was fitted to the natural logarithm of the rates, $y = \alpha + \beta x + \varepsilon$, where $y = \ln (rate)$ and x = calender year, and then the APC was calculated as $100 \times (e^\beta - 1)$. We also calculated the relative contributions for rate changes which provide us for determining the contributions from different kinds of myopia made to the overall trends [22]. All analyses (except when noted) were performed using SPSS statistics 22.0 (SPSS Inc., Chicago, Illinois, USA) and Graphpad Prism software, version 5.0 (Graphpad software Inc., SanDiego, CA, USA). A P value of less than 0.05 was considered statistically significant.

Results
Characteristics of the study population
Basic characteristics of the study population were summarized in Table 1. A total of 43,858 high school students were enrolled from 2001 to 2015, including 21,843 (49.8%) males and 22,015 (50.2%) females. Those who had a history of traumas, eye diseases or refractive surgeries were excluded from the analysis. The average age of the subjects was 18.46 ± 0.69 years old.

Changes in refractive error
During the 15 years period, the mean SER significantly increased both in the right eye (from – 2.5 ± 2.0 D to – 3.4 ± 2.3 D) and in the left eye (from – 2.4 ± 2.0D to – 3.2 ± 2.3D). Spearman's correlation analysis indicated that the refractive error (RE) was closely related between the right and left eyes (Table 2). Representative results presented in our study were from the worse eye of each subject.

Prevalence of myopia
From 2001 to 2015, the prevalence of overall myopia increased from 79.5% to 87.7% (P < 0.05, Fig. 1). Compared between the five groups, the prevalence of non-myopia (20.5% to 12.4%) and low myopia (32.7% to 24.4%) significantly decreased, with a significant increase in the prevalence of moderate myopia (38.8% to 45.7%), high myopia (7.9% to 16.6%) and very high myopia (0.08% to 0.92%).

Fig 2 and Table 3 showed the time trend of myopia prevalence in each subgroup during 2001 to 2015. The annual percent change (APC) was 0.59% (95%CI: 0.41 to

Table 1 Basic characteristics of the study population and difference in myopia prevalence between females and males in Fenghua city, eastern China, 2001 to 2015

Year	N (%)	Age	Gender Female/Male	Myopia prevalence Female/Male	OR	95% CI	P value
2001	2418	18.50 ± 0.65	1084/1334	81.1/78.3	1.19	0.98 to 1.46	0.087
2002	2324	18.52 ± 0.59	997/1327	86.0/81.8	1.37	1.09 to 1.71	0.007
2003	2462	18.51 ± 0.64	1062/1400	88.7/79.4	2.04	1.62 to 2.57	0.000
2004	2654	18.61 ± 0.68	1247/1407	87.7/79.0	1.90	1.53 to 2.35	0.000
2005	3072	18.48 ± 0.72	1436/1636	85.7/78.2	1.68	1.39 to 2.02	0.000
2006	2974	18.49 ± 0.73	1454/1520	85.8/78.2	1.69	1.40 to 2.05	0.000
2007	3014	18.34 ± 0.57	1497/1517	89.0/78.8	2.19	1.79 to 2.69	0.000
2008	3055	18.64 ± 0.74	1481/1574	89.5/80.7	2.03	1.65 to 2.50	0.000
2009	2930	18.56 ± 0.73	1517/1413	89.0/81.0	1.89	1.54 to 2.33	0.000
2010	3276	18.46 ± 0.70	1801/1475	89.7/84.0	1.65	1.35 to 2.03	0.000
2011	3079	18.51 ± 0.69	1655/1424	89.1/82.9	1.69	1.38 to 2.09	0.000
2012	3283	18.46 ± 0.71	1794/1489	90.1/82.2	1.97	1.60 to 2.41	0.000
2013	3234	18.41 ± 0.65	1755/1479	88.8/83.0	1.62	1.32 to 1.98	0.000
2014	3151	18.39 ± 0.62	1671/1480	90.9/85.3	1.72	1.38 to 2.14	0.000
2015	2932	18.31 ± 0.60	1564/1368	90.8/84.1	1.87	1.49 to 2.34	0.000

OR odds ratio, CI confidence interval, female vs male, Chi-square test

Table 2 Correlation of refractive error between the right and left eyes

Year	Right		Left		P value[a]	Spearman r
	Mean ± SD	Median (IQR)	Mean ± SD	Median (IQR)		
2001	−2.5 ± 2.0	−3.0(−4.0,-2.0)	−2.4 ± 2.0	−3.0(−4.0,-2.0)	0.021	0.90
2002	−2.7 ± 2.0	−3.0(−4.0,-2.0)	−2.6 ± 2.0	−3.0(−4.0,-2.0)	0.020	0.89
2003	−2.8 ± 2.0	−3.0(−4.5,-2.0)	−2.7 ± 2.0	−3.0(−4.0,-2.0)	0.011	0.89
2004	−2.8 ± 2.0	−3.0(−4.0,-2.0)	−2.7 ± 2.0	−3.0(−4.0,-2.0)	0.006	0.90
2005	−2.6 ± 2.1	−3.0(−4.0,-2.0)	−2.5 ± 2.1	−3.0(−4.0,-2.0)	0.004	0.90
2006	−2.7 ± 2.0	−3.0(−4.0,-2.0)	−2.6 ± 2.0	−3.0(−4.0,-2.0)	0.010	0.92
2007	−2.9 ± 2.0	−3.5(−4.0,-2.0)	−2.8 ± 2.0	−3.0(−4.0,-2.0)	0.037	0.91
2008	−3.0 ± 2.1	−3.5(−4.5,-2.0)	−2.9 ± 2.1	−3.5(−4.5,-2.0)	0.007	0.92
2009	−3.1 ± 2.2	−3.5(−5.0,-2.0)	−3.0 ± 2.2	−3.5(−4.5,-2.0)	0.022	0.93
2010	−3.1 ± 2.2	−3.5(−5.0,-2.25)	−3.0 ± 2.2	−3.5(−4.5,-2.0)	0.012	0.90
2011	−3.2 ± 2.1	−3.5(−5.0,-2.5)	−3.0 ± 2.2	−3.5(−4.75,-2.0)	0.011	0.92
2012	−3.2 ± 2.2	−3.5(−5.0,-2.5)	−3.1 ± 2.2	−3.5(−5.0,-2.0)	0.007	0.93
2013	−3.2 ± 2.1	−3.5(−5.0,-2.5)	−3.1 ± 2.2	−3.5(−5.0,-2.25)	0.010	0.91
2014	−3.3 ± 2.2	−3.5(−5.0,-2.5)	−3.1 ± 2.2	−3.5(−5.0,-2.25)	0.006	0.91
2015	−3.4 ± 2.3	−3.5(−5.0, −1.75)	−3.2 ± 2.3	−3.25(−5.0, −1.5)	0.000	0.93

RE refractive error, *IQR* interquartile range, [a] Mann Whitney test

0.77, $P = 0.000$). Significant decreasing trend was observed in low myopia subgroup (APC = − 1.73, 95%CI: -2.23 to − 1.24, $P = 0.000$), while significant increasing trend was found in moderate myopia (APC = 0.78, 95%CI: 0.36 to 1.20, $P = 0.001$), high myopia (APC = 5.48, 95%CI: 4.40 to 6.54, $P = 0.000$), especially in very high myopia (APC = 14.59, 95%CI: 7.33 to 22.34, $P = 0.001$). As shown in Table 4, high myopia (contribution rate 27.00%) and very high myopia (contribution rate 69.07%) contributed the major part of the increasing trend of myopia prevalence.

Males versus females

Compared between genders, the prevalence of overall myopia was higher in females than males (Chi-squared test, $P < 0.005$; except for 2001, $P = 0.087$, Table 1, Fig. 3). From 2001 to 2015, the prevalence of myopia increased 9.7% in female students (81.1% to 90.8%, mean = 88.1 ± 2.6%, $P < 0.001$) and 5.8% in male students (78.3% to 84.1%, mean = 81.1 ± 2.4%, P < 0.001), respectively. The odds ratio (OR) was 1.87 (95%CI: 1.49 to 2.34, $P = 0.000$) in 2015.

Meta-analysis of myopia prevalence

A meta-analysis was conducted to evaluate myopia prevalence in young adults. The search strategy identified 125 unique articles, from which 12 full-text articles were retrieved for final review after screening titles and abstracts. Characteristics of the included studies were summarized and shown in Table 5. No significant

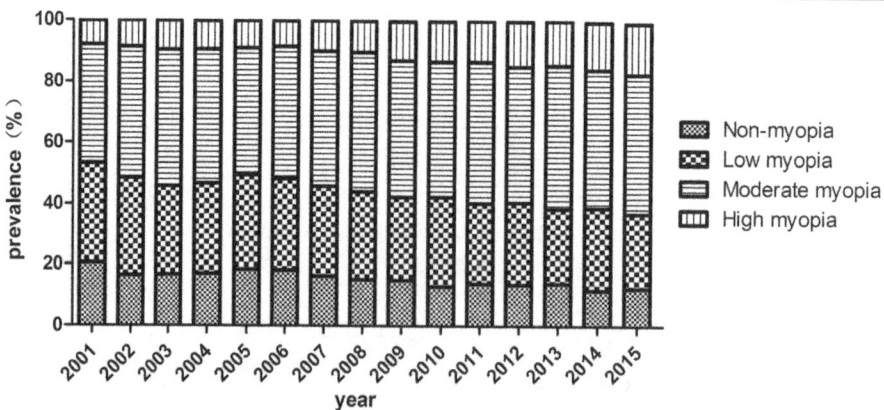

Fig. 1 Proportional distribution of refractive error among young adults in Fenghua city, eastern China, from 2001 to 2015

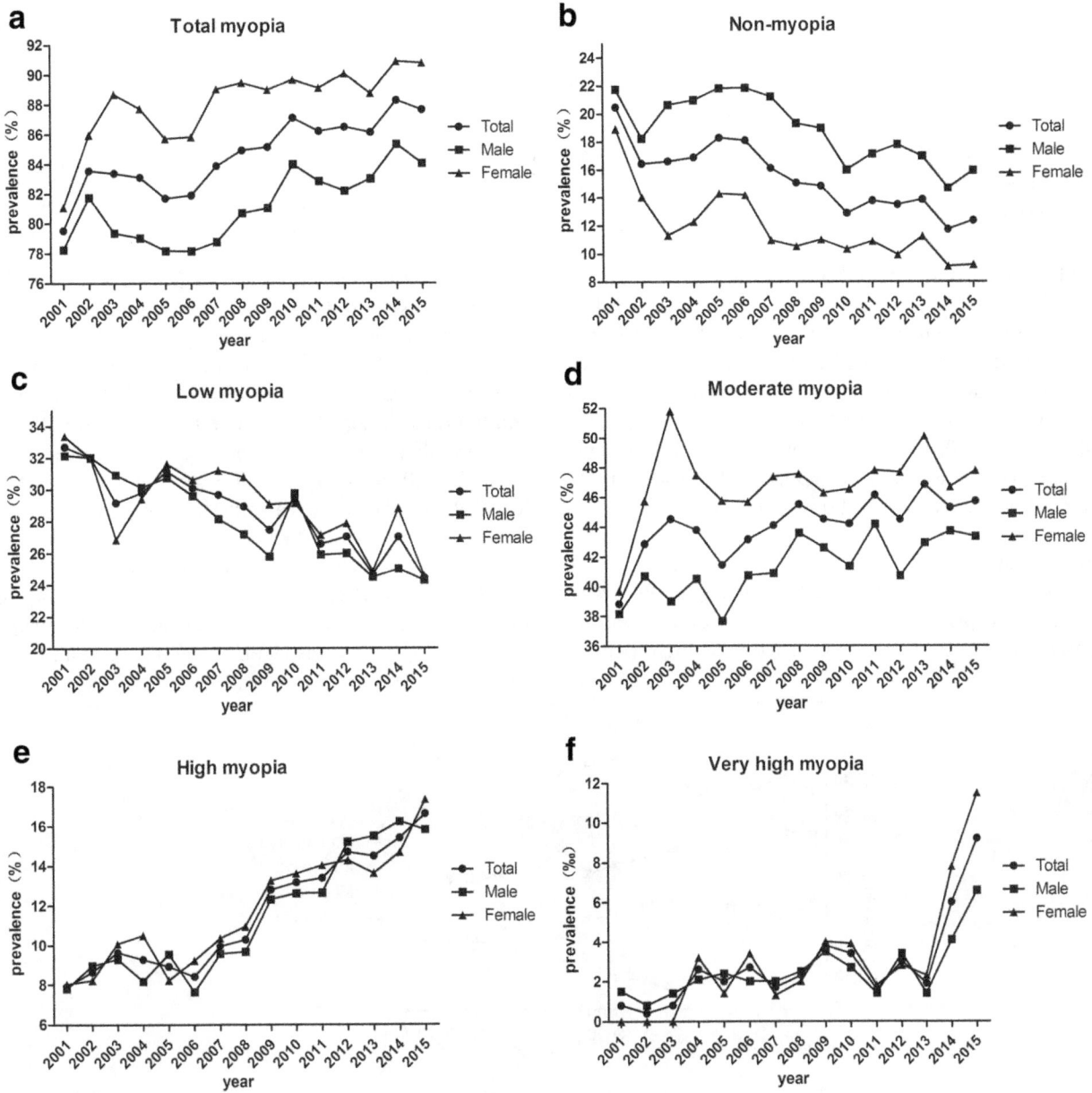

Fig. 2 Trends in myopia prevalence among young adults in Fenghua city, eastern China, from 2001 to 2015. (**a**) Total myopia group; (**b**) Non-myopia subgroup; (**c**) Low myopia subgroup; (**d**) Moderate myopia subgroup (**e**) High myopia subgroup and (**f**) Very high myopia subgroup

Table 3 Trends in myopia prevalence among high school students in Fenghua city, eastern China, during 2001 to 2015

	2001		2015		APC (%)	95%CI	P value
	N	Prevalence (%)	N	Prevalence (%)			
Total myopia	1923	79.53	2570	87.65	0.59	0.41, 0.77	0.000
Low myopia	791	32.71	716	24.42	−1.73	−2.23, −1.24	0.000
Moderate myopia	939	38.83	1340	45.70	0.78	0.36, 1.20	0.001
High myopia	191	7.90	487	16.61	5.48	4.40, 6.54	0.000
Very high myopia	2	0.08	27	0.92	14.59	7.33, 22,34	0.001

APC annual percent change, CI, confidence interval, Annual percent change between 2001 and 2015 was calculated by the myopia prevalence

Table 4 The relative contributions of decreasing and increasing trend of myopia prevalence among high school students in Fenghua city during 2001 to 2015

	Decreasing trend		Increasing trend	
	β	Contribution rate (%)	β	Contribution rate (%)
Low myopia	−0.02	100		
Moderate myopia			0.008	3.93
High myopia			0.053	27.00
Very high myopia			0.136	69.07

publication bias was found among the included studies (Begg's $P = 0.23$, Egger's $P = 0.34$). Sensitivity analysis showed that no individual study affected the pooled incidence, both in myopia and high myopia group. Forest plot for included studies showed the prevalence of myopia (Fig. 4 a, incidence 69.9, 95%CI = 49.5–90.3%, $I^2 = 100\%$, $P = 0.000$) and high myopia (Fig. 4 b, incidence 11.6, 95%CI = 7.6–15.6%, $I^2 = 99.9\%$, $P = 0.000$) in the random-effects model (Additional files 1).

Discussion

Our study showed a remarkable increase in the prevalence of myopia among high school students in eastern China over a 15-year period, especially high (APC = 5.48%) and very high myopia (APC = 14.59%). Females were more likely to develop myopia than males.

During the past decades, multiple population-based surveys from different areas of the world have provided comparative data on the prevalence of myopia in young adults (Table 5, Fig. 4 a). In our study, the overall myopia prevalence in high school students increased from 79.5% in 2001 to 87.7% in 2015. In Taiwan, the prevalence of myopia in 18-year-old children increased from 74% in 1983 to 84% in 2004 [23]. In Singapore, the overall myopia prevalence in young males increased from 79.2% in 1996–1997 to 81.6% in 2009–2010 [14]. In Korea, the prevalence of myopia and high myopia among young males was significantly higher in an urban

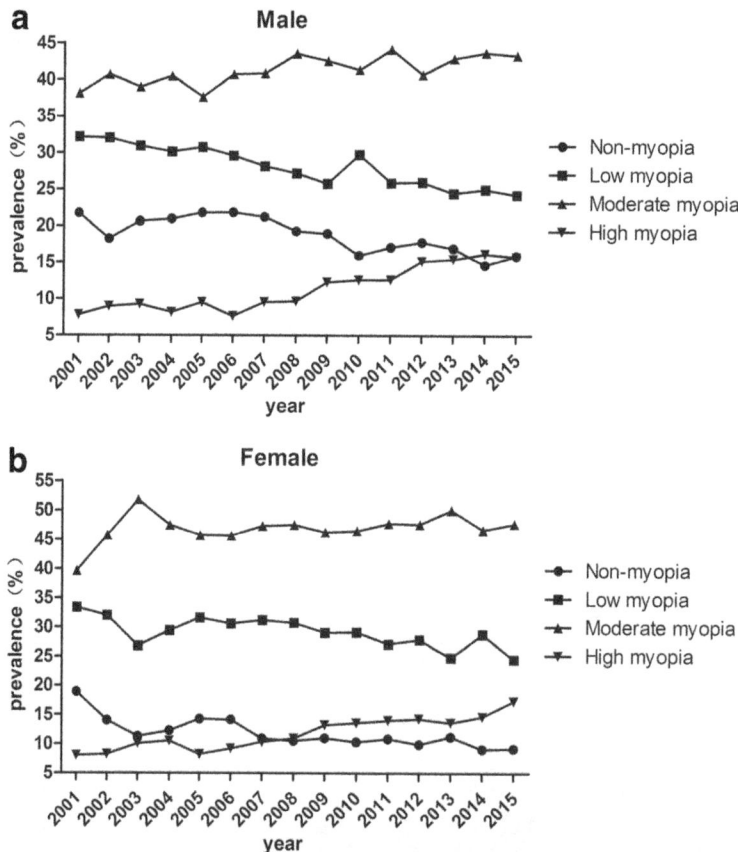

Fig. 3 The prevalence of myopia including subgroups in male (**a**) and female (**b**) subjects in Fenghua city, eastern China, from 2001 to 2015

Table 5 Summary and meta-analysis of recent studies on myopia and high myopia prevalence among young adults

Author (Year)	Location	Population-based?	N	Refraction method	Myopia definition	Mean Age	Prevalence (%)		Ref
							Myopia	High myopia	
Jung (2012)	Seoul, Korea	No[a]	23,616	CAR	< −0.5D	19	96.5	21.61	Ref 8
Sun (2012)	Shanghai, China	Yes	5083	NCAR	< −0.5D	20	95.5	19.5	Ref11
Lee (2013)	Taiwan, China	No[a]	5145	NCAR	< −0.5D	21.6	86.1	NA	Ref 9
Lin (2004)	Taiwan, China	Yes	45,345	CAR	<−0.25D	18	84	16	Ref17
Lee (2013)	Jeju, Korea	No[a]	2805	CAR	< −0.5D	19	83.3	6.8	Ref18
Koh (2014)	Singapore	No[a]	28,908	NCAR	< −0.5D	19.5	81.6	14.7	Ref10
Wu (2013)	Shandong, China	Yes	6364	NCAR	≤ −0.5D	17	80	14	Ref12
You (2014)	Beijing, China	Yes	16,771	NCAR	≤ −0.5D	18	74.2	1.8	Ref19
Li (2017)	Beijing, China	Yes	37,424	CAR	≤ −0.5D	15.25	66.48	6.69	Ref13
Matamoros (2015)	France	Yes	100,429	NCAR	≤ −0.5D	38.5	39.1	3.4	Ref19
Dayan (2005)	Israel	Yes	919,929	NCAR	≤ −0.5D	17	28.3	NA	Ref14
Mcknight (2014)	Western Australia	Yes	1344	CAR	< −0.5D	20.1	23.7	NA	Ref21
Meta-analysis[b]	–	–	–	–	–	–	70 (49–90)	12 (8–16)	–

[a]data from male conscripts; *NA* not available, *Ref* reference *NCAR* non-cycloplegic autorefraction, *CAR* cycloplegic autorefraction. [b] pooled prevalence and 95% confidence interval of myopia and high myopia by meta-analysis

population (96.5% and 21.6% in Seoul) [4] than in a rural population (83.3% and 6.8% in Jeju) [24], which indicated that environmental factors may play an important role in the development of myopia [24]. In contrast, the incidence of myopia in Western countries varies significantly between different ethnic groups, with a rate of 39.1% (2012–2013) in France [25], 72% (2007–2008) in Canada [26], 23.7% (2014) in Western Austria [27] and 33.1% (1999–2004) in the United States [28]. In general, myopia prevalence among young adults in East Asia is much higher than in Western countries.

Another remarkable change shown by our survey was that the proportion of high myopia (7.9% to 16.6%), especially very high myopia (0.08% to 0.92%) significantly increased during a 15-year period. Similar results have been reported previously (Table 5, Fig. 4 b). In the Taiwan study, the prevalence of high myopia among 18-year-old students increased from 10.9% in 1983 to 21% in 2000. The highest prevalence of high myopia was in Seoul (21.61% in 2012) [4], followed by Shanghai (19.5% in 2012) [6], Zhejiang (15.4% in 2014), Shandong (14% in 2013) [7],Beijing (6.69% in 2015) [29] and Jeju (6.8% in 2013) [5]. A recent systematic review predict that by 2050 there will be 4758 million people with myopia (49.8% of the world population) and 938 million people with high myopia (9.8% of the world population) [10]. It has been reported that high myopia is associated with several ocular disorders such as glaucoma, cataract, maculopathy, choroidal neovascularization, macular hole and retinal detachment [11]. The increasing prevalence of high myopia and very high myopia may therefore result in a series of associated complications and become a serious public health problem. Future prevention efforts should be strengthened to control the increasing prevalence of high and very high myopia.

The etiology of myopia still remains unclear. However, genetic and environmental factors are widely believed to play an important role [13]. Near work is one of the important environmental factors [30]. In China, the school system, especially the National College Entrance Examination is becoming more and more competitive. All students aged 16 to 18 years usually spend much time in study and expect to achieve high scores in this important examination. Lack of outdoor activity is very common in Chinese students. For example, 12.5% of students did not take part in any outdoor activity, and 11.2% of high school students did not participate in any physical education classes [31]. Associated factors, such as increasing educational pressures, higher school achievement, more near work and less time in sports activity, may contribute to the increasing prevalence of myopia [32]. Compared between genders, female students usually spend more time with reading and work-related issues, with less outdoor activities, making them more vulnerable to developing myopia [33]. A significantly higher prevalence of myopia in female subjects was observed in our survey, which was consistent with the results of previous studies [6, 34, 35].

Our study has several strengths. First, this was a population-based large scale study including 43,858 participants of similar age, which provided the status of myopia prevalence in this age group. Second, this was a long time period survey, which described a secular change and time trend of myopia prevalence during the past 15 years. However, several methodological

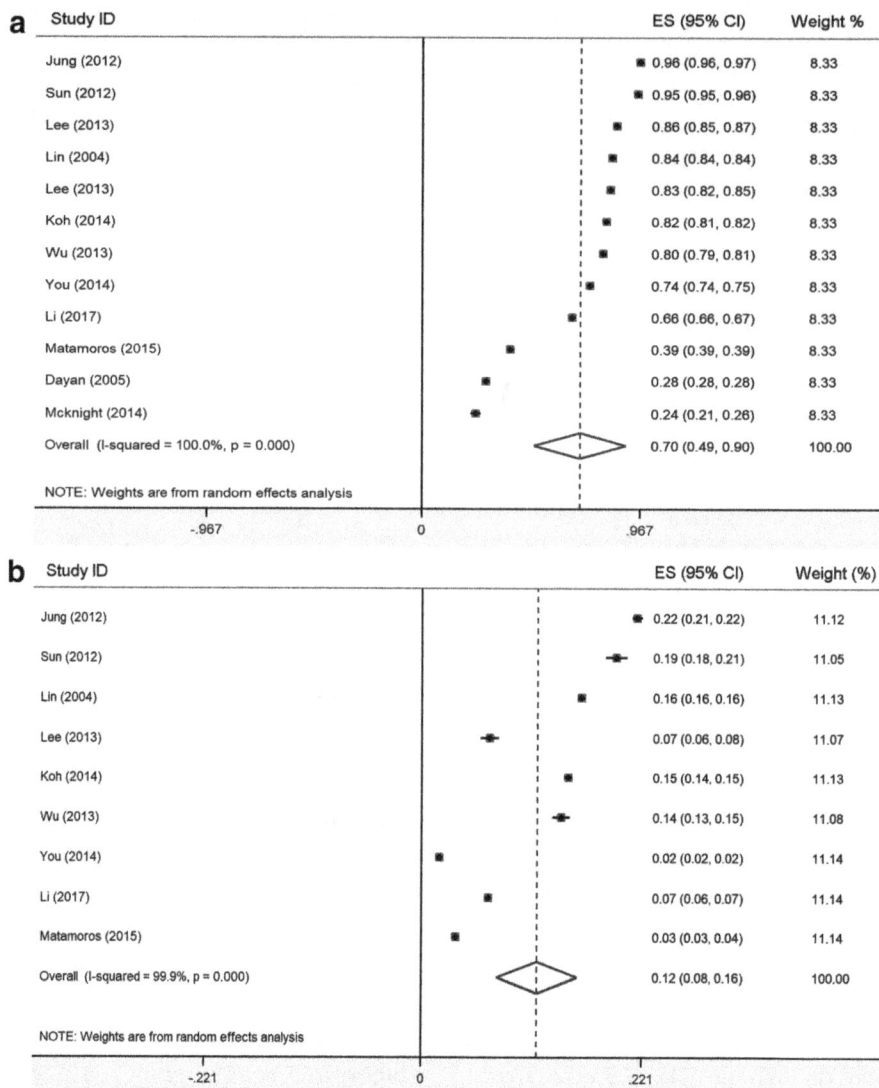

Fig. 4 Meta-analysis of the included studies evaluating the prevalence of myopia (**a**) and high myopia (**b**) in young adults, based on random-effects model

limitations should be acknowledged. First, cycloplegia was not used in our survey and it is well known that cycloplegic refraction yields better results than non-cycloplegic autorefraction. Non-cycloplegic auto-refraction can result in overestimation of myopia [36]. However, because this was a large scale physical examination, cycloplegic refraction was difficult to apply in each subject due to limited resources. Second, questionnaires and face-to-face interviews were not applied in the study and we have no access to the demographic factors (e.g., race/ ethnicity/ genetic background/ socioeconomic status and so on). Therefore, only descriptive analysis was presented and no multivariate analysis to evaluate the risk factors that account for the increasing prevalence.

Conclusion

In conclusion, there was a remarkable increase in the prevalence of myopia among high school students in eastern China over the past 15 years, especially high and very high myopia. Females were more likely to develop myopia than males. More attention should be paid to prevention and control of myopia in the future, especially high and very high myopia.

Abbreviations
APC: annual percentage change; BCVA: best-corrected visual acuity; CAR: cycloplegic autorefraction; CI: confidence interval; NCAR: non-cycloplegic autorefraction; RE: refractive error; SER: spherical equivalent refraction; VA: visual acuity

Acknowledgements
The authors thank the Colleges of Ophthalmology department (Fenghua people's hospital) and the participants involved in this study as well as the schools where the research was conducted.

Funding
This study was supported by the National Natural Science Foundation of China (No.81700829) and the Fundamental Research Funds for the Central Universities.

Authors' contributions
M C, AM W and KJ W designed research; AM W and LN Z conducted research; M C and W W analyzed data; XY C and XN Y performed statistical analysis; M C and KJ W wrote the draft of the manuscript. All authors read, reviewed and approved the final manuscript.

Competing interests
The authors declare that they have no competing interests.

Author details
[1]Eye Center, the 2nd Affiliated Hospital, Medical College of Zhejiang University, Hangzhou, China. [2]Zhejiang Provincial Key Lab of Ophthalmology, Hangzhou, China. [3]Department of Ophthalmology, Fenghua People's Hospital, Fenghua, Zhejiang, China. [4]Department of Ophthalmology, Lishui People's Hospital, Lishui, Zhejiang, China.

References
1. Morgan IG, Ohno-Matsui K, Saw SM. Myopia. Lancet. 2012;379(9827):1739–48.
2. Wong YL, Saw SM. Epidemiology of Pathologic myopia in Asia and worldwide. Asia Pac J Ophthalmol (Phila). 2016;5(6):394–402.
3. Morgan IG, He M, Rose KA. EPIDEMIC OF PATHOLOGIC MYOPIA: what can laboratory studies and epidemiology tell us? Retina. 2017;37(5):989–97.
4. Jung SK, Lee JH, Kakizaki H, Jee D. Prevalence of myopia and its association with body stature and educational level in 19-year-old male conscripts in Seoul, South Korea. Invest Ophthalmol Vis Sci. 2012;53(9):5579–83.
5. Lee YY, Lo CT, Sheu SJ, Lin JL. What factors are associated with myopia in young adults? A survey study in Taiwan military conscripts. Invest Ophthalmol Vis Sci. 2013;54(2):1026–33.
6. Sun J, Zhou J, Zhao P, Lian J, Zhu H, Zhou Y, Sun Y, Wang Y, Zhao L, Wei Y, Wang L, Cun B, Ge S, Fan X. High prevalence of myopia and high myopia in 5060 Chinese university students in shanghai. Invest Ophthalmol Vis Sci. 2012;53(12):7504–9.
7. Wu JF, Bi HS, Wang SM, Hu YY, Wu H, Sun W, Lu TL, Wang XR, Jonas JB. Refractive error, visual acuity and causes of vision loss in children in Shandong, China. The Shandong children eye study. PLoS One. 2013;8(12):e82763.
8. Bar Dayan Y, Levin A, Morad Y, Grotto I, Ben-David R, Goldberg A, Onn E,
Avni I, Levi Y, Benyamini OG. The changing prevalence of myopia in young adults: a 13-year series of population-based prevalence surveys. Invest Ophthalmol Vis Sci. 2005;46(8):2760–5.
9. Vitale S, Sperduto RD, Ferris FL 3rd. Increased prevalence of myopia in the United States between 1971-1972 and 1999-2004. Arch Ophthalmol. 2009;127(12):1632–9.
10. Holden BA, Fricke TR, Wilson DA, Jong M, Naidoo KS, Sankaridurg P, Wong TY, Naduvilath TJ, Resnikoff S. Global prevalence of myopia and high myopia and temporal trends from 2000 through 2050. Ophthalmology. 2016;123(5):1036–42.
11. Ikuno Y. Overview of the complications of high myopia. Retina. 2017;37(12):2347–51.
12. Leo SW. Scientific Bureau of World Society of Paediatric O, strabismus. Current approaches to myopia control Curr Opin Ophthalmol. 2017;28(3):267–75.
13. Hopf S, Pfeiffer N. Epidemiology of myopia. Ophthalmologe. 2017;114(1):20–3.
14. Koh V, Yang A, Saw SM, Chan YH, Lin ST, Tan MM, Tey F, Nah G, Ikram MK. Differences in prevalence of refractive errors in young Asian males in Singapore between 1996-1997 and 2009-2010. Ophthalmic Epidemiol. 2014;21(4):247–55.
15. Yu X, Lyu D, Dong X, He J, Yao K. Hypertension and risk of cataract: a meta-analysis. PLoS One. 2014;9(12):e114012.
16. Higgins JP, Thompson SG, Deeks JJ, Altman DG. Measuring inconsistency in meta-analyses. BMJ. 2003;327(7414):557–60.
17. DerSimonian R, Kacker R. Random-effects model for meta-analysis of clinical trials: an update. Contemporary clinical trials. 2007;28(2):105–14.
18. Egger M, Davey Smith G, Schneider M, Minder C. Bias in meta-analysis detected by a simple, graphical test. BMJ. 1997;315(7109):629–34.
19. Begg CB, Mazumdar M. Operating characteristics of a rank correlation test for publication bias. Biometrics. 1994;50(4):1088–101.
20. Li N, Chen YL, Li J, Li LL, Jiang CZ, Zhou C, Liu CX, Li D, Gong TT, Wu QJ, Huang YH. Decreasing prevalence and time trend of gastroschisis in 14 cities of Liaoning Province: 2006-2015. Sci Rep. 2016;6:33333.
21. Hankey BF, Ries LA, Kosary CL, Feuer EJ, Merrill RM, Clegg LX, Edwards BK. Partitioning linear trends in age-adjusted rates. Cancer Causes Control. 2000;11(1):31–5.
22. Xiang YB, Zhang W, Gao LF, Liu ZW, Xu WH, Liu EJ, Ji BT. Methods for time trend analysis of cancer incidence rates. Zhonghua Liu Xing Bing Xue Za Zhi. 2004;25(2):173–7.
23. Lin LL, Shih YF, Hsiao CK, Chen CJ. Prevalence of myopia in Taiwanese schoolchildren: 1983 to 2000. Ann Acad Med Singap. 2004;33(1):27–33.
24. Lee JH, Jee D, Kwon JW, Lee WK. Prevalence and risk factors for myopia in a rural Korean population. Invest Ophthalmol Vis Sci. 2013;54(8):5466–71.
25. Matamoros E, Ingrand P, Pelen F, Bentaleb Y, Weber M, Korobelnik JF, Souied E, Leveziel N. Prevalence of myopia in France: a cross-sectional analysis. Medicine (Baltimore). 2015;94(45):e1976.
26. Hrynchak PK, Mittelstaedt A, Machan CM, Bunn C, Irving EL. Increase in myopia prevalence in clinic-based populations across a century. Optom Vis Sci. 2013;90(11):1331–41.
27. McKnight CM, Sherwin JC, Yazar S, Forward H, Tan AX, Hewitt AW, Pennell CE, McAllister IL, Young TL, Coroneo MT, Mackey DA. Myopia in young adults is inversely related to an objective marker of ocular sun exposure: the western Australian Raine cohort study. Am J Ophthalmol. 2014;158(5):1079–85.
28. Vitale S, Ellwein L, Cotch MF, Ferris FL 3rd, Sperduto R. Prevalence of refractive error in the United States, 1999-2004. Arch Ophthalmol. 2008;126(8):1111–9.
29. Li Y, Liu J, Qi P. The increasing prevalence of myopia in junior high school students in the Haidian District of Beijing, China: a 10-year population-based survey. BMC Ophthalmol. 2017;17(1):88.
30. French AN, Ashby RS, Morgan IG, Rose KA. Time outdoors and the prevention of myopia. Exp Eye Res. 2013;114:58–68.
31. Ji CY, Chen TJ. Working group on obesity in C. Empirical changes in the prevalence of overweight and obesity among Chinese students from 1985 to 2010 and corresponding preventive strategies. Biomed Environ Sci. 2013;26(1):1–12.

32. Rose KA, Morgan IG, Smith W, Burlutsky G, Mitchell P, Saw SM. Myopia, lifestyle, and schooling in students of Chinese ethnicity in Singapore and Sydney. Arch Ophthalmol. 2008;126(4):527–30.

33. You QS, Wu LJ, Duan JL, Luo YX, Liu LJ, Li X, Gao Q, Wang W, Xu L, Jonas JB, Guo XH. Prevalence of myopia in school children in greater Beijing: the Beijing childhood eye study. Acta Ophthalmol. 2014;92(5):e398–406.

34. Guo YH, Lin HY, Lin LL, Cheng CY. Self-reported myopia in Taiwan: 2005 Taiwan National Health Interview Survey. Eye (Lond). 2012;26(5):684–9.

35. Ferraz FH, Corrente JE, Opromolla P, Padovani CR, Schellini SA. Refractive errors in a Brazilian population: age and sex distribution. Ophthalmic Physiol Opt. 2015;35(1):19–27.

36. Sanfilippo PG, Chu BS, Bigault O, Kearns LS, Boon MY, Young TL, Hammond CJ, Hewitt AW, Mackey DA. What is the appropriate age cut-off for cycloplegia in refraction? Acta Ophthalmol. 2014;92(6):e458–62.

16

Comparison of two techniques for toric intraocular lens implantation: hydroimplantation versus ophthalmic viscosurgical devices

Yueqin Chen, Qian Cao, Chunyan Xue[*] and Zhenping Huang[*]

Abstract

Background: To compare the results between hydroimplantation of a single-piece, acrylic foldable toric intraocular lens (IOLs) and conventional implantation using an ophthalmic viscosurgical device (OVD).

Methods: In this study, 60 eyes with cataract and preexisting regular corneal astigmatism of 1.0 to 3.0 diopters (D) underwent the implantation of the AcrySof toric IOLs (Alcon Laboratories, Inc.). The patients were randomly assigned to a conventional implantation technique with an OVD or a hydroimplantation technique. Comparison of preoperative and postoperative parameters was performed using paired Student t tests, and independent Student t test was used to compare between the two groups.

Results: Three months postoperatively, the mean subjective astigmatism was 0.45 D ± 0.24 (SD) in the OVD group and 0.49 ± 0.29 D in the hydroimplantation group ($P = 0.492$). The mean endothelial cell density (ECD) loss was 7.54% ± 0.82% and 7.32% ± 0.59%, respectively ($P = 0.117$). The mean absolute IOL rotation was 4.77 ± 2.32 degrees and 4.70 ± 1.95 degrees, respectively ($P = 0.334$). The mean time for IOL implantation was 71.50 ± 8.10 s and 37.60 ± 3.90 s, respectively ($P < 0.001$). Two hours, 1 day, 1 week, 1 month, and 3 months postoperatively, there was no significant difference in IOP between the two groups ($P > 0.05$), although IOP two hours postoperatively seemed to be a little higher in the OVD group.

Conclusions: Compared with the use of OVDs for toric IOLs implantation, the hydroimplantation technique provided advantages of increased efficiency, reduced surgical time and cost, and no concerns of OVD-induced elevated IOP.

Trial registration: Current Controlled Trials ISRCTN55696872, Retrospectively registered.

Keywords: Endothelial cell density, Hydroimplantation, Intraocular pressure, Ophthalmic viscosurgical device, Toric intraocular lens

* Correspondence: xuechunyancn@163.com; hzpjlyy@hotmail.com
Department of Ophthalmology, Jinling Hospital, School of Medicine, Nanjing University, 305 East Zhongshan Road, Nanjing, People's Republic of China

Background

It is estimated that 25% to 40% of cataract patients have astigmatism more than 1.0 diopters (D) [1, 2]. With the increasing demands for good refractive outcomes after cataract surgery, toric intraocular lenses (IOLs) have been widely used to correct preoperative corneal astigmatism during surgery. Many studies have shown that the toric IOL implantation offers a predictable and stable procedure for the correction of preexisting corneal astigmatism, and induces a low amount of higher-order aberration [1, 3–6]. The key to achieve a good reduction of astigmatism is the precise alignment of the toric IOL axis on the planned meridian. In the standard procedure, after the injection of the toric IOL, the ophthalmic viscosurgical device (OVD) should be aspirated from the anterior chamber, including from behind the lens. This procedure is crucial for the toric IOL axis being finally positioned on the planned meridian. And it could be especially difficult when one haptic of the toric IOL is located adjacent to the main incision.

Hydroimplantation,implantation of a foldable IOL without an OVD, was introduced by Tak [7], and adopted and modified by other surgeons later [8–12]. To our knowledge, there has not been any study about comparison between hydroimplantation and conventional technique for the implantation of toric IOLs. However, the hydroimplantation technique can make the toric IOL implantation much easier by skipping two steps of rotation, and the toric IOL could be rotated to its final meridian directly.

The aim of this study was to evaluate and compare the clinical results between the OVD group and the hydroimplantation group for the implantation of a single-piece, acrylic foldable toric IOL.

Methods

Patient population

This randomized prospective study comprised 60 eyes with cataract and preexisting regular corneal astigmatism between 1.0 and 3.0 diopters (D) who had implantation of an AcrySof toric IOL (Alcon Laboratories, Inc.). The surgeries were performed between Jan 2012 and May 2014 by one experienced surgeon (Dr. Chunyan Xue) at the Refractive Center, Department of Ophthalmology, Jinling Hospital, Nanjing, China. The eyes were randomized prospectively into two groups (the OVD group and the hydroimplantation group) according to the statistical random table. The study protocol was approved by the Ethical Committee of Jinling Hospital. All patients were fully informed of the details and possible risks of the procedure, and written informed consents were obtained from all the patients. Described research adhered to the tenets of the Declaration of Helsinki.

Inclusion criteria were age-related cataract with preoperative corneal astigmatism between 1.0 and 3.0 D

and nucleus sclerosis up to grade 3. Preoperative corneal astigmatism was measured by keratometry (IOLMaster, Zeiss Humphrey, Carl Zeiss Meditec, Inc., Dublin, CA 94568). Exclusion criteria were history of previous ocular surgery, pupil size less than 7.5 mm after dilatation, anterior chamber less than 2.25 mm, compromised endothelial cell function, corneal disorder, complicated cataract, glaucoma, pseudoexfoliation, severe myopia, and diabetic retinopathy.

Preoperative assessment

Preoperative evaluations included subjective refraction, uncorrected visual acuity (UCVA), best corrected visual acuity (BCVA) (Snellen or "E" chart), keratometry (IOLMaster, Zeiss Humphrey, Carl Zeiss Meditec, Inc., Dublin, CA 94568), corneal topography (Humphrey ATLAS Corneal Topography System, Carl Zeiss Meditec, Inc., Dublin, CA 94568), intraocular pressure (IOP) (Computerized Tonometer CT-80A, Topcon Corp. Tokyo, Japan), endothelial cell density (ECD) (SP-3000P, Topcon Corp. Tokyo, Japan), slitlamp examination (PS-11E, Topcon Corp. Tokyo, Japan), and indirect fundus examination.

Intraocular Lens

The AcrySof toric IOL SN6ATT (Alcon Laboratories, Inc., Fort Worth, TX, USA) has open-loop modified L-haptics with 3 reference dots on each side that mark the axis of the cylinder on its posterior surface. The IOL can filter ultraviolet and blue light and is a single-piece IOL made of hydrophobic acrylic material with a refractive index of 1.55, a 6.0-mm optic diameter, and a 13.0-mm overall length. The spherical IOL power was calculated using the IOLMaster (Carl Zeiss Meditec AG) and the SRK/T formula. The cylinder power and the alignment axis were calculated using the Acrysof toric calculator available from Alcon Laboratories (www.acrysoftoriccalculator.com). The main incision was created at 135° and the surgical induced astigmatism was set as 0.5 D at 45° according to the data of previous operations of the same surgeon.

Surgical technique

Preoperatively, limbal reference marks of the astigmatic axis were made under a slit lamp directly [13]. The patients were sitting at the slit lamp and instructed to look at a distant target at head height with the fellow eye. The slit light was centered on the apex of the cornea and turned in the steep astigmatic meridian in the orthograde position using the rotator switch of the slit light. Then, two points of the astigmatic meridian at the limbus were marked with a marking pen. All of the markings were done by the surgeon.

5% Tropicamide with 5% phenylephrine eye drops were used for preoperative pupillary dilation. The surgery was performed using the Infiniti Vision System (Alcon Laboratories, Inc.). In both groups, after topical anesthesia with oxybuprocaine hydrochloride 0.4% eye drops, a 2-step superior clear corneal incision with an approximate 2.0 mm chord length was created with a 2.2 mm Intrepid dual-bevel slit knife (Alcon Laboratories, Inc.), and a side port was created at 2 o'clock at the limbus using a paracentesis knife (Alcon Laboratories, Inc.). After the anterior chamber was filled with DiscoVisc OVD (Alcon Laboratories, Inc.), a continuous curvilinear capsulorhexis measuring 5.0 to 5.5 mm in diameter was generated using capsular forceps. Hydrodissection and hydrodelineation were performed. Following in-the-bag phacoemulsification using the quick-chop technique, the rest of the cortex was removed by irrigation/aspiration using the Intrepid silicone-sleeved coaxial system (Alcon Laboratories, Inc.).

In the OVD group, the anterior chamber and the capsular bag was filled with DiscoVisc (Alcon Laboratories, Inc.). The toric IOL was placed in the cartridge which was lubricated with DiscoVisc. The IOL was then implanted into the capsular bag using a D cartridge mounted on a Monarch II injector (Alcon Laboratories, Inc.) by the surgeon. The injector was held with the left hand and rotated for advancement of the IOL with the other hand. After the IOL was injected into the capsular bag, gross alignment was achieved by rotating the IOL clockwise until it was placed 20–30 degrees short of the planned axis. After the DiscoVisc was thoroughly removed from the eye and from behind the IOL, the IOL was rotated to its final position by exactly aligning the reference marks on the toric IOL with the alignment axis marks. A final check was made after the anterior chamber was filled and the incisions were hydrated.

In the hydroimplantation group, following the removal of any residual cortical material, balanced salt solution (BSS) (Alcon Laboratories, Inc.) was used to maintain the anterior chamber shape instead of the DiscoVisc. To implant the IOL, the irrigation cannula was inserted into the anterior chamber through the left side port. The IOL was gradually injected into the eye through the tip of the cartridge with the assistance of an assistant who screwed the end of the injector, and the tip of the irrigation cannula could be used to guide the IOL into the capsular bag. With the help of the irrigation cannula tip and the small tip of a cyclodialysis spatula, the IOL was rotated to its final position by exact alignment of the reference marks on the toric IOL with the alignment axis marks. Finally, the incisions were hydrated (Fig. 1).

Tobramycin-dexamethasone ointment was applied to the eye at the end of the surgery. Postoperatively, tobramycin and dexamethasone eye drops were applied topically every hour. The eye drops were tapered after 1 week and then discontinued after 2 weeks.

Postoperative assessment

Postoperative IOP were performed at 2 h, 1 day, 1 week, 1 month, and 3 months after surgery. Postoperative UDVA, ECD, refractive astigmatism (keratometry: IOLMaster, Zeiss Humphrey, Carl Zeiss Meditec, Inc., Dublin, CA 94568), IOL rotation were also evaluated after surgery. The time for the IOL implantation was recorded during the surgery. Rotation of the toric IOL was evaluated by a slit lamp: A thin slit beam was rotated to the axis markings of the IOL, and then the orientation of the IOL was estimated in 1-degree steps [14]. Astigmatism vector analysis was performed using Thibos and Horner's power vector notation [15].

Statistical analysis

The results were analyzed using SPSS software (version 17.0, SPSS, Inc.). Data were presented as Mean ± SD. Visual acuity was converted to logarithm of the minimum angle of resolution (logMAR) before statistical analysis. For quantitative variables, independent Student t test was used to compare between the two groups. Comparison of preoperative and postoperative parameters was performed using paired Student t tests. A normal distribution check (Kolmogorov-Smirnov test) was performed to validate the use of a Student t test. Qualitative variables were analyzed using the *Chi-square* test. A P value less than 0. 05 was considered statistically significant.

Results

Sixty eyes were included in this study. All the eyes had successful operations with total surgical time less than 20 min, and no eye had posterior capsule rupture or other complications during the surgery. Table 1 shows the demographic data. No statistically significant differences in age, sex, UCVA, BCVA, IOP, ECD, or refractive astigmatism were observed between the two groups before surgery ($P > 0.05$).

Visual acuity

After surgery, UCVA improved significantly in all the patients ($P < 0.001$). Three months postoperatively, the mean UCVA was 0.19 ± 0.11 logMAR (range 0.00 to 0. 40 logMAR) in the OVD group and 0.19 ± 0.12 logMAR (range 0.00 to 0.40 logMAR) in the hydroimplantation group. There was no statistically significant difference in UCVA between the two groups ($P = 0.550$).

Refractive outcomes

There was a significant reduction of refractive astigmatism in the two groups after surgery ($P < 0.001$). Three months postoperatively, the mean refractive astigmatism was 0.45 ± 0.24 D (range 0.14 to 1.01 D) in the OVD group and 0.49 ± 0.29 D (range 0.12 to 1.28 D) in the hydroimplantation group. There was no statistically significant difference in refractive astigmatism between

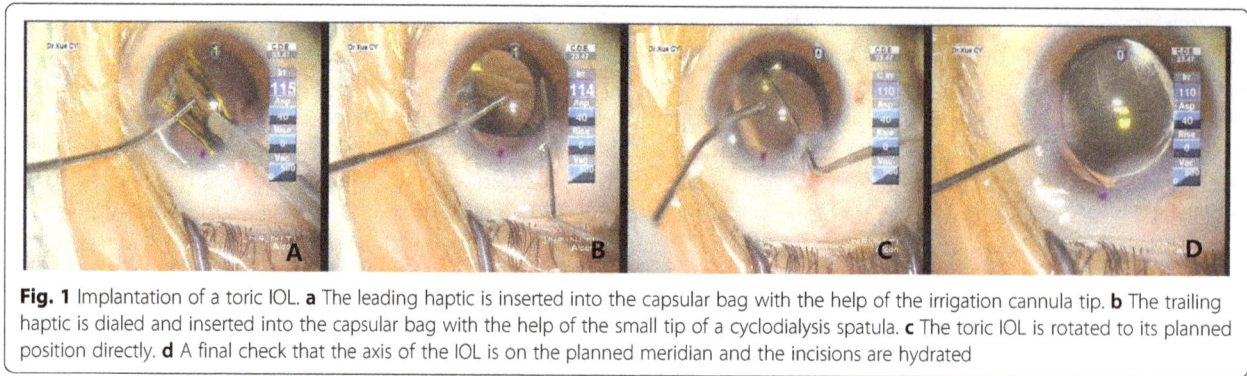

Fig. 1 Implantation of a toric IOL. **a** The leading haptic is inserted into the capsular bag with the help of the irrigation cannula tip. **b** The trailing haptic is dialed and inserted into the capsular bag with the help of the small tip of a cyclodialysis spatula. **c** The toric IOL is rotated to its planned position directly. **d** A final check that the axis of the IOL is on the planned meridian and the incisions are hydrated

the two groups ($P = 0.492$). Figures 2 and 3 show the linear regression about the expected vs achieved spherical equivalent (SE) 3 months postoperatively in the 2 groups, and 28 eyes (93.3%) in the OVD group and 27 eyes (90.0%) in the hydroimplantation group were within ±1.50 D of target refraction.

Figure 4 shows the postoperative astigmatism power vector in both groups. Three months postoperatively, the mean Jackson cross-cylinder at J0 and J45 was 0.08 ± 0.19 D (range – 0.26 to 0.43 D) and 0.08 ± 0.14 D (range – 0.20 to 0.41 D) respectively in the OVD group, and 0.00 ± 0.23 D (range – 0.62 to 0.46 D) and 0.09 ± 0.15 D (range – 0.25 to 0.49 D) respectively in the hydroimplantation group. There was no statistically significant difference in J0 ($P = 0.287$) or J45 ($P = 0.992$) between the two groups.

Endothelial cell density

Three months after surgery, the mean ECD was 2235.50 ± 294.33 cells/mm^2 (range 1723.4 to 2765.8 cells/mm^2) in the OVD group and 2343.59 ± 287.43 cells/mm^2 (range 1712.6

to 2699.4 cells/mm^2) in the hydroimplantation group. The mean ECD loss was $7.54\% \pm 0.82\%$ and $7.32\% \pm 0.59\%$, respectively ($P = 0.117$).

Intraocular pressure

Table 2 shows the IOP in 2 h, 1 week, 1 month, and 3 months after surgery. There was no significant difference in IOP between the two groups during the follow up ($P > 0.05$), although IOP two hours postoperatively seemed to be a little higher in the OVD group.

Intraocular lens rotation

Three months postoperatively, the mean absolute IOL rotation relative to the intended meridian was 4.77 ± 2.32 degrees (range 1 to 10 degrees) in the OVD group and 4.70 ± 1.95 degrees (range 2 to 10 degrees) in the hydroimplantation group. There was no statistically significant difference in IOL rotation between the two groups ($P = 0.334$) (Fig. 5).

Table 1 Demographic data at baseline

Variables	OVD group	Hydroimplantation group	P value
Number	30	30	
Gender (M/F)	10/15	11/17	0.480
Age (years)	69.53 ± 10.33	67.53 ± 9.14	0.513
UCVA (logMAR)	0.93 ± 0.25	0.81 ± 0.14	0.536
BCVA (logMAR)	0.67 ± 0.24	0.68 ± 0.22	0.483
ECD (cells/mm^2)	2418.66 ± 322.97	2529.71 ± 317.50	0.939
IOP (mmHg)	16.15 ± 2.48	15.29 ± 2.31	0.803
Refractive astigmatism (D)	2.29 ± 0.44	2.10 ± 0.42	0.804
Toric IOL model, n (%)			
T3	9 (30.0)	11 (36.7)	
T4	9 (30.0)	8 (26.7)	
T5	11 (36.7)	10 (33.3)	
T6	1 (3.3)	1 (3.3)	

OVD ophthalmic viscosurgical device, *UCVA* uncorrected visual acuity, *BCVA* best-corrected visual acuity, *ECD* endothelial cell density, *IOP* intraocular pressure, *D* diopters

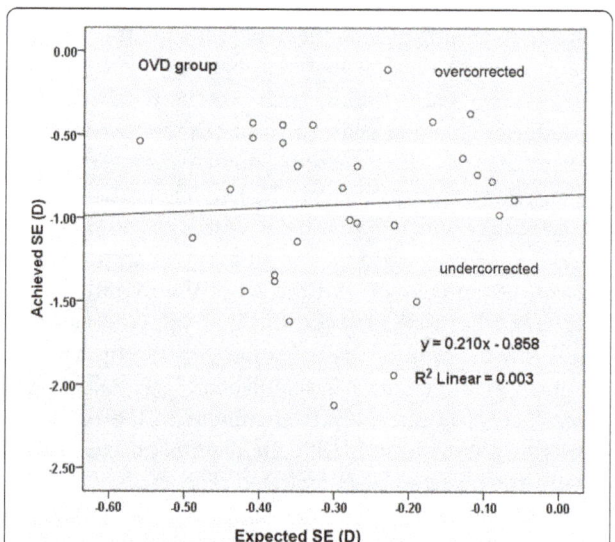

Fig. 2 Achieved SE correction versus expected SE correction 3 months postoperatively in OVD group. (*SE* spherical equivalent, *OVD* ophthalmic viscosurgical device)

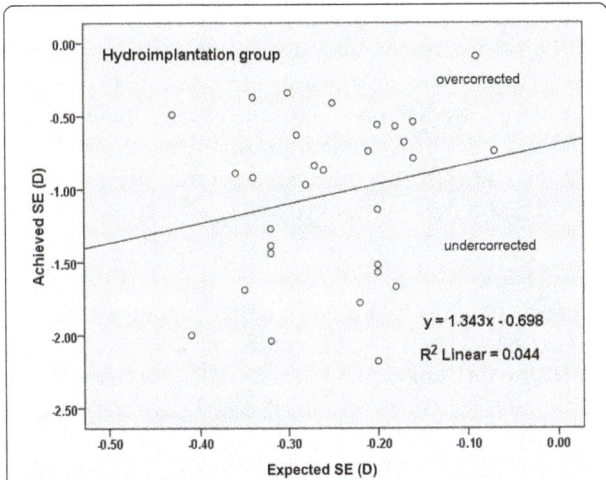

Fig. 3 Achieved SE correction versus expected SE correction 3 months postoperatively in hydroimplantation group. (*SE* spherical equivalent)

Time for intraocular lens implantation

The time for the IOL implantation was calculated from the end of complete removal of the cortex to the beginning of incision hydrated. The mean time for the toric IOL implantation was 71.50 ± 8.10 s in the OVD group and 37.60 ± 3.90 s in the hydroimplantation group. The time for the IOL implantation was much less in the hydroimplantation group ($P < 0.001$).

Discussion

There are many studies about foldable IOLs implantation using anterior chamber infusion, but no comparison study

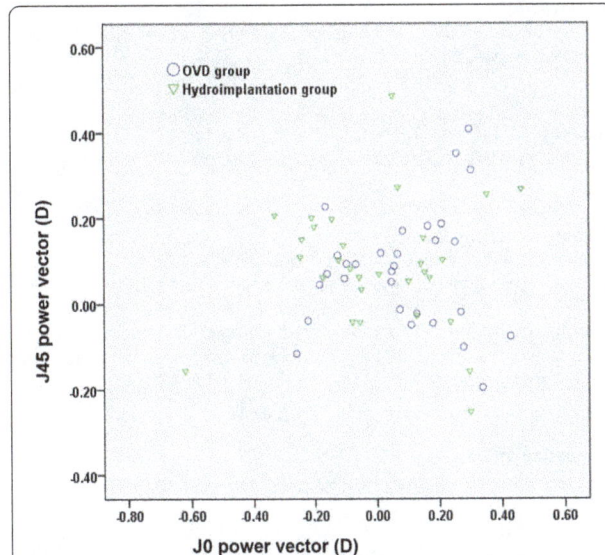

Fig. 4 Astigmatism vectors. The x-axes represent the J0 power vector (D). The y-axes represent the J45 power vector (D). (*OVD* ophthalmic viscosurgical device, *J0* Jackson cross-cylinder, axes at 0 degree and 90 degree, *J45* Jackson cross-cylinder, axes at 45 degree and 135 degree)

Table 2 Mean IOP change (mmHg) postoperatively

Time	OVD group	Hydroimplantation group	P value
2 h	16.25 ± 3.38	14.79 ± 3.02	0.830
1 day	14.98 ± 3.52	14.13 ± 2.83	0.119
1 week	13.45 ± 2.56	13.56 ± 2.35	0.609
1 month	14.15 ± 1.72	13.47 ± 1.78	0.715
3 months	14.70 ± 1.99	14.08 ± 1.93	0.981

IOP intraocular pressure, *OVD* ophthalmic viscosurgical device

about toric IOLs implantation. In this study, we find that the advantages of the hydroimplantation over OVDs are increased efficiency and reduced cost [16]. During the IOL implantation, the IOL can be rotated to its final position directly, skipping two steps of rotation using hydroimplantation compared with OVDs. Therefore, the hydroimplantation technique leads to deceased surgery time and increased efficiency, which is important in high-volume surgical centers. In our study, the mean time for the toric IOL implantation was 71.50 s in the OVD group and 37.60 s in the hydroimplantation group. The time for the IOL implantation was much less in the hydroimplantation group. Additionally, if smaller sized OVD syringes become available in the future, the hydroimplantation technique may reduce costs. And the manufacturer may produce OVD with smaller size and less cost.

UCVA and refractive astigmatism are important parameters of success for cataract patients with preoperative corneal astigmatism undergone implantation of toric IOLs. Three months after surgery, UDVA and refractive astigmatism were improved in both groups, and there were no significant differences between the two groups in UDVA or in refractive astigmatism. Three months postoperatively, the mean absolute IOL rotation relative to the intended meridian was 4.77 degrees with a range from 1 to 10 degrees in the OVD group and 4.70 degrees with a

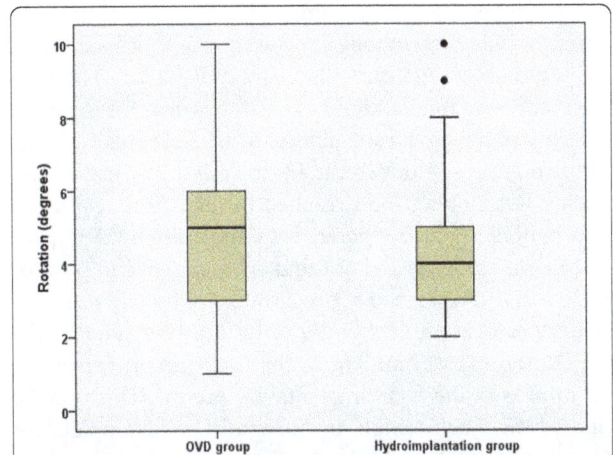

Fig. 5 Absolute axis rotation between the two groups three months postoperatively. (OVD = ophthalmic viscosurgical device)

range from 2 to 10 degrees in the hydroimplantation group. The rotation of the IOL was similar between the two groups. Complete IOL fixation on the posterior capsule is another advantage of hydroimplantation [10], which is more important for AcySof toric IOL. The stability of AcySof toric IOL in our study is inferior to the findings by Waltz, Hirnschall, and Lee et al. with the mean rotation from 2.2 to 4.1 degrees [17–20]. This result may be related to the evaluation method, preoperative marking, axis placement during surgery, and complete removal of the OVD or using hydroimplantation method.

In this study, BSS was used with a modification of Michael Blumenthal's AC chamber maintainer to maintain the anterior chamber and expand the bag [21]. Nonetheless, this study was carried out on normal corneas and foldable acrylic IOLs. Besides, the technique has limitations in compromised anterior chamber stability compared with OVDs. Therefore, we must be careful to abandon OVDs only when we can safely expand the bag, and it should be evaluated whether it could be applicable for diseased corneas and other IOLs. We do not recommend this technique for novice ophthalmologists. Mackool suggests using this technique in normal cases and to keep the OVD implantation technique for IOLs that open abruptly and complicated cases such as posterior capsular rupture, torn anterior capsulorhexis, and floppy-iris syndrome [9].

In the hydroimplantation method, the irrigation cannula was inserted into the anterior chamber through the left side port with the surgeon's left hand and the injector held with the other hand. It was not a 2-handed technique when the IOL was implanted using a manual Monarch injector. The IOL was injected into the eye with the aid of an assistant who screwed the end of the injector. If a motorized IOL injector was used, the injection procedure with hydroimplantation would be a 2-handed technique [22]. Furthermore, this procedure would be easy and safe when the eye was stabilized by the irrigation cannula in the side port.

As Lee reported that using BSS for maintaining the anterior chamber without OVD during IOL implantation did not cause a significant difference in ECD loss 3 months after surgery, our study showed the same results [11]. There was no significant difference in ECD loss between the two groups in our study. Lee revealed that use of BSS during IOL implantation resulted in reduction in postoperative IOP spike compared with the use of OVD [11]. But in our study, we did not find any difference in postoperative IOP between the two groups, although IOP two hours postoperatively seemed to be a little higher in the OVD group (16.25 mmHg in the OVD group versus 14.79 mmHg in the hydroimplantation group). This may be due to the small sample in our study or incomplete removal of the OVD in Lee's study. Of note, previously vitrectomized eyes were included in Lee's study which were absent in our study. The study by Studeny et al.

found no influence of the implantation technique (OVD or hydroimplantation) on postoperative IOP changes, which was comparable to our study [9]. However, larger studies may be needed to evaluate the influence of the two techniques on postoperative IOP, especially at different time point on the first postoperative day.

Conclusion

In conclusion, the hydroimplantation technique provides comparable outcomes to the conventional technique using OVDs for the implantation of toric IOLs, however, it has the advantages of increased efficiency, reduced surgical time and cost (if smaller size of OVD is available), and no concerns of OVD-induced elevated IOP. Furthermore, this technique is useful for the alignment of toric IOLs during the surgery, and the stability of the toric IOLs after surgery. However, the hydroimplantation cannot completely replace the OVD technique since this technique has advantages in complex cases. Importantly, this technique is only recommended to experienced surgeon, for novice ophthalmologists may cause some tough intraoperative complications. Thus, hydroimplantation technique may be an alternative method for the implantation of a single-piece, acrylic foldable toric IOL in some cases.

Abbreviations

BBS: Balanced salt solution; BCVA: Best-corrected visual acuity; ECD: Endothelial cell density; IOLs: Intraocular lens; IOP: Intraocular pressure; LogMAR: Logarithm of the minimum angle of resolution; OVD: Ophthalmic viscosurgical device; SE: Spherical equivalent; UCVA: Uncorrected visual acuity

Acknowledgements

The authors would like to acknowledge all members of the Department of Ophthalmology of Jinling Hospital.

Funding

The whole study was performed without any funding.

Authors' contributions

YC participated in the analysis of the data and drafting the manuscript. QC retrieved information from medical records and supplied technical support. CX planned the study, performed the surgeries, and retrieved information from medical records. ZH participated in the study design, interpretation of the data, and the revision of the manuscript. All authors read and approved the final manuscript.

Competing interests

The authors declare that they have no competing interests.

References

1. Leon P, Pastore MR, Zanei A, Umari I, Messai M, Negro C, et al. Correction of low corneal astigmatism in cataract surgery. Int J Ophthalmol. 2015;8:719–24.
2. Bachernegg A, Ruckl T, Strohmaier C, Jell G, Grabner G, Dexl AK. Vector analysis, rotational stability, and visual outcome after implantation of a new aspheric Toric IOL. J Refract Surg. 2015;31:513–20.

3. Bissen-Miyajima H, Negishi K, Hieda O, Kinoshita S. Microincision hydrophobic acrylic aspheric Toric intraocular Lens for astigmatism and cataract correction. J Refract Surg. 2015;31:358–64.

4. Farooqui JH, Koul A, Dutta R, Shroff NM. Management of moderate and severe corneal astigmatism with AcrySof(R) toric intraocular lens implantation - our experience. Saudi J Ophthalmol. 2015;29:264–9.

5. Nagpal R, Sharma N, Vasavada V, Maharana PK, Titiyal JS, Sinha R, et al. Toric intraocular lens versus monofocal intraocular lens implantation and photorefractive keratectomy: a randomized controlled trial. Am J Ophthalmol. 2015;160:479–86. e2

6. Toto L, Vecchiarino L, D'Ugo E, Cardone D, Mastropasqua A, Mastropasqua R, et al. Astigmatism correction with toric IOL: analysis of visual performance, position, and wavefront error. J Refract Surg. 2013;29:476–83.

7. Tak H. Hydroimplantation: foldable intraocular lens implantation without an ophthalmic viscosurgical device. J Cataract Refract Surg. 2010;36:377–9.

8. Bohm P. Usefulness of hydroimplantation technique for foldable IOL implantation. J Cataract Refract Surg. 2010;36:1623–4.

9. Mackool RJ. Hydroimplantation. J cataract refract Surg. 2010;36:1801. author reply 1801

10. Studeny P, Hyndrak M, Kacerovsky M, Mojzis P, Sivekova D, Kuchynka P. Safety of hydroimplantation: a foldable intraocular lens implantation without the use of an ophthalmic viscosurgical device. Eur J Ophthalmol. 2014;24(6):850.

11. Lee HY, Choy YJ, Park JS. Comparison of OVD and BSS for maintaining the anterior chamber during IOL implantation. Korean J Ophthalmol. 2011;25:15–21.

12. Carifi G, Pitsas C, Zygoura V, Kopsachilis N. Hydroimplantation of intraocular lenses. J Cataract Refract Surg. 2013;39:1281–2.

13. Bayramlar H, Dag Y, Sadigov F. Comments on corneal astigmatic marking methods. J Cataract Refract Surg. 2013;39:966.

14. Zuberbuhler B, Signer T, Gale R, Haefliger E. Rotational stability of the AcrySof SA60TT toric intraocular lenses: a cohort study. BMC Ophthalmol. 2008;8:8.

15. Thibos LN, Horner D. Power vector analysis of the optical outcome of refractive surgery. J Cataract Refract Surg. 2001;27:80–5.

16. Shingleton BJ, Mitrev PV. Anterior chamber maintainer versus viscoelastic material for intraocular lens implantation: case-control study. J Cataract Refract Surg. 2001;27:711–4.

17. Waltz KL, Featherstone K, Tsai L, Trentacost D. Clinical outcomes of TECNIS toric intraocular lens implantation after cataract removal in patients with corneal astigmatism. Ophthalmology. 2015;122:39–47.

18. Hirnschall N, Maedel S, Weber M, Findl O. Rotational stability of a single-piece toric acrylic intraocular lens: a pilot study. Am J Ophthalmol. 2014;157:405–11.

19. Lee JY, Kang KM, Shin JP, Kim IT, Kim SY, Park DH. Two-year results of AcrySof toric intraocular lens implantation in patients with combined microincision vitrectomy surgery and phacoemulsification. Br J Ophthalmol. 2013;97:444–9.

20. Ferreira TB, Almeida A. Comparison of the visual outcomes and OPD-scan results of AMO Tecnis toric and Alcon Acrysof IQ toric intraocular lenses. J Refract Surg. 2012;28:551–5.

21. Grinbaum A, Blumenthal M, Assia E. Comparison of intraocular pressure profiles during cataract surgery by phacoemulsification and extracapsular cataract extraction. Ophthalmic Surg Lasers Imaging. 2003;34:182–6.

22. Khokhar S, Sharma R, Patil B, Aron N, Gupta S. Comparison of new motorized injector vs manual injector for implantation of foldable intraocular lenses on wound integrity: an ASOCT study. Eye (Lond). 2014;28:1174–8.

17

Awareness of retinopathy of prematurity among pediatricians

Mohammad T. Akkawi[1], Jamal A. S. Qaddumi[2*], Hala R. M. Issa[2] and Liana J. K. Yaseen[2]

Abstract

Background: Retinopathy of prematurity (ROP) is a disorder of the developing retina of preterm infants due to defective vasculogenesis. The aim of the study was to analyze the level of awareness, knowledge, attitude and practice of pediatricians about ROP in the West Bank, Palestine.

Methods: A questionnaire was designed on the knowledge, attitude, and practice (KAP) pattern. The questionnaire included questions about pediatrician's educational and practicing profile, knowledge of screening guidelines, risk factors for ROP, referral facilities and barriers for referral. The questionnaire was given to70 practicing specialists and residents in hospitals having neonatal intensive care units in the West Bank, Palestine. It was a self-administered questionnaire, collected between November 2016 and February 2017.

Results: A total of 70 pediatricians from 11 different hospitals without ROP screening service participated in the study. The mean age of the participants was 33.04 ± 7.74. Of which, 62.9% were males and 37.1% were females. Fifty-nine (84.3%) answered that ROP is preventable, while 11 (15.7%) responded that ROP is not preventable. Nine (12.9%) pediatricians had no idea as to which part of the eye is affected in ROP. Among the participants, 29 (41.4%) did not know when ROP screening should be started. Sixty-three (90%) pediatricians were sure that ROP is treatable. Regarding barriers for ROP screening, 'ophthalmologist not available' reason was expressed by 37.1% (26/70), 'discharge person not writing' by 20% (14/70) and 'parents not agreeing' by 18.6% (13/70) of the participants. Knowledge on the use of laser as a treatment modality of ROP was shown by 39 (55.7%) participants, and the use of anti-VEGF was shown by 6 (8.6%) participants, whereas 25 (35.7%) of the participants didn't know about the treatment modalities.

Conclusion: The study findings suggest that a large majority of pediatricians were aware of ROP as a preventable disease, but had less information about ROP screening guidelines and service delivery. The study suggests the need to increase the awareness of pediatricians by dissemination of information about ROP and creating a close coordination between them and ophthalmologists to address barriers for service delivery in Palestine.

Keywords: Awareness, Pediatricians, Retinopathy of prematurity

* Correspondence: Jamal9877@najah.edu
[2]An-Najah National University, Nablus, Palestine
Full list of author information is available at the end of the article

Background

Retinopathy of prematurity (ROP), previously called retro-lental fibroplasias, is a vasoproliferative disorder of the retina which occurs principally in premature children due to defective vasculogenesis as a result of exposure to risk factors [1]. It mainly affects premature babies born at or before 32 weeks and weighing 1500 g or less at birth [2]. However, larger and more mature infants can develop severe ROP in countries with low/ moderate levels of development compared with highly developed countries [3]. Several risk factors have been found to be associated with the development of ROP. The most identified are low gestational age, low birth weight, poor postnatal growth, inadequately administered oxygen supplementation, respiratory distress and blood transfusion. Most studies show the most significant factors to be low gestational age and low birth weight [4, 5]. A significant improvement of the standards in neonatal intensive care units (NICUs) and perinatal care has increased the survival rate for the premature babies over the last decades. Consequently, the incidence of ROP has increased in parallel [6].

Retinal examination in preterm infants should be performed by an ophthalmologist with a sufficient knowledge and experience in order to identify accurately the location and sequential retinal changes of ROP [7]: Screening would be undertaken in the neonatal unit for babies who are still in-patients. Discharged babies can be examined in the neonatal unit during follow up, or in eye departments. Revised guidelines for screening have been suggested by the American Academy of Pediatrics, the American Association for Pediatric Ophthalmology and Strabismus and the American Academy of Ophthalmology. Those recommend screening for ROP in all infants with birth weight < 1500 g or gestational age of 32 weeks or less [8]. In contrast, the British Association for Perinatal Medicine and the College of Ophthalmologists recommend screening only infants < 1500 g at birth [9]. Timing of the initial examination is based on both postmenstrual age (PMA) and chronological age (CA) and is undertaken to detect 99% of infants at risk of a poor visual outcome. The first examination is conducted between four and nine weeks CA, depending on PMA at birth. Subsequent studies have confirmed the efficacy of conducting the first examination at four weeks CA in more mature infants [10]. These criteria only apply to these high income settings, wider criteria are used in less well resourced settings and less developed countries to ensure that all babies at risk are examined [3].

The current gold standard in treating sever, Type 1 ROP is still panretinal laser photocoagulation. However, ongoing studies in premature infants have been investigating the safety and efficacy of antiangiogenic therapies, especially anti-VEGF drugs. This seems to provide valuable and encouraging information for ROP treatment in the near future, though the long-term ocular and systematic safety of Anti-VEGF agents is not yet known [11]. A study was done in South India showed that awareness of ROP is poor among pediatricians. The same study mentioned that reports from other developing countries like China, Thailand and Vietnam also show a similar trend [12]. A study was done in 2013 in Nigeria to determine the level of awareness of the screening protocols for ROP among pediatricians, concluded that although majority of pediatricians are aware of ROP, they are poorly informed on the management and screening of the condition, and they need to be educated to be aware in order to prevent this treatable cause of blindness in children [13]. Another study was conducted in India 2011 to evaluate the prevailing practices for screening and referral scheme among Indian pediatricians for ROP concluded that only 14.5% were following international recommendations for ROP referral and that the screening remains poor due to the non-availability of trained ophthalmologists as well as inconsistent screening guidelines [14].

Retinopathy of prematurity is emerging as an important cause of avoidable blindness in both developed and developing countries [15]. Proper screening and referral practices will help saving sight for a more productive life. This is vital as number of blind years in a child increases the burden of care upon the family affected and the society as a whole [16, 17]. To the best of our knowledge, no studies were done in Palestine concerning ROP screening or awareness among pediatricians. This study was conducted to assess knowledge, attitude and practice patterns (KAP) of pediatricians about ROP.

Methods

The study was a cross-sectional non-interventional descriptive study. It was conducted in eleven different Palestinian hospitals (private and governmental) in the West Bank that contain neonatal intensive care units (NICUs) and have no ophthalmology departments. Pediatricians usually consult a specialized ophthalmologist from outside to screen cases with high risk for ROP, any intervention was undergone in a specialized hospital. We invited seventy pediatricians (specialists and residents) who are in direct contact with neonatal care who all participated in the study. The data were collected between November 2016 and February 2017. A self-administered semi-structured questionnaire was formed on the knowledge, attitude and practice (KAP) pattern. It was gathered and modified from other questionnaires of similar published researches to assess knowledge, screening, referral barriers and treatment of ROP [12].

The study was approved by An-Najah National University IRB committee. Also, informed consent was taken from each participant, explained clearly that participants' privacy was insured.

Results

Seventy pediatricians participated in the study. The demographic details are given in Table 1. The mean age of the participants was 33.04 + − 7.74 years, range 25 to 59 years. 44 (62.5%) were males. There were 31 (44.3%) qualified pediatricians, while residents in training were 39 (55.7%). 16 (22.6%) had been practicing for more than 10 years, 14 (19.9%) had about 5 to 10 years of practice experience and 40 (57.2%) had less than 5 years practice experience. Most of the respondents, 67(95.7%) were governmentally employed.

Fifty nine (84.3%) pediatricians said that ROP is preventable, 3 (4.3%) responded that ROP is not preventable, and 8 (11.4%) did not know. Twenty-four (34.3%) participants thought that blindness due to ROP is reversible, 35 (50.0%) said it is irreversible, whereas 11 (15.7%) did not know (Table 2).

Regarding ROP identification, 61 (87.1%) mentioned that it is identified by examining the retina and 9 (12.9%) did not know. Table 2 shows pediatrician's awareness about who performs screening for ROP.

Table 3 shows percentages of pediatricians with respect to their idea on the period of first eye test for ROP screening, that is, when to refer to ophthalmologist for ROP screening.

Referral for ROP screening was routinely undertaken by 67 (95.7%) respondents. The major two methods of referral among those were writing a discharge slip (60%) or informing the parents verbally (42.8%). The main reason given for not screening for ROP was the unavailability of an ophthalmologist in the same hospital among 26 (37.1%). Other contributing reason had to do with the discharging doctor not writing a screening referral order in 14 participants (20%).

Sixty-three (90.0%) pediatricians were sure that ROP is treatable, while 7 (10.0%) thought the opposite. Knowledge on the use of laser or anti-VEGF injection as a treatment modality of ROP was recorded in 39 (55.7%)

Table 1 Demographic details of the participants

Variable	Category	Frequency	Percent
Gender	Male	44	62.5
	Female	26	37.1
Age (years)	25–35	48	68.6
	36–45	16	22.9
	46–55	5	7.1
	56–65	1	1.4
Educational qualification	Specialist	31	44.3
	Resident	39	55.7

Table 2 Awareness of participants regarding risk factors of retinopathy of prematurity and who performs screening for retinopathy of prematurity

Variable	Category	Frequency	Percent
Causes of ROP	Low gestational age	2	2.9
	Weight less than 1800 g	5	7.1
	Sick require oxygen	2	2.9
	All the above	60	85.7
	Don't know	1	1.4
Eye test to be performed By	Retina specialist	21	30.0
	Pediatric ophthalmologist	48	68.6
	Don't know	1	1.4

and 6 (8.6%) participants respectively. 22 (31.4%) did not know how ROP is treated. In response to the question regarding the participants' opinion on how successful the treatment of ROP is in preventing blindness, only 26 (37.1%) thought it is good, 17 (24.3%) said very good, 26 (37.1%) considered it satisfactory, while only one (1.4%) thought it is poor.

Only 16 (22.9%) pediatricians were satisfied with their current status of awareness and knowledge on ROP, while 30 (42.9%) were not satisfied, 24 (34.3%) had no idea about the current status on the awareness and knowledge.

Discussion

Retinopathy of prematurity, when severe can result in permanent visual disability, causing a high financial burden for the community and the individual. Guidelines have been established in some countries to enhance early identification and prompt treatment of babies with ROP. Pediatricians who are the primary caregivers of premature babies ought to be aware of the risk factors, screening and referral protocols, as well as treatment modalities and outcomes. This will lead to improvement in the quality of care of these babies, and thus saving their sight, along with the inherent costs of blindness to the individual and community [13].

In our study, although the majority of pediatricians had knowledge about some of the risk factors for ROP, a significant number of them were not aware of the correct timing of ROP screening. This may be due to the lack of clear established screening protocols for ROP in

Table 3 Awareness of participants regarding timing of ROP screening

Variable	Category	Frequency	Percent
Period for first eye test	4–6 weeks	41	58.6
	Depend on the gestational age	25	35.7
	Don't know	3	4.3
	Other	1	1.4

Palestine, and so it may contribute to a delayed detection of the problem.

The American Academy of ophthalmology clarified that indications for screening are region dependent. Thus, it is advisable to develop more researches about possible risk factors and screening criteria specific to country, instead of relaying merely on the criteria published by developed countries. Gilbert [3] advised those who did not have local screening guidelines for ROP to use wide screening criteria.

Identifying barriers for referral is vital for formulating any successful model. In our study the major reason given for not screening for ROP was the unavailability of an ophthalmologist in the same hospital according to over a third of the participants. In a study done by Mohammad et al. from the United States about barriers for ROP screening or follow-up eye care after discharge from the NICU, it was found that infants who were not screened for ROP in the NICU had a greater risk for missing follow-up eye care compared to those who had their first retinal examination in the NICU [18]. This highlights the importance of screening taking place in the NICU and disseminating information about ROP in our hospitals.

Unfortunately, some of the participants in our study were sure that ROP is not treatable. This may affect their willing to refer cases for screening, and thus prevents early detection and treatment of such a preventable issue.

The role of the nursing staff is critical to a successful prevention of ROP- induced blindness as they help in monitoring oxygen saturation targets during the whole period of treatment. They are responsible for feeding and temperature control and play a vitally important role in preventing late sepsis, they participate actively in the recommendations to the patient's family regarding follow up examinations after discharge [19].Apart from this, many cases of prematurity are babies of multiple gestations after IVF as their parents complained of infertility for years, so there might be a need to raise awareness among obstetricians and parents who are contemplating IVF as well.

In our study, only 16 (22.9%) pediatricians were satisfied with their current status on awareness and knowledge on ROP. Up to now, there are no studies concerning KAP for ROP among pediatricians published in Palestine. We hope this study to be a step in enhancing knowledge among pediatricians, as well as establishing clear protocols concerning referral and screening of ROP.

Our study had some limitations, as with all self-reported questionnaires, the data could not be validated as their practices were not observed. It did not include other health care providers i.e. nurses in the NICU, Also a question about the place where the babies are usually screened was not included in the questionnaire.

In order to improve the awareness of ROP among pediatricians, nurses, obstetricians, and parents we recommend appropriate coordination between pediatricians and ophthalmologists, as well as dissemination of information through publishing articles and seminars in medical conferences, medical journals and health education materials for parents so local multidisciplinary workshops to highlight this issue is recommended.

Conclusion

The study findings suggest that a large majority of specialists and residents were aware of ROP as a disease, but had less information about ROP screening guidelines, service delivery and treatment modalities. The study suggests the need to create close coordination between pediatricians and ophthalmologists to address screening guidelines and barriers for service delivery in our country. The vital role of pediatricians in any screening program supports the need to enlighten them and increase their awareness by dissemination of information about ROP through seminars and literature, as well as spreading awareness among key members involved in preterm baby care.

Abbreviations

CA: Chronological age; GA: Gestational age; KAP: Knowledge, attitude, and practice; NICU: Neonatal intensive care unit; PMA: Postmenstrual age; ROP: Retinopathy of prematurity

Acknowledgments
The Authors would like to thank all participants without whom there would be no study.

Funding
This work has been entirely been made by the efforts and the financial support of the authors. No fund or financial assistance has been provided from other resources.

Authors' contributions
MA has made substantial contributions to the conception and design of the study, the acquisition of data, the analysis and interpretation of the data, and the drafting of the manuscript. JQ has made substantial contributions to design, data analysis and interpretation, and to drafting the manuscript. HI has made substantial contributions to the conception and design of the study, the acquisition of data, the analysis and interpretation of the data, and the drafting of the manuscript. LY has made substantial contributions to the conception and design of the study, the acquisition of data, the analysis and interpretation of the data, and the drafting of the manuscript. All authors have given final approval of the version to be published.

Competing interests
The authors declare that they have no competing interests.

Author details
[1]Department of Special Surgeries, Faculty of Medicine and Health Sciences, An-Najah National University Hospital, An-Najah National University, Nablus, Palestine. [2]An-Najah National University, Nablus, Palestine.

References

1. Terry TL. Extreme prematurity and fibroblastic overgrowth of persistent vascular sheath behind each crystalline lens: I. Preliminary report. Am J Ophthalmol. 1942;25(2):203–4.
2. Waheeb S, Alshehri K. Incidence of retinopathy of prematurity at two tertiary centers in Jeddah, Saudi Arabia. Saudi J Ophthalmol. 2016;30(2):109–12.
3. Gilbert C. Characteristics of Infants with Severe Retinopathy of Prematurity in Countries with Low, Moderate, and High Levels of Development: Implications for Screening Programs. Pediatrics. 2005;115(5) https://doi.org/10.1542/peds.2004-1180.
4. Kim TI, Sohn J, Pi SY, Yoon YH. Postnatal risk factors of retinopathy of prematurity. Paediatr Perinat Epidemiol. 2004;18(2):130–4.
5. Akkoyun I, Oto S, Yilmaz G, Gurakan B, Tarcan A, Anuk D, Akgun S, Akova YA. Risk factors in the development of mild and severe retinopathy of prematurity. J AAPOS. 2006;10(5):449–53.
6. Abdel HA, Mohamed GB, Othman MF. Retinopathy of prematurity: a study of incidence and risk factors in NICU of Al-Minya University Hospital in Egypt. J Clin Neonatol. 2012;1(2):76.
7. Fierson WM, Saunders RA, Good W, Palmer EA, Phelps D, Reynolds J, Chiang MF, Ruben JB, Granet DB, Blocker RJ, Bradford GE. Screening examination of premature infants for retinopathy of prematurity. Pediatrics. 2013;131(1):189–95.
8. Section on Ophthalmology American Academy of Pediatrics, American Academy of Ophthalmology; American Association for Pediatric Ophthalmology and Strabismus. Screening examination of premature infants for retinopathy of prematurity. Pediatrics. 2006;117(2):572–6.
9. Wilkinson AR, Clark D, Fielder A, Marlow N, Schulenburg WE, Weindling AM. Retinopathy of prematurity: guidelines for screening and treatment. The report of a joint working party of the Royal College of Opthalmologists and the British Association of Perinatal Medicine. Early Hum Dev. 1996;46(3):239–58.
10. Jefferies AL. Retinopathy of prematurity: recommendations for screening. Paediatr Child Health. 2010;15(10):667.
11. Mutlu FM, Sarici SU. Treatment of retinopathy of prematurity: a review of conventional and promising new therapeutic options. Int J Ophthalmol. 2013;6(2):228.
12. Sathiamohanraj SR, Shah PK, Senthilkumar D, Narendran V, Kalpana N. Awareness of retinopathy of prematurity among pediatricians in a tier two city of South India. Oman J Ophthalmol. 2011;4(2):77–80.
13. Uhumwangho OM, Israel-Aina YT. Awareness and screening for retinopathy of prematurity among paediatricians in Nigeria. J West Afr Coll Surg. 2013;3(3):33.
14. Patwardhan SD, Azad R, Gogia V, Chandra P, Gupta S. Prevailing clinical practices regarding screening for retinopathy of prematurity among pediatricians in India: a pilot survey. Indian J Ophthalmol. 2011;59(6):427.
15. Blencowe H, Lawn JE, Vazquez T, Fielder A, Gilbert C. Preterm-associated visual impairment and estimates of retinopathy of prematurity at regional and global levels for 2010. Pediatric Res. 2013;74(S1):35.
16. Rani PK, Jalali S. Knowledge, attitude, practice study of retinopathy of prematurity amongst pediatricians attending a neonatal ventilation workshop in South India. World J Retina Vitreous. 2011;1:9–13.
17. Jalali S, Anand R, Kumar H, Dogra MR, Azad R, Gopal L. Programme planning and screening strategy in retinopathy of prematurity. Indian J Ophthalmol. 2003;51(1):89.
18. Attar MA, Gates MR, Iatrow AM, Lang SW, Bratton SL. Barriers to screening infants for retinopathy of prematurity after discharge or transfer from a neonatal intensive care unit. J Perinatol. 2005;25:36–40.
19. Kalyan G, Moxon S. The role of neonatal nurses in the prevention of retinopathy of prematurity. Indian Pediatr. 2016;53(Suppl.2):S143–50.

18

Pseudophakic mini-monovision: high patient satisfaction, reduced spectacle dependence, and low cost

Debora Goetz Goldberg[1][*][iD], Michael H. Goldberg[2], Riddhi Shah[1], Jane N. Meagher[2] and Haresh Ailani[2]

Abstract

Background: Cataract surgery with pseudophakic mini-monovision has lower out-of-pocket patient expense than premium multifocal intraocular lenses (IOL). The purpose of this study was to evaluate patient-reported satisfaction and spectacle dependence for key activities of daily living after cataract surgery with pseudophakic mini-monovision. The study also examined statistical relationships between patient demographic variables, visual acuity and satisfaction.

Methods: Prospective cohort study of 56 patients (112 eyes) who underwent bilateral cataract surgery with pseudophakic mini-monovision. Mini-monovision corrects one eye for distance vision and the other eye is focused at near with -0.75 to -1.75 D of myopia. All patients with 1 diopter or greater of corneal astigmatism had a monofocal toric IOLs implanted or limbal relaxing incision. The main study outcomes were assessed at the last follow-up appointment and included refraction, visual acuity, patient reported spectacle use, and patient satisfaction. Descriptive statistics, correlation matrixes and Pearson's chi-square tests were examined.

Results: Uncorrected visual acuity was significantly better post-operatively. Most patients reported the surgery met their expectations for decreased dependence on spectacles (93%). Most patients report little or no use of spectacles post-operatively for computer use (93%), distance viewing (93%) and general use throughout the day (87%). A small number of patients report spectacle use for reading (9%) and night driving (18%). There were no relationships detected between demographic variables and visual acuity or patient satisfaction.

Conclusions: Aging of the population presents one of the biggest challenges in the health sector, which includes a rising number of individuals with chronic vision impairment and increased demand for accessible treatment strategies. Cataract surgery with pseudophakic mini-monovision results in high patient satisfaction and considerable reduction in spectacle dependence. Pseudophakic mini-monovision technique is a low-cost, valuable option for patients who would like to reduce dependence on spectacles post-operatively and should be considered along with premium multifocal IOLs in options available for patients based on their needs, preferences and clinical indicators. Reducing spectacle dependence with the pseudophakic mini-monovision technique could improve the functionality, independence and quality of life for many patients who are unsuitable or are unable to pay additional fees associated with premium multifocal IOLs.

* Correspondence: dgoldbe4@gmu.edu
[1]Department of Health Administration and Policy, George Mason University
Peterson Family Health Sciences Hall, 4400 University Drive, MS: 1J3, Fairfax,
Virginia 22030, USA
Full list of author information is available at the end of the article

Background

Decreased spectacle dependence with a minimum of optical disturbances has become a major refractive goal of cataract surgery. However, patients with traditional cataract surgery are often dependent on spectacles post-operatively. Several surgical options exist for reducing spectacle dependence including bilateral diffractive multifocal intraocular lenses (IOLs) and traditional monofocal IOLs with pseudophakic mini-monovision. Multifocal IOLs are increasingly used to reduce spectacle dependence, although these IOLs may not be a feasible option for many patients due to additional out-of-pocket expense patients may incur for facility and physician charges attributable to multifocal IOLs [1].

Monovision using traditional monofocal IOLs is a surgical option that corrects distance vision in the dominant eye; the non-dominant eye focuses intentionally for near to mid-range vision. This leads to the process of neuroadaptation where the brain can use the distance image from the dominant eye and the near image from the non-dominant eye to achieve a wider range of functional vision [2]. In this surgery the amount of intended myopia can vary, with full monovision defined as the reading eye exhibits a residual refractive error of − 2.50 diopters or more. Modified monovision or "mini-monovision" requires a smaller interocular diopteric power difference between eyes than traditional monovision, typical calculations of the near eye are anywhere between −.75 and − 1.75 diopters of myopia. Patients with significant astigmatism can also undergo mini-monovision surgery along with toric IOL implants or limbal relaxing incisions. Previous research has found that IOLs implanted bilaterally using the mini-monovision approach result in few optical side effects and exceptional distance and intermediate visual outcomes. Concerns remain regarding near visual outcomes that require some patients to wear spectacles for reading fine print or computer work [3].

Both multifocal IOLs and monofocal IOLs with mini-monovision technique have been found to significantly improve uncorrected visual acuity and spectacle independence [4–8]. A few studies comparing multifocal IOLs with the mini-monovision technique found similar results between the groups on visual acuity [5, 7] and spectacle independence [6, 9]. However, challenges remain after cataract surgery with multifocal IOLs due to visual aberrations such as halos, glare, shadows, waxy vision, and difficulty reading in dim light [2, 4, 5, 9–11]. These unwanted visual symptoms following multifocal IOL surgery are common; previous research has found between 30 and 65% of patients report visual aberrations [10]. One study found that up to 10% of patients reported that the glare and halos were debilitating, with many of those patients requiring a lens exchange to correct their symptoms [2].

In the United States, there is economic incentive for surgeons to use multifocal IOLs in lieu of mini-monovision with monofocal IOLs because the physician can legally make a surcharge to the patient for the use of a premium multifocal IOL, which is typically an out-of-pocket expense for patients [7]. High patient out-of-pocket expenses for premium multifocal IOLs is common in many counties. Physicians may also be able to charge additional fees for necessary testing prior to cataract surgery for mini-monovision; however, these fees run considerably less than charges for the premium multifocal IOLs.

The National Academy of Medicine promotes research on approaches to reduce vision impairment that are focused on patient-centered care and low-cost treatment strategies [12]. Mini-monovision is a low-cost, effective option for management of presbyopia and has fewer side effects than multifocal IOLs [4, 5]. Patients often are drawn by the financial savings of mini-monovision with traditional IOLs compared with multifocal IOLs. However, few studies have evaluated patient reported satisfaction with spectacle dependence following mini-monovision with traditional IOLs. The main purpose of this study was to determine if mini-monovision cataract surgery fulfilled patients' expectations and decreased dependence on spectacle correction for distance, midrange and near functions. A secondary objective of the study was to determine if patient characteristics, such as age and gender, are related to visual acuity or patient satisfaction following surgery.

Methods

This prospective cohort study was a partnership between Eye Consultants of Northern Virginia (ECNV) and George Mason University, College of Health and Human Services. The ECNV and George Mason University Internal Review Board approved the study protocols. Study outcomes include clinical measures of uncorrected visual acuity and patient-reported data obtained through a questionnaire completed by patients at the 3-month post-operative follow up exam. The questionnaire consisted of 6 items measuring spectacle use for near, mid-range and distance functions such as driving at night, using the computer, and reading. The questionnaire also asked patients to rate their overall satisfaction with mini-monovision cataract surgery for reduction of spectacle dependence. Chart reviews were conducted by ECNV ophthalmologists and ophthalmic technicians to extract patient demographic data and measures of visual function.

Patient sample

The sample was drawn from all patients at ECNV in need of bilateral cataract extraction who chose the mini-monovision cataract surgery option, which included 63 consecutive patients between 2012 and 2015. Patients who experienced major ocular pathology such as corneal dystrophy, degeneration or macular pathology were excluded from the study. There were 56 patients (112 eyes) who fully completed the questionnaire on spectacle use and satisfaction, resulting in an 89% response rate. All patients provided informed consent prior to surgery and before completion of the questionnaire.

Preoperative examination

All patients had a complete preoperative ophthalmic examination including subjective and objective refraction, biomicroscopy of the anterior and posterior eye segments, intraocular pressure (IOP), macular optical coherence tomography (OCT), automated and manual keratometry, optical biometry, and immersion A-scan.

Surgical technique

Pseudophakic mini-monovision was chosen for this study because the gradual difference between the two eyes is more tolerable by patients than full monovision. For purposes of this study, the definition of mini-monovision is the near eye calculated between − 1.25 and − 1.50 diopters spherical equivalent. In all patients the dominant eye was corrected for distance vision. Toric IOLs or limbal relaxing incision were used on patients who had corneal astigmatism greater than 1 diopters. Two patients who previously wore monovision contact lenses, the refractive outcome was calculated for − 2.00 diopters. The same experienced surgeon (M.G.) performed all of the surgeries under topical anesthesia using a standard phacoemulsification procedure. All patients were treated with aspheric IOL implants (AcrySof®IQ IOL or the AcrySof® Toric/IQ IOL).

Postoperative examination

Routine postoperative examinations were performed 1 day, 3 weeks and 3 months (up to 6 months) after surgery. The exam included testing for visual acuity, visual aberrations, IOP, subjective and objective refraction and biomicroscopy of the anterior segment. The main study outcomes were assessed at the last follow-up visit. Outcomes included visual acuity, visual aberrations, patient reported questionnaire data on spectacle usage for common Activities of Daily Living (ADLs), and patient satisfaction with reduction of spectacle dependence following the mini-monovision technique.

Statistical analysis

Statistical analyses were performed using STATA 14 software. Measures of central tendency and dispersion are provided on patient demographic variables and responses to survey questions. Correlation matrixes and Pearson's chi-square tests were examined to determine associations between patient demographic variables, visual acuity, and overall patient satisfaction with reduction of spectacle dependence following surgery. The paired-samples t-test was performed to compare pre- and postoperative visual acuity means (converted to logMAR units) to test for statistical significance. A P value of less than .05 was considered statistically significant for this study.

Results

This study included 112 eyes of 56 patients. Cataract surgery was uneventful in all cases and there were no intraoperative complications. All patients completed the questionnaire on spectacle dependence and attended the last follow-up visit. The sample comprised of 39 female and 17 male patients between the ages of 55 and 80.

Patient demographic information and surgical procedures are presented in Table 1. Additional procedures were performed on patients to correct astigmatism. This included 10 eyes treated with limbal relaxing incision. Two patients who had previous refractive surgery underwent IOL exchange on the dominant eye to achieve the desired post-operative refraction.

Visual acuity

The preoperative and postoperative visual acuity are reported in Table 2 in logMAR units. The postoperative uncorrected near and distance visual acuities were significantly better than preoperative measurements in the patient sample ($P < .001$). The target refraction for the distance eye was plano and the near eye was − 1.25

Table 1 Patient Sample Demographics ($n = 56$)

Demographic Variable	% (n)
Participant Age	
55–64	14.3 (8)
65–74	64.3 (36)
75+	21.4 (12)
Gender	
Male	30.4 (17)
Female	69.6 (39)
Additional Procedures	
Limbal Relaxing Incision OD	8.9 (5)
Limbal Relaxing Incision OS	8.9 (5)
IOL Exchange OD	1.8 (1)
IOL Exchange OS	1.8 (1)

Table 2 Pre and Post Surgery Visual Acuity Characteristics (n = 56)

Pre-Surgical Measurements	Mean ± SD (logMAR units)
Uncorrected Vision OD	0.95 ± 0.45
Uncorrected Vision OS	0.9 ± 0.44
Post-Surgical Measurements	Mean ± SD (logMAR units)
Uncorrected Vision Distance Eye	0.09 ± 0.09
Uncorrected Vision Near Eye	0.15 ± 0.14

to − 1.50. Fifty-one patients (91%) were within ±.50 diopters of the intended spherical equivalent for the distance eye. Fifty-two patients (93%) were within ±.50 diopters of the target range for the near eye. There were no patient reports of meaningful glare or halos for near or distance functions.

Patient reported satisfaction and spectacle use

All patients completed a questionnaire on spectacle use and satisfaction, see Table 3. One question asked patients if the mini-monovision technique met their expectations for decreased dependence on spectacles. This satisfaction scale ranged from 1 to 10, with 1 representing the lowest level of satisfaction and 10 representing the highest level of satisfaction. The research findings show most patients reported cataract surgery with mini-monovision technique met their expectations for decreased dependence on spectacles. On this question 51 (93%) patients reported 7 or higher on a 10-point satisfaction scale, with only one (2%) patient reporting a 3 or less on their level of satisfaction.

Questions on spectacle use were based on a frequency scale from 0 to 10, with 0 representing never wearing spectacles and 10 representing always wearing spectacles. Overall, patients reported low use of spectacles for specific activities for distance, mid-range and near functions. Patient report of spectacle use was lowest for computer use, distance viewing, and for general use throughout the day. The majority of patients 51 (93%) reported low scores (0, 1, 2 or 3) for the amount of time they wear spectacles while working on a computer. Likewise, most patients, 51 (93%), also reported low scores (0, 1, 2 or 3) for the amount of time they wear spectacles for distance viewing. Slightly fewer patients, 48 (87%), reported low scores (0, 1, 2 or 3) for the amount of time they wear spectacles throughout the day.

The highest reported use of spectacles was for reading and for driving at night. Most patients, 41 (73%), reported low scores (0, 1, 2, 3) for wearing spectacles for reading, with 5 (9%) patients reported high scores (7, 8, 9, 10). Similarly, 42 patients (76%) reported low scores (0, 1, 2, 3) for wearing spectacles for night driving; however, 11 (18%) patients reported high scores (7, 8, 9, 10) for wearing spectacles for driving at night. The study findings indicate that for most patients cataract surgery with the mini-monovision technique relieved their need for spectacles for distance, mid-range and near functions. Nevertheless, a small number of patients need vision correction with spectacles for reading and driving at night.

Additional analysis

Correlation matrixes and Pearson's chi-square tests were examined to determine associations between patient demographic variables, visual acuity and satisfaction. No associations were found between gender and post-operative uncorrected visual acuity in the distance eye (Pearson chi2 2.54, $P = .467$) or near eye (Pearson chi2 3.44, $P = .486$). No association was found between age and post-operative uncorrected visual acuity in the distance eye (Pearson chi2 54.10, $P = .780$). However, a statistically significant positive association was found between age and post-operative uncorrected visual acuity in the near eye (Pearson chi2 117.66, $P = .009$). No associations were found between patient age and patient satisfaction (Pearson chi2 127.24, $P = 0.452$), nor were there associations between patient gender and satisfaction (Pearson chi2 7.69, $P = 0.262$). A statistically significant positive association was found between post-surgery uncorrected visual acuity and patient satisfaction, indicating that patients with better vision were more satisfied with cataract surgery involving the mini-monovision technique (Pearson chi2 30.32, $P = .034$).

Table 3 Patient Reported Spectacle Use and Satisfaction (n = 56)

Patient Survey Question	Mode	Mean	Std Dev
1. Time Wearing Glasses for Reading	0	2.4	2.8
2. Time Wearing Glasses at Computer	0	0.9	2.0
3. Time Wearing Glasses for Distance	0	0.7	1.7
4. Time Wearing Glasses for Driving at Night	0	2.1	3.8
5. Time Wearing Glasses throughout the Day	0	1.6	1.6
6. Mini-Monovision Surgery Met Patient Expectations for Decreased Dependence on Glasses	10	9.3	1.6

Note: Questions 1–5 based on a 0 to 10 scale and question 6 based on a 1 to 10 scale

Discussion

Results of this study found that cataract surgery with the mini-monovision technique significantly improved patients' uncorrected visual acuity and reduced their spectacle dependence. Almost all patients in the study reported that cataract surgery with the mini-monovision technique met their expectations for decreasing dependence on spectacles, with most patients reporting little or no use of spectacles post-operatively. Patients reported low use of spectacles for computer work, distance viewing, and general activities throughout the day. The quality and levels of light and/or the distance from the object may be related to the need for a small number of patients to wear spectacles postoperatively for reading and driving at night. Previous research has found that patients who receive either monofocal or multifocal IOL for cataract surgery have issues with night driving [13]. Other studies found that patients undergoing cataract surgery with multifocal IOLs experience more difficulties with night vision and night driving than patients undergoing cataract surgery with monovision [14].

Study results also found a positive relationship between post-surgery uncorrected visual acuity and patient satisfaction, indicating that patients with better vision were more satisfied with cataract surgery involving the mini-monovision technique. While there was significant improvement in visual acuity postoperatively, patients with poorer outcomes were less satisfied with pseudophakic mini-monovision for spectacle dependence. It is also possible that postoperative astigmatism interferes with near, mid-range and distance visual acuity, and therefore with patient satisfaction and spectacle dependence.

Results of this study, along with other research [15], indicate that cataract surgery with pseudophakic mini-monovision is a successful option to lessen patient dependence on spectacles for near, midrange and distance functions after cataract surgery. Cataract surgery with multifocal IOLs has also been shown to be an effective method for reducing dependence on spectacles. For many patients, multifocal IOLs are an appropriate and valuable service. Nevertheless, many previous studies have shown that some patients experience optical side effects, such as glare, halos, and dysphotopsia, which can cause patient discomfort and decreased satisfaction [10]. The dissatisfaction from multifocal IOLs often cannot be improved with spectacles and instead requires additional surgery such as IOL exchange to a monofocal IOL. In contrast, patient dissatisfaction with the pseudophakic mini-monovision technique is mostly related to the refractive outcome, which can be corrected with spectacles or contact lenses and does not require additional surgery. A systematic review of research on quality outcomes revealed that patients with multifocal IOLs are more likely than patients with pseudophakic

mini-monovision technique to undergo IOL exchange due to dissatisfaction with image quality [16].

The decision to opt for either cataract surgery with multifocal IOLs or cataract surgery with the mini-monovision technique should be based on consideration of patient motivation to achieve spectacle independence [11], patient ADLs [15, 17], treatment costs, and ability to cope with possible side effects. An understanding of the benefits and risks of both pseudophakic mini-monovision and multifocal IOLs is critical for patients to be informed decision makers. The move toward patient-centered care supports the need for patient engagement and informed decisions about treatment options. Patient-centered care is "providing care that is respectful of and responsive to individual patient preferences, needs, and values, and ensuring that patient values guide all clinical decisions" [18]. Informed consent, one component of patient-centered care, includes discussion of: the illness and the natural consequences of no treatment; detailed information on the proposed operation, including commonly known complications; and alternative forms of treatment [19]. Physicians should advise their patients on all possible options for reducing dependency on spectacles with cataract surgery including potential side effects and additional out-of-pocket costs. Providing patients with complete information about expected benefits and risks, and expected costs, will lead individuals to be more confident in the recommended choice [20].

Results of this study should be considered along with study limitations, which include a small sample size, limited number of ADLs assessed in the questionnaire, and the lack of comparison data on patient satisfaction outcomes with other options to reduce patient dependence on spectacles following cataract surgery. Future studies should focus on assessment of spectacle dependence when performing ADLs with technologies such as cellular messaging and cellular entry search [17]. Future studies should also consider healthcare practitioner assessment of ADLs following cataract surgery with mini-monovision. Additional Randomized Controlled Trials are needed to compare efficacy of the mini-monovision technique with cataract surgery using multifocal IOLs [21]. There is also a need for research on the role of costs in patient decision making for selecting techniques to reduce dependence on spectacles.

Conclusion

Aging of the population presents one of the biggest challenges in the health sector, which includes a rising number of individuals with chronic vision impairment and increased demand for accessible treatment strategies. Pseudophakic mini-monovision is a low-cost option for patients who would like to reduce dependence on spectacles post-operatively and should be considered along with multifocal IOLs in options available for patients based on their needs, preferences and clinical indicators. Reducing spectacle dependence with the mini-monovision technique could improve the functionality, independence and quality of life for many patients who are unsuitable for multifocal IOLs or are unable to pay additional fees associated with multifocal IOLs.

Abbreviations
ADLs: Activities of daily living; ECNV: Eye Consultants of Northern Virginia; IOLs: Intraocular lens; IOP: Intraocular pressure; OCT: Optical coherence tomography; RCT: Randomized Controlled Trials; Std dev: Standard Deviation

Acknowledgements
None.

Funding
No external funding sources to disclose.

Authors' contributions
DG –Study design, statistical analysis, drafting, critical revision and final approval of the manuscript. MG – Study design, data collection, critical revision and final approval of the manuscript. RS – Development of study database, literature review, drafting, critical revision and final approval of the manuscript. JM – Study design, data collection, critical revision and final approval of the manuscript. HA – Study design, literature review, critical revision and final approval of the manuscript.

Competing interests
All investigators on this project declare no competing interest or relationships with commercial entities related to the research or clinical activities in this report.

Author details
[1]Department of Health Administration and Policy, George Mason University Peterson Family Health Sciences Hall, 4400 University Drive, MS: 1J3, Fairfax, Virginia 22030, USA. [2]Eye Consultants of Northern Virginia, 8134 Old Keene Mill Rd., Ste. 300, Springfield, VA 22152, USA.

References
1. Centers for Medicare and Medicaid Services. Implementation of the centers for Medicare & Medicaid Services (CMS) ruling 05–01 regarding presbyopia-correcting intraocular lenses (IOLs) for Medicare beneficiaries. Available at: https://www.cms.gov/Outreach-and-Education/Medicare-Learning-Network-MLN/MLNMattersArticles/downloads/mm3927.pdf. (2005). Accessed 7 July 2017.
2. Greenstein S, Pineda R. The quest for spectacle Independence: a comparison of multifocal intraocular lens implants and pseudophakic monovision for patients with presbyopia. Semin Ophthalmol. 2017;32(1):111–5.
3. Ito M, Shimizu K, Niida T, Amano R, Ishikawa H. Binocular function in patients with pseudophakic monovision. J Cataract Refract Surg. 2014;40(8):1349–54.
4. Zhang F, Sugar A, Jacobsen G, Collins M. Visual function and spectacle independence after cataract surgery: bilateral diffractive multifocal intraocular lenses versus monovision pseudophakia. J Cataract Refract Surg. 2011;37(3):446–53.
5. Labiris G, Giarmoukakis A, Patsiamanidi M, Papadopoulos Z, Kozobolis VP. Mini-monovision versus multifocal intraocular Lens implantation. J Cataract Refract Surg. 2015;41:53–7.
6. Chen M, Atebara N, Chen TT. A comparison of a monofocal Acrysoft IOL using the "blended monovision" formula with the multifocal array IOL for glasses independence after cataract surgery. Ann Ophthalmo. 2007;39:237.
7. Wilkins MR, Allan BD, Rubin GS, et al. Randomized trial of multifocal intraocular lenses versus monovision after bilateral cataract surgery. Ophthalmology. 2013;120:2449–55.
8. Mahrous A, Ciralsky JB, Lai EC. Revisiting monovision for presbyopia. Curr Opin Ophthalmol. 2018;29(4):313–7.
9. Mu J, Chen H, Li Y. Comparison study of visual function and patient satisfaction in patients with monovision and patients with bilateral multifocal intraocular lenses. Zhonghua Yan Ke Za Zhi. 2014;50:95–9.
10. Woodward MA, Randleman J, Stulting R. Dissatisfaction after multifocal intraocular lens implantation. J Cataract Refract Surg. 2009;35(6):992–7.
11. de Silva SR, Evans JR, Kirthi V, Ziaei M, Leyland M. Multifocal versus monofocal intraocular lenses after cataract extraction. Cochrane Database Syst Rev. 2016;12:CD003169. https://www.cochranelibrary.com/cdsr/doi/10.1002/14651858.CD003169.pub4/full. Accessed 22 Oct 2018.
12. National Academies of Sciences, Engineering, and Medicine. Making eye health a population health imperative: Vision for Tomorrow. Washington, D. C.: The National Academies Press; 2016. http://www.nationalacademies.org/hmd/Reports/2016/making-eye-health-a-population-health-imperative-vision-for-tomorrow.aspx. Accessed 7 July 2017
13. Dick HB, Krummenauer F, Schwenn O, Krist R, Pfeiffer N. Objective and subjective evaluation of photic phenomena after monofocal and multifocal intraocular lens implantation. Ophthalmology. 1999;106(10):1878–86.
14. Stock R, Thumé T, Paese L, Bonamigo E. Subjective evaluation of uncorrected vision in patients undergoing cataract surgery with (diffractive) multifocal lenses and monovision. Clin Ophthalmol. 2017;11:1285–90.
15. Labiris G, Toli A, Perente A, Ntonti P, Kozobolis VP. A systematic review of pseudophakic monovision for presbyopia correction. Int J Ophthalmol. 2017;10(6):992–1000.
16. Wang S, Stem M, Oren G, Shtein R, Lichter P. Patient-centered and visual quality outcomes of premium cataract surgery: a systematic review. Eur J Ophthalmol. 2017;27(4):387–401.
17. Labiris G, Ntonti P, Patsiamanidi M, Sideroudi H, Georgantzoglou K, Kozobolis V. Evaluation of activities of daily living following pseudophakic presbyopic correction. Eye Vis. 2017;4:2.
18. Institute of Medicine, Committee on quality of health Care in America. Crossing the quality chasm: a new health system for the 21st century. Washington, DC: National Academies Press; 2001.
19. American College of Surgeons. Statements on Principles. Available at: https://www.facs.org/about-acs/statements/stonprin. (2016). Accessed 7 July 2017.
20. Krumholz HM. Informed consent to promote patient-centered care. JAMA. 2010;303(12):1190–1.
21. Lidija K, Hrvoje B, Mladen B, Ivan C, Vladimir T. Monovision versus Multifocality for presbyopia: systematic review and meta-analysis of randomized controlled trials. Adv Ther. 2017;34:1815–39.

19

Evaluation of Scheimpflug imaging parameters in blepharospasm and normal eyes

Huina Zhang[1†], Hongjie Zhou[2†], Tiepei Zhu[1] and Juan Ye[1*]

Abstract

Background: To investigate changes in corneal elevation, pachymetry, and keratometry in discriminating between normal and blepharospasm eyes, as measured by the Pentacam rotating Scheimpflug camera.

Methods: This was a prospective, cross-sectional study. A total of 47 consecutive patients with a range of blepharospasm severity and 40 age- and sex- matched healthy subjects were included, one eye of each subject was randomly chosen for data analysis. Blepharospasm severity was evaluated using the Jankovic scale and categorized as mild, moderate, or severe. Corneal parameters were measured by the Pentacam rotating Scheimpflug camera to derive corneal tomography information. Various parameters regarding keratometry, elevation at the anterior and posterior corneal surface, pachymetric data, final D value, and topometric indices from the Pentacam software were recorded, and the relationship between the blink rate and corneal parameters was analyzed. Intraclass correlation coefficients (ICCs) were assessed to evaluate the repeatability of intraobserver.

Results: Increased topographic asymmetry was observed in moderate and severe blepharospasm. Front K1and front Km were significantly higher in cases of mild ($P < 0.05$), moderate ($P < 0.0001$), and severe ($P < 0.0001$) blepharospasm as compared with controls. Front K2, back K1, back K2, and back Km were significantly higher in cases of moderate ($P < 0.01$) and severe ($P < 0.001$) blepharospasm as compared with controls. For corneal topometric indices, both ISV and IVA were significantly increased in severe blepharospasm ($P < 0.05$). Radii minimum were significantly increased in cases of moderate and severe blepharospasm ($P < 0.05$).There were no differences in corneal elevation and corneal pharcymetric parameters among the four groups, except for front BFS, which was significantly different in blepharospasm groups ($P < 0.05$). Final D values were significantly higher in the severe blepharospasm ($P < 0.01$) group than that among controls. There were significant correlations between the blink rate and most corneal tomographic parameters. All parameters showed high reproducibility (ICC: 0.921–0.996) for normal and blepharospasm subjects.

Conclusions: Blepharospasm may lead to a redistribution of the pressure applied by the lids over the cornea and, consequently, may result in corneal shape changes, which can be documented through corneal topography.

Keywords: Blepharospasm, Pentacam, Corneal curvature Corneal topography

---

* Correspondence: yejuan@zju.edu.cn
†Huina Zhang and Hongjie Zhou contributed equally to this work.
[1]Department of Ophthalmology, the Second Affiliated Hospital, Zhejiang University School of Medicine, Hangzhou, Zhejiang, China
Full list of author information is available at the end of the article

Background

Benign essential blepharospasm is one of the most common neuromuscular disorders. In cases of blepharospasm, a grumbling facial expression, the fluttering of the eyelids, an increased frequency of blinking, and chronic involuntary contractions are the main signs [1].It is well-known that the corneal surface is susceptible to eyelid pressure [2–4].Moon et al. [5] reported corneal astigmatism changes in patients with blepharospasm or hemifacial spasm after the injection of botulinum toxin (BTX). Thus, in addition to the cosmetic problems involved in eyelid appearance, blepharospasm may also lead to a redistribution of the pressure applied by the lids over the cornea and, consequently, may result in corneal shape changes, which can be documented through corneal topography.

Placido disk-based corneal topography and biomicroscopic examination are widely used in the clinical diagnosis of cornea diseases. However, the corneal topography study only yields the measurement of anterior corneal surface and cannot reflect the alteration of the entire corneal architecture. It has been shown that corneal curvature measurements performed via the Pentacam have excellent repeatability [6]. The Pentacam (Oculus, Inc., Wetzlar, Germany) is a piece of equipment that uses a rotating Scheimpflug camera to image the anterior segment (including both the anterior and posterior corneal surfaces) [7, 8].It measures 25,000 data points from 50 meridians over the cornea in less than 2 s [9]. Although previous research using Scheimpflug photography has investigated astigmatism of the posterior corneal surface, the curvature of the cornea was only measured along 6 meridians [10]. The magnitude and axis of the astigmatism obtained in these studies may not be as accurate as those obtained via the Pentacam.

To the best of our knowledge, no studies have been conducted regarding corneal parameter differences between normal and blepharospasm eyes, as measured by Scheimpflug imaging. Therefore, the aim of present study is to prospectively determine the efficacy of corneal elevation, pachymetry, and keratometry in discriminating between normal and blepharospasm eyes with respect to Jankovic Rating scale stage [11],with a view to contributing to our understanding of the specific corneal structural alterations that occur in blepharospasm.

Methods

Subjects and clinical evaluations

This prospective, case-control study included 47 patients with blepharospasm (10 male and 37 female eyes, mean age: 58.64 ± 9.03 years old) and 40 normal subjects (candidates for cataract surgery with normal corneas, 13 male and 27 female eyes, mean age: 59.18 ± 10.05 years old), one eye of each subject was randomly chosen for data analysis.

Before study enrollment, all patients provided informed consent to participate in the research. The research protocol followed the tenets of the Declaration of Helsinki and was approved by the ethics committee of the Second Affiliated Hospital, Zhejiang University School of Medicine, from August 2016 through December 2016.A diagnosis of blepharospasm was established via the Jankovic Rating scale [12] (0 = no spasm; 1 = mild spasm, barely noticeable; 2 = mild spasm, without functional impairment; 3 = moderate spasm, with moderate functional impairment; 4 = severe, incapacitating spasm), categorizing the eyes as mild(12 eyes), moderate(20 eyes), or severe(15 eyes). All patients must have had the symptoms of blepharospasm for over six months according to this classification system.

Ophthalmic examinations consisted of best-corrected visual acuity measurements, slit-lamp examination, and extraocular movements. Patients with the following conditions were excluded from the study: a history of ocular or eyelid surgery; glaucoma; blepharoptosis; strabismus; significant hyperopia (> + 1 diopter); corneal abnormalities due to other factors, such as trauma, keratoconus, chronic eye rubbing, and vernal keratoconjunctivitis; and anyone who was unable to cooperate with the examinations. The participants who wore soft contact lenses were asked to stop for at least 2 weeks,and those who wore rigid contact lenses were asked to stop using them for 5 weeks before this assessment.

The blink rate was measured via direct observation [13]. Two investigators sat in the room during a lecture and secretly counted the blinks of each subject for 1 min using a mechanical counter, repeated for two times. The data were pooled, and the results were expressed as the means ±standard deviations based on four independent experiments. Subjects were unaware of the blink measurements.

Corneal tomography

We followed the methods of Zhu et al.2017 [14]. A Pentacam HR system (Oculus, Wetzlar, Germany) was used to evaluate the anterior and posterior corneal surfaces. The measurements were performed in the automatic release mode by the same experienced examiner, and 25 rotating Scheimpflug images were obtained for each eye within 2 s. Image quality was checked, and for each eye, only one high-quality examination was recorded. The sagittal curvature, front elevation, corneal thickness, back elevation, and Belin/Ambrósio Enhanced Ectasia Display were evaluated. Elevation data were measured in a standardized fashion relative to a reference best-fit sphere (BFS) that was calculated at a fixed optical zone of 8.0 mm.

The following data were obtained with this instrument: (1) keratometric values: flat keratometry (K1), steep keratometry (K2), mean keratometry (Km), astigmatism altitude, and axis for the central 3.0 mm of cornea;(2) topometric indices: index of surface variance (ISV), index of vertical asymmetry

(IVA), keratoconus-index (KI), center keratoconus-index (CKI), index of height decentration (IHD), index of height asymmetry (IHA), and radii minimum (RM); (3) variables in elevation map: diameter of BFS, elevation at apex point, maximum elevation, and elevation at the thinnest point within the central 4.0 mm zone; (4) corneal pachymetric parameters: corneal thickness at the thinnest point and at the apex, the difference of thickness between these two points (apex/thinnest difference), the thinnest location, pachymetric progression indices, and Ambrósio's relational thickness (ART); and (5) final D-value.

The astigmatism value of both corneal surfaces was converted into the rectangular forms of Fourier notation (J0 [Jackson cross-cylinder with axes at 180° and 90°] and J45 [Jackson cross-cylinder with axes at 45° and 135°]) for power vector analysis using the following equations: $J0 = (-C/2)\sin2\alpha$ and $J45 = (-C/2)\cos2\alpha$, where C was the corneal astigmatism magnitude, and α was the meridian of steep keratometry [15].

Statistical analysis

Statistical analysis was performed with a one-way ANOVA, followed by the Dunnett multiple-comparisons test (GraphPad Prism 5 software; GraphPad Software, San Diego, CA). A p-value of < 0.05 was considered to be statistically significant. All results were compared between investigators by using the intraclass correlation coefficient (ICC). Results from one investigator were reported in this study as the mean and standard deviation for all eyes. Additionally, spearman correlation analyses were used to define the correlation between the blink rate and Pentacam parameters. All statistical analyses were performed using the Statistical Package for the Social Science, Version 20.0 (SPSS Inc., Chicago, IL). A p-value of < 0.05 was considered statistically significant.

Results

The characteristics of the study subjects are presented in Table 1. There were no age-, disease duration-, or sex-related statistical differences between patients with blepharospasm

and control subjects. The average blink rate was significantly increased in each blepharospasm subgroup ($p < 0.0001$).

Keratometric parameters

Table 2 provides the keratometric parameters in the blepharospasm and control groups. Front K1and front Km were significantly higher in cases of mild ($p < 0.05$), moderate ($p < 0.0001$), and severe ($p < 0.0001$) blepharospasm. Front K2, back K1, back K2, and back Km were significantly higher in cases of moderate ($p < 0.01$) and severe ($p < 0.001$) blepharospasm. However, there were no significant differences among the four groups in terms of front J0, front J45, front astigmatism magnitude (front Astig), back J0, back J45, and back Astig.

Corneal topometric indices

Among corneal topometric indices, both ISV and IVA were significantly increased in cases of severe blepharospasm ($p < 0.05$). Radii minimum were significantly increased in cases of moderate and severe blepharospasm ($p < 0.05$). No significant changes in keratoconus index, central keratoconus index, index of height asymmetry or index of height decentration were noted among the four groups (P>0.05) (Table 3).

Corneal elevation and corneal pharcymetric parameters

In the elevation maps, no statistically significantly differences between the variables were noted among the four groups in terms of elev front apex, elev front thinnest, elev front max 4.0 mm, elev back apex, elev back thinnest, elev back max 4.0 mm, and back BFS, whereas front BFS diameter was significantly lower in blepharospasm groups than in the control group ($p < 0.05$, Table 4).

As illustrated in Table 5,the corneal pharcymetric parameters in the eyes with blepharospasm, including apex thickness, thinnest thickness, apex/thinnest difference, thinnest location, min PI, max PI, average PI, max ART, and average ART, did not differ from those of controls (P >0.05, Table 5).

Table 1 Comparison of baseline characteristics between control and blepharospasm groups

	Control	Blepharospasm		
		Mild	Moderate	Severe
Age (yrs)	59.18 ± 10.05	54.07 ± 8.67	60.05 ± 8.51	60.4 ± 9.32
Male (n, %)	13 (32.5%)	4 (33.3%)	5 (25%)	2 (13.3%)
Subjects (n)	40	12	20	15
Jankovic Rating Scale	0	1 or 2	3	4
Disease duration (mean yrs. + SD)	N	3.9 ± 2.7	4.4 ± 3.2	3.4 ± 3.2
Blink Rate (blinks/min)	17.56 ± 3.62	30.64 ± 5.41****	39.54 ± 5.99****	52.45 ± 7.79****

Jankovic Rating Scale: 0 = no spasm; 1 = mild spasm, barely noticeable; 2 = mild spasm, without functional impairment; 3 = moderate spasm, with moderate functional impairment;4 = severe, incapacitating spasm
Data are mean standard deviation unless otherwise indicated
****P < 0.0001, versus controls

Table 2 Comparison of keratometric parameters between control and blepharospasm groups

	Control	Blepharoptosis		
		Mild	Moderate	Severe
Front K1 (D)	42.24 ± 1.26	43.28 ± 0.89*	44.58 ± 1.42****	44.51 ± 1.37****
Front K2 (D)	43.32 ± 1.41	43.96 ± 1.35	44.86 ± 1.83***	45.55 ± 1.09****
Front Km (D)	42.82 ± 1.32	43.94 ± 0.86*	44.56 ± 1.77****	44.99 ± 1.05****
Front Astig (D)	1.21 ± 0.60	1.03 ± 0.57	0.81 ± 0.30	1.05 ± 1.38
Front J0 (D)	0.05 ± 0.39	0.09 ± 0.46	− 0.06 ± 0.22	0.18 ± 0.52
Front J45 (D)	0.01 ± 0.42	− 0.10 ± 0.38	−0.02 ± 0.25	0.11 ± 0.67
Back K1 (D)	− 6.04 ± 0.22	− 6.03 ± 0.15	− 6.36 ± 0.29****	−6.34 ± 0.24***
Back K2 (D)	− 6.37 ± 0.26	−6.44 ± 0.19	−6.61 ± 0.29**	−6.68 ± 0.14***
Back Km (D)	− 6.19 ± 0.23	−6.22 ± 0.15	−6.48 ± 0.29****	−6.50 ± 0.14****
Back Astig(D)	0.32 ± 0.16	0.38 ± 0.13	0.26 ± 0.11	0.32 ± 0.23
Back J0 (D)	0.03 ± 0.15	− 0.08 ± 0.10	−0.03 ± 0.09	0.02 ± 0.16
Back J45 (D)	−0.01 ± 0.09	−0.02 ± 0.13	−0.002 ± 0.10	−0.02 ± 0.12

Astig astigmatism magnitude, D diopter
Data are mean standard deviation unless otherwise indicated
*$p < 0.05$, **$P < 0.01$, ***$P < 0.001$ and ****$P < 0.0001$ versus controls

Final D,the correlations of blink rate with corneal parameters and ICC

As shown in Fig. 1, the mean final D values were significantly higher in the severe blepharospasm (1.72 ± 0.67, $p < 0.01$) group than among controls (1.01 ± 0.66). Figure 2 shows the correlations between blink rate with corneal parameters. Blink rate was significantly and negatively correlated with back K1 ($R^2 = 0.246$, $p < 0.001$), back K2 ($R^2 = 0.224$, $p < 0.001$), back Km ($R^2 = 0.266$, $p < 0.001$), and RM ($R^2 = 0.165$, $p < 0.001$). A significant positive correlation was also found between blink rate and front K1 ($R^2 = 0.344$, $p < 0.001$), front K2 ($R^2 = 0.292$, $p < 0.001$), front Km ($R^2 = 0.335$, $p < 0.001$) and final D ($R^2 = 0.078$, $p = 0.009$). Table 6 summarises ICC, indicating that corneal curvature measurements performed via the Pentacam had good repeatability (ICC: 0.921–0.996).

Discussion

The corneal surface is vulnerable to eyelid pressure [2]. Using the Pentacam system, Zhu et al. [14] indicated that congenital blepharoptosis not only induced corneal asymmetry and irregularity, but also affected corneal tomography, such as increased corneal elevation in blepharoptosis eyes with more than moderate severity and even focalized corneal thinning in severe cases. Changes in corneal topography and corneal astigmatism induced by eyelid surgeries were also observed after gold-weight implant, ptosis, ectropion, and eyelid mass surgeries [16, 17].Such changes may be explained by the anatomical proximity between the eyelids and the cornea and by the pressure exerted by the eyelids on the corneal surface, resulting in corneal deformation [17].

There have been relatively few reports in the literature on the effect of blepharospasm on corneal curvatures. Using corneal topography, Osaki has demonstrated that

Table 3 Comparison of corneal topometric indices between control and blepharospasm

	Control	Blepharospasm		
		Mild	Moderate	Severe
Index of surface variance	20.9 ± 13.4	20.83 ± 11.5	18.1 ± 5.26	29.67 ± 11.7*
Index of vertical asymmetry	0.16 ± 0.10	0.16 ± 0.05	0.15 ± 0.06	0.23 ± 0.09*
Keratoconus index	1.02 ± 0.03	1.02 ± 0.02	1.02 ± 0.03	1.04 ± 0.03
Central keratoconus index	1.002 ± 0.01	1.01 ± 0.01	1.001 ± 0.01	1.007 ± 0.01
Index of height asymmetry	6.13 ± 4.69	7.07 ± 5.28	6.05 ± 5.58	9.46 ± 8.42
Index of height decentration	0.01 ± 0.01	0.01 ± 0.01	0.01 ± 0.01	0.02 ± 0.01
Radii minimum	7.63 ± 0.64	7.32 ± 0.15	7.31 ± 0.37*	7.18 ± 0.20**

Data are mean standard deviation unless otherwise indicated
*$P < 0.05$, ** $P < 0.01$, versus controls

Table 4 Comparison of corneal elevation parameters between control and blepharospasm

| | Control | Blepharoptosis | | |
		Mild	Moderate	Severe
Elev front apex (μm)	1.48 ± 1.43	1.17 ± 1.12	1.10 ± 1.59	1.87 ± 1.77
Elev front thinnest (μm)	1.05 ± 2.56	0.42 ± 1.44	1.10 ± 1.59	1.40 ± 2.13
Elev front max 4.0 mm (μm)	4.74 ± 2.99	3.08 ± 0.79	3.90 ± 2.12	4.47 ± 2.50
Front BFS (mm)	7.82 ± 0.24	7.62 ± 0.16*	7.62 ± 0.31**	7.58 ± 0.12**
Elev back apex (μm)	2.68 ± 2.52	3.25 ± 4.73	1.90 ± 2.53	2.87 ± 2.56
Elev back thinnest (μm)	5.08 ± 3.50	4.67 ± 4.29	4.70 ± 3.37	5.40 ± 4.31
Elev back max 4.0 mm (μm)	9.90 ± 4.30	9.25 ± 3.93	9.00 ± 4.11	8.47 ± 4.45
Back BFS (mm)	6.45 ± 0.39	6.41 ± 0.12	6.29 ± 0.30	6.26 ± 0.12

BFS = diameter of best fit sphere in 8.0-mm area; Elev = elevated; Max = maximum; mm = millimeter; μm = micrometer
Data are mean standard deviation unless otherwise indicated
*$P < 0.05$, **$P < 0.01$, versus controls

patients treated with BTX-A for hemifacial spasm developed significant eyelid and corneal changes on the affected eyes during the toxin's period of action. The results showed a statistically significant decrease in steep K and astigmatism 2 months after BTX-A treatment [18]. In the present study, a significant difference in corneal astigmatism magnitude was found between the control and blepharospasm groups, including front K1, front K2, front Km, back K1, back K2, and back Km, and the curvature change is positively proportional to the severity of the disease. Additionally, we found the radii minimum were significantly decreased in the moderate and severe groups, indicating the decrease of the smallest radius of curvature in the entire field of measurements, further confirming corneal curvature change in the blepharospasm groups.

The Pentacam system could also provide several topometric indices that only consider the anterior corneal surface. These changes may be related to either the restoration of symmetry in the upper and lower lid apposition on the cornea or the rearrangement of the tear film

[17]. We found a significant difference between ISV and IVA in the severe group. These results indicate that blepharospasm may increase the asymmetry and irregularity of the anterior corneal surface in cases of severe blepharospasm.

Among the properties of the corneal surface, elevation provides the most accurate representation of its shape. However, the Pentacam system have two reference database in Belin/Ambrósio Enhanced Ectasia Display, including Myopia/Normal and Hyperopia/Mixed Cyl, previous clinical observations indicated that there is an increased variability in the posterior elevation in hyperopic eyes on tomographic evaluation [19]. If this is true, it would lead to false positives when compared against a myopic biased normative database. Therefore, we exclude patients with significant hyperopia (> + 1 diopter). Corneal topographers can be categorized into two groups based on whether they can measure the elevation of the anterior and posterior surfaces of the cornea (front BFS and back BFS). However, to our knowledge, no study has reported on changes in corneal elevation in

Table 5 Comparison of corneal pharcymetric parameters between control and blepharospasm

| | Control | Blepharoptosis | | |
		Mild	Moderate	Severe
Apex thickness (μm)	542.2 ± 35.59	567.6 ± 28.46	542.6 ± 28.37	543.9 ± 36.10
Thinnest thickness (μm)	537.8 ± 34.82	561.4 ± 29.31	536.3 ± 26.85	538.8 ± 37.60
Apex/Thinnest difference (μm)	5.20 ± 5.15	4.17 ± 3.19	6.25 ± 5.63	5.13 ± 3.81
Thinnest location (mm)	0.71 ± 0.31	0.72 ± 0.24	0.92 ± 0.69	0.79 ± 0.34
Min PI	0.71 ± 0.19	0.57 ± 0.22	0.59 ± 0.65	0.71 ± 0.19
Max PI	1.33 ± 0.25	1.13 ± 0.15	1.82 ± 2.63	1.46 ± 0.73
Avg PI	1.00 ± 0.15	0.90 ± 0.10	0.94 ± 0.24	0.93 ± 0.31
Max ART (μm)	424.2 ± 92.24	483.8 ± 55.06	437.9 ± 39.00	448.9 ± 114.8
Avg ART (μm)	548.0 ± 98.61	621.3 ± 104.8	545.0 ± 60.51	571.1 ± 122.4

ART Ambrósio's relational thickness, Avg average, Max maximum, Min minimum, mm millimeter, PI progression index, μm micrometer
Data are mean standard deviation unless otherwise indicated

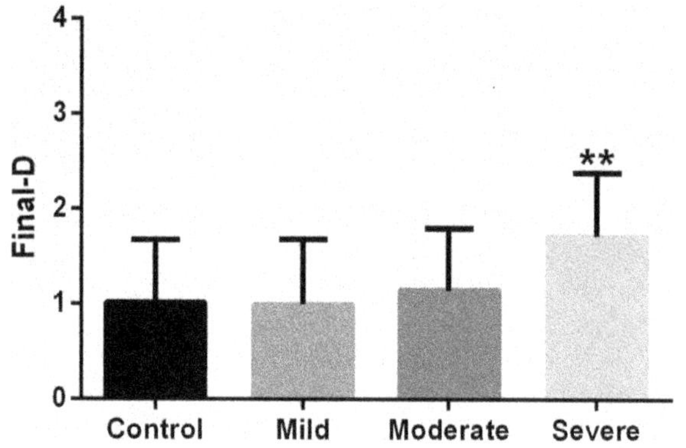

Fig. 1 The distribution of final D values in healthy controls and blepharospasm groups. The final D value increased with increasing severity of blepharospasm. *p < 0.05, one-way ANOVA with the Dunnett's multiple comparison test

blepharospasm eyes. In our study, no significant difference in most corneal elevation parameters was found between the control and blepharospasm groups, except for front BFS, which was significantly different in the severe group. The diagnostic value of front BFS was suggested by Lim et al. [20], who found that front BFS was significantly higher among cases of keratoconus. However, to our knowledge of the seindices, their variability, as well as their value in reflecting the shape of the cornea are limited, and much research is still required before they can be applied with confidence and certainty.

An increased frequency of blinking was one of the main symptoms of blepharospasm. The normal blink rate is about 12 blinks/min [21], but a mean blink rate of 24.8 blinks/min has also been reported [22]. In the present study, the normal blink rate was about $17.56 \pm$

3.62blinks/min, while blepharospasm patients had rates of 30.64 ± 5.41blinks/min or higher. Rapid blinking is associated with worse ocular surface disease and tear stability [23], and we found a correlation between blink rate and several corneal parameters, including front K1, front K2, front Km, back K1, back K2, back Km, final D, and radii minimum, indicating that rapid blinking also increases the mechanical pressure on the surface of the cornea and changes the corneal curvature.

The final D index from the Belin/Ambrósio Enhanced Ectasia Display is amultimetric combination parameter composed of keratometric, pachymetric, pachymetric progression, and back elevation parameters. It is suggested that the final D index could be used as the sole parameter to identify early corneal ectasia [24]. Using a final D value greater than 2.61 as a cut off value may help to identify the majority of keratoconus suspects who truly have the disease [25]. In the present study, we found that final D values were significantly higher in the severe blepharospasm group than among controls, which indicated a high risk of subclinical keratoconus-like changes in severely blepharospastic eyes.

The limitations of this study should be noted as well. Firstly, all included subjects were Chinese. Because the anatomy of the eyelids and orbits differ between Asians and other races, the accurate definition and classification of blepharospasm also differ between these groups [26, 27]. Secondly, the sample size of our study was small, and the parameters must be investigated in a larger patient group. Third, it is a single-center study, which may make our results prone to a hospital-based bias. Finally, it is important to be aware of the predictive limitations of our cross-sectional study. Although the cross-sectional design

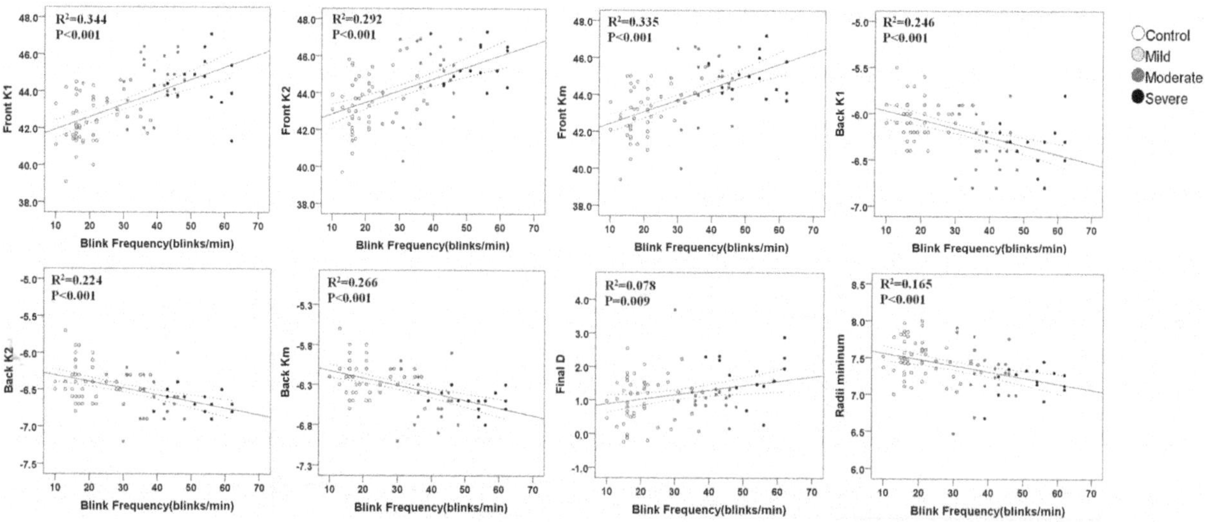

Fig. 2 Correlations between blink rate (blinks/min) and corneal parameters, including front K1, front K2, front Km, back K1, back K2, back Km, final D and radii minimum. Spearman rank correlation coefficients (R^2 value) are shown with statistical significance of the correlations. The linear regression line is shown with the 95% confidence intervals of mean

Table 6 Intraclass correlation coefficient of parameters between control and blepharospasm

	Control	Blepharoptosis		
		Mild	*Moderate*	*Severe*
Anterior				
Keratometric (K1, K2, Km)	0.991–0.994	0.984–0.998	0.992–0.996	0.981–0.992
Topometric (ISV, IVA, KI, CKI, IHD, IHA)	0.982–0.989	0.972–0.994	0.987–0.994	0.946–0.978
Elevation	0.975–0.985	0.964–0.991	0.943–0.965	0.923–0.967
Posterior				
Keratometric (K1, K2, Km)	0.967–0.995	0.981–0.995	0.942–0.987	0.921–0.965
Elevation	0.932–0.985	0.946–0.979	0.921–0.954	0.934–0.981
Pachymetry				
Pachymetry parameters	0.945–0.967	0.945–0.967	0.923–0.956	0.943–0.956
(Apex thickness, Min PI, Max PI)	0.978–0.981	0.954–0.976	0.925–0.975	0.932–0.967

K1 flat keratometry, *K2* steep keratometry, *Km* mean keratometry, *ISV* index of surface variance, *IVA* index of vertical asymmetry, *KI* keratoconus-index, *CKI* center keratoconus-index, *IHD* index of height decentration, *IHA* index of height asymmetry, *PI* progression index

allowed us to provide evidence of corneal tomography differences between blepharospasm patients and the control group, longitudinal design studies are necessary to establish a true cause-and-effect relationship.

Conclusions

In summary, this study measured the corneal architecture with a Pentacam rotating Scheimpflug camera, and proved that the pressure applied by the lids over the cornea may result in corneal shape changes in blepharospasm patients, particularly in severe cases, which may play a critical role in everyday diagnostic procedures and the pre-operative screening of patients seeking refractive surgery.

Abbreviations

ART: Ambrósio's relational thickness; BFS: Best-fit sphere; BTX: Botulinum toxin; CKI: Center keratoconus-index; Front Astig: Front astigmatism magnitude; IHA: Index of height asymmetry; IHD: Index of height decentration; ISV: Index of surface variance; IVA: Index of vertical asymmetry; K1: Flat keratometry; K2: Steep keratometry; KI: Keratoconus-index; Km: Mean keratometry; PI: Progression index; RM: Radii minimum

Funding

Supported by project foundation: 1. The Medical and Health Science and Technology Program of Zhejiang Province (2018242126) 2. National Natural Science Foundation of China (81670888) 3. The National Key Research and Development Program of China (2016YFC1100403).

Authors' contributions

HZ: Conception and design the research, draft the manuscript. HZ: Acquisition of data, analysis and interpretation of data. TZ: Revise the manuscript critically for important intellectual content. JY: Design the research and give final approval of the version to be published. All authors read and approved the final manuscript.

Competing interests

The authors declare that they have no competing interests.

Author details

[1]Department of Ophthalmology, the Second Affiliated Hospital, Zhejiang University School of Medicine, Hangzhou, Zhejiang, China. [2]Hangzhou Hospital for the Prevention and Treatment of Occupational Diseases, Hangzhou, Zhejiang, China.

References

1. Malinovsky V. Benign essential blepharospasm. J Am Optom Assoc. 1987;58: 646–51.
2. Read SA, Collins MJ, Carney LG. The influence of eyelid morphology on normal corneal shape. Invest Ophthalmol Vis Sci. 2007;48:112–9.
3. Shaw AJ, Collins MJ, Davis BA, Carney LG. Corneal refractive changes due to short-term eyelid pressure in downward gaze. J Cataract Refract Surg. 2008; 34:1546–53.
4. Shaw AJB: Eyelid pressure on the Cornea. 2009.
5. Moon NJ, Lee HI, Kim JC. The changes in corneal astigmatism after botulinum toxin-a injection in patients with blepharospasm. J Korean Med Sci. 2006;21:131–5.
6. Shankar H, Taranath D, Santhirathelagan CT, Pesudovs K. Anterior segment biometry with the Pentacam: comprehensive assessment of repeatability of automated measurements. J Cataract Refract Surg. 2008;34:103–13.
7. Konstantopoulos A, Hossain P, Anderson DF. Recent advances in ophthalmic anterior segment imaging: a new era for ophthalmic diagnosis? Br J Ophthalmol. 2007;91:551–7.
8. Barkana Y, Gerber Y, Elbaz U, Schwartz S, Ken-Dror G, Avni I, et al. Central corneal thickness measurement with the Pentacam Scheimpflug system, optical low-coherence reflectometry pachymeter, and ultrasound pachymetry. J Cataract Refract Surg. 2005;31:1729–35.
9. Buehl W, Stojanac D, Sacu S, Drexler W, Findl O. Comparison of three methods of measuring corneal thickness and anterior chamber depth. Am J Ophthalmol. 2006;141:7–12.
10. Dubbelman M, Sicam VA, Van der Heijde GL. The shape of the anterior and posterior surface of the aging human cornea. Vis Res. 2006;46:993–1001.
11. Jankovic J, Kenney C, Grafe S, Goertelmeyer R, Comes G. Relationship between various clinical outcome assessments in patients with blepharospasm. Mov Disord. 2009;24:407–13.
12. Jankovic J, Schwartz K. Botulinum toxin injections for cervical dystonia. Neurology. 1990;40:277–80.
13. Patel S, Henderson R, Bradley L, Galloway B, Hunter L. Effect of visual display unit use on blink rate and tear stability. Optom Vis Sci. 1991;68:888–92.

14. Zhu T, Ye X, Xu P, Wang J, Zhang H, Ni H, et al. Changes of corneal tomography in patients with congenital blepharoptosis. Sci Rep. 2017;7:6580.
15. Thibos LN, Wheeler W, Horner D. Power vectors: an application of Fourier analysis to the description and statistical analysis of refractive error. Optom Vis Sci. 1997;74:367–75.
16. Mavrikakis I, Beckingsale P, Lee E, Riaz Y, Brittain P. Changes in corneal topography with upper eyelid gold weight implants. Ophthal Plast Reconstr Surg. 2006;22:331–4.
17. Detorakis ET, Ioannakis K, Kozobolis VP. Corneal topography in involutional ectropion of the lower eyelid: preoperative and postoperative evaluation. Cornea. 2005;24:431–4.
18. Osaki T, Osaki MH, Osaki TH, Hirai FE, Nallasamy N, Campos M. Influence of involuntary eyelid spasms on corneal topographic and eyelid morphometric changes in patients with hemifacial spasm. Br J Ophthalmol. 2016;100:963–70.
19. Kim JT, MC MWB, Jr RA, Khachikian SS. Tomographic normal values for corneal elevation and Pachymetry in a hyperopic population. J Clin Exp Ophthalmol. 2011;2
20. Lim L, Wei RH, Chan WK, Tan DT. Evaluation of keratoconus in Asians: role of Orbscan II and Tomey TMS-2 corneal topography. Am J Ophthalmol. 2007;143:390–400.
21. Carney LG, Hill RM. The nature of normal blinking patterns. Acta Ophthalmol. 1982;60:427–33.
22. Collins M, Seeto R, Campbell L, Ross M. Blinking and corneal sensitivity. Acta Ophthalmol. 1989;67:525–31.
23. Rahman EZ, Lam PK, Chu CK, Moore Q, Pflugfelder SC. Corneal sensitivity in tear dysfunction and its correlation with clinical parameters and blink rate. Am J Ophthalmol. 2015;160:858–66. e5
24. Muftuoglu O, Ayar O, Hurmeric V, Orucoglu F, Kilic I. Comparison of multimetric D index with keratometric, pachymetric, and posterior elevation parameters in diagnosing subclinical keratoconus in fellow eyes of asymmetric keratoconus patients. J Cataract Refract Surg. 2015;41:557–65.
25. Belin MW, Villavicencio OF, Ambrosio RR, Jr. Tomographic parameters for the detection of keratoconus: suggestions for screening and treatment parameters. Eye & contact lens 2014; 40:326–330.
26. Paik JS, Jung SK, Han KD, Kim SD, Park YM, Yang SW. Obesity as a potential risk factor for Blepharoptosis: the Korea National Health and nutrition examination survey 2008-2010. PLoS One. 2015;10:e0131427.
27. Griepentrog GJ, Diehl NN, Mohney BG. Incidence and demographics of childhood ptosis. Ophthalmology. 2011;118:1180–3.

20

Therapeutic effects of 3% diquafosol ophthalmic solution in patients with short tear film break-up time-type dry eye disease

Yongseok Mun[1†], Ji-Won Kwon[2†] and Joo Youn Oh[1,3*]

Abstract

Background: To investigate therapeutic effects of topical diquafosol tetrasodium 3% ophthalmic solution in patients with short tear film break-up time (TFBUT)-type dry eye (DE).

Methods: The prospective study was performed in 70 eyes of 70 patients with short TFBUT-type DE. Diagnosis of short TFBUT-type DE was made based on the presence of DE symptoms, TFBUT value ≤ 5 s, corneoconjunctival staining score ≤ 2 (on a scale of 0 to 4), and Schirmer I value > 5 mm. Patients with systemic immunologic disorders or ocular graft-versus-host disease were excluded. Before and after instillation of 3% diquafosol ophthalmic solution six times per day for 4 weeks, subjective DE symptoms, TFBUT, corneoconjunctival staining score, and Schirmer I value were examined and compared. Also, demographic factors were compared between patients who showed improvement in each DE parameter by treatment and those who did not.

Results: Four-week treatment with 3% diquafosol ophthalmic solution significantly improved DE symptoms ($p < 0.0001$), increased TFBUT ($p < 0.0001$), and reduced corneoconjunctival staining scores ($p < 0.0001$). Schirmer I values were not changed by treatment. The age of patients who showed improvement in subjective DE symptoms after treatment was significantly lower than that of patients who did not (53.4 ± 27.5 vs. 63.3 ± 13.9 years, $p = 0.012$). Ocular side effects developed in 3 patients (4.3%), including conjunctival chemosis ($n = 1$) and persistent stinging sensation ($n = 2$).

Conclusions: Diquafosol tetrasodium 3% ophthalmic solution is effective in improving subjective symptoms and tear film stability in short TFBUT-type DE patients.

Keywords: Diquafosol tetrasodium 3%, Dry eye disease, Short tear film break-up time-type dry eye

* Correspondence: jooyounoh77@gmail.com
†Yongseok Mun and Ji-Won Kwon contributed equally to this work.
[1]Department of Ophthalmology, Seoul National University Hospital, 101, Daehak-ro, Jongno-gu, Seoul 03080, South Korea
[3]Laboratory of Ocular Regenerative Medicine and Immunology, Biomedical Research Institute, Seoul National University Hospital, 101 Daehak-ro, Jongno-gu, Seoul 03080, South Korea
Full list of author information is available at the end of the article

Background

Dry eye disease (DED) is a multifactorial disease of the ocular surface, which is associated with various conditions such as tear film instability and hyperosmolarity, ocular surface inflammation and damage, or neurosensory abnormalities [1]. For etiopathogenic classification of DED, the TFOS DEWS II Definition and Classification Subcommittee reinforced the two major etiological categories of DED: aqueous deficient and evaporative [1]. Aqueous deficient dry eye (ADDE) is due to a failure of lacrimal tear production, and evaporative dry eye (EDE) is associated with increased evaporation of the tear film in the presence of normal lacrimal secretion. Importantly, ADDE and EDE are not mutually exclusive and commonly overlapping, [1] both leading to tear film instability which can be measured by the tear break-up time (TFBUT). Recently, a new concept of short tear film break-up time (TFBUT)-type dry eye (DE) has emerged as a potentially new type of DED [2, 3].

The short TFBUT-type DE is characterized by a short TFBUT and DE symptoms without ocular surface damage and tear deficiency [2, 3]. This type of DE has been shown to be associated with visual display terminal (VDT) work and contact lens (CL) wear [4–7], and therefore, the prevalence of short TFBUT-type DE is rising with the widespread use of VDT and CL [8, 9]. For the treatment, a few studies in a small number of patients showed the efficacy of 3% diquafosol ophthalmic solution in improving subjective symptoms and TFBUT in patients with short TFBUT-type DE [10–12].

Diquafosol is an agonist for $P2Y_2$ purinergic receptor which exists in conjunctival epithelial cells, goblet cells, and epithelium of meibomian glands [13–16]. By activating $P2Y_2$ receptors on the ocular surface, diquafosol stimulates both fluid secretion from conjunctival epithelial cells and mucin secretion from goblet cells, thereby stabilizing the tear film and hydrating the ocular surface, independent of tear secretion from lacrimal glands [13–16]. Hence, it is possible that diquafosol ophthalmic solution has therapeutic potential in short TFBUT-type DE patients. In this study, we investigated the therapeutic effects of topical application of diquafosol tetrasodium 3% ophthalmic solution in patients with short TFBUT-type DE.

Methods

Patients

The study was approved by the Institutional Review Board of Seoul National University Hospital (IRB No. 1402–058-557) on February 25, 2014 and performed in accordance with the tenets of the Declaration of Helsinki. The patients with short TFBUT-type DE were prospectively enrolled with informed consent in Seoul National University Hospital from March 14, 2014 to December 19, 2014 and followed-up for 4 weeks. The

diagnosis of short TFBUT-type DE was made based upon the presence of DE symptoms, TFBUT value ≤5 s, corneoconjunctival staining score ≤ 2 (on a scale of 0 to 4), and Schirmer I test value > 5 mm/5 min. Patients with systemic immune-mediated diseases such as secondary Sjögren's syndrome or graft-versus-host disease were excluded. Also, patients who were on topical medication(s) for treatment of ocular diseases other than DED such as glaucoma or allergic conjunctivitis were excluded.

Treatment and examination

The subjective DE symptoms, TFBUT, corneoconjunctival staining scores, and Schirmer I values were examined before and after 4 weeks of instillation of diquafosol tetrasodium 3% ophthalmic solution (Diquas®, Santen Pharmaceutical Co., Ltd., Osaka, Japan) six times per day. Other topical medications than Diquas® were discontinued during the study period. Demographic factors including age and gender were compared between patients who showed improvement in each DE parameter after treatment and those who did not show any change. Systemic or ocular side effects were recorded.

The criteria for subjective DE symptom scoring are as follows: 0 (no symptom), 1 (mild symptoms of ocular dryness, occasional and not interfering with daily life), 2 (moderate symptoms, occasional or chronic, but not interfering with daily life), 3 (severe frequent or constant, but not interfering with daily life), and 4 (severe, constant and disabling). The corneoconjunctival staining score was assessed by fluorescein staining as follows: 0 (no staining), 1 (mild conjunctival and corneal staining), 2 (moderate conjunctival and corneal staining), 3 (moderate to severe conjunctival staining and marked central corneal staining), and 4 (severe conjunctival staining and severe, diffuse corneal punctate erosions).

TFBUT measurements were performed as previously recommended [2]. In brief, after instillation of a small quantity of 1% fluorescein dye into the inferior conjunctival sac, patients were instructed to blink several times to ensure mixing of the dye with the tear. Under a cobalt blue filter and slit lamp biomicroscope, the interval between the last complete blink and appearance of the first corneal black spot in the stained tear film was measured [2]. The measurements were made three times for each eye by the same doctor, and the mean value of the three measurements was calculated.

The Schirmer I test was done by putting the Schirmer paper strip at the junction of the middle and lateral thirds of the lower eyelid of patients without anesthesia. Patients were then instructed to close their eyes for 5 min, and the wetting length of the strip was recorded in mm.

The primary outcome was the mean change from baseline in TFBUT at 4 weeks after treatment and the secondary outcome measures were the changes in the subjective DE symptom scores and Schirmer I test results.

Statistical analysis

The power analysis was performed to justify the number of patients using G*Power 3.1.9.2. A sample size of 80 patients was determined to provide the study with 80% statistical power to detect 30% mean difference in TFBUT between control and treatment groups under the assumption that data would be missing in 15% of patients.

The GraphPad Prism® (GraphPad Software, Inc., La Jolla, CA) was used for statistical analysis. The change between pre and post-treatment values in each patient was assessed for significant difference by two-tailed paired t test. The comparisons of demographic factors between patients who showed improvement in each DE parameter after treatment and those who did not were made by two-tailed t test. Statistical significance was defined as p value < 0.05.

Results

Initially, 80 eyes of 80 patients with short TFBUT-type DE were enrolled. In case of bilateral involvement, the eye with shorter TFBUT at baseline was included for analysis. Three eyes were withdrawn from the study because of ocular side effects and 7 eyes excluded because of follow-up loss. Therefore, a total of 70 eyes completed the study, from which data were analyzed.

Demographic data and baseline ocular characteristics were shown in Table 1. The subjects included 9 men and 61 women, and the mean age was 55.8 ± 14.1 years (range 22 to 83 years). At the time of enrollment, 27 patients (38.6%) were using artificial tears containing hyaluronic acid on irregular basis without symptomatic relief. The subjective DE symptom score was 2.84 ± 0.65 at baseline, and TFBUT was 2.72 ± 0.94 s. The corneoconjunctival staining score was 1.17 ± 0.61, and Schirmer I value was 9.34 ± 2.60 mm. Patients were instructed to

Table 1 Patient demographics and baseline ocular characteristics ($n = 70$)

Demographics	
Gender (male: female)	9: 61
Age (years in mean ± SD, range)	55.8 ± 14.1 (22–83)
Diabetes mellitus	4 (5.7%)
Use of topical medication(s)	
Artificial tears (hyaluronic acid-based)	27 (38.6%)
Ocular characteristics	
Dry eye symptom score (range)	2.84 ± 0.65 (1–4)
Tear film break-up time (sec, range)	2.72 ± 0.94 (1–5)
Ocular staining score (range)	1.17 ± 0.61 (0–2)
Schirmer I test (mm, range)	9.34 ± 2.60 (6–18)

discontinue any eye drops and start using 3% diquafosol ophthalmic solution alone.

After 4 weeks of treatment with 3% diquafosol ophthalmic solution, the subjective DE symptom improved in 55 eyes (78.6%) compared to before treatment, and TFBUT increased in 46 eyes (65.7%) (Table 2). The corneoconjunctival staining score was reduced in 44 eyes (62.8%) by treatment (Table 2). Quantitative analysis showed that the diquafosol treatment significantly reduced DE symptom scores in patients from 2.84 ± 0.65 to 1.63 ± 1.19 ($p < 0.0001$) and increased TFBUT from 2.72 ± 0.94 s to 4.13 ± 1.62 s ($p < 0.0001$) (Fig. 1). Also, the corneoconjunctival staining scores decreased from 1.17 ± 0.61 to 0.42 ± 0.63 after treatment ($p < 0.0001$) (Fig. 1). However, the Schirmer I values were not changed by treatment (9.34 ± 2.60 mm before treatment vs. 9.59 ± 2.88 mm after treatment, $p = 0.6013$).

Additionally, demographic factors were compared between patients who showed improvement in each DE parameter and those who did not show any improvement with 3% diquafosol sodium. Of note was the finding that the age of patients whose DE symptoms improved after treatment was significantly lower than that of patients whose symptoms did not change (53.4 ± 27.5 vs. 63.3 ± 13.9 years, $p = 0.012$) (Table 3). No significant changes were found in the age between patients who had improvement in TFBUT or ocular staining score and those who did not (Table 3).

Ocular side effects developed in 3 patients (4.3%) that included persistent stinging sensation in two patients and conjunctival chemosis in one. Conjunctival chemosis disappeared after cessation of diquafosol and application of fluorometholone eye drops (Flarex®, Alcon Laboratories, Inc. Fort Worth, TX). The stinging sensation completely resolved in all patients after discontinuing 3% diquafosol.

Discussion

Since 3% diquafosol ophthalmic solution (Diquas®) was launched and approved in South Korea (in 2011) and in Japan (in 2010), it has been widely used in clinic for treatment of DE. As a $P2Y_2$ purinergic receptor agonist, diquafosol has novel mechanisms of action including stimulation

Table 2 The percentage of patients who showed changes in dry eye symptoms and ocular signs after 4 weeks of topical 3% diquafosol ophthalmic solution administration

Changes after treatment	No. patients (%)		
	Improved	No change	Worsened
Subjective dry eye symptom	55 (78.6)	15 (21.4)	0 (0)
Tear film break-up time[a]	46 (65.7)	22 (31.4)	2 (2.9)
Ocular staining score	44 (62.8)	23 (32.9)	3 (4.3)

[a]An increase in tear film break-up time after treatment was defined as "Improved, and a decrease as "Worsened". The same values of tear film break-up time before and after treatment were defined as "No change"

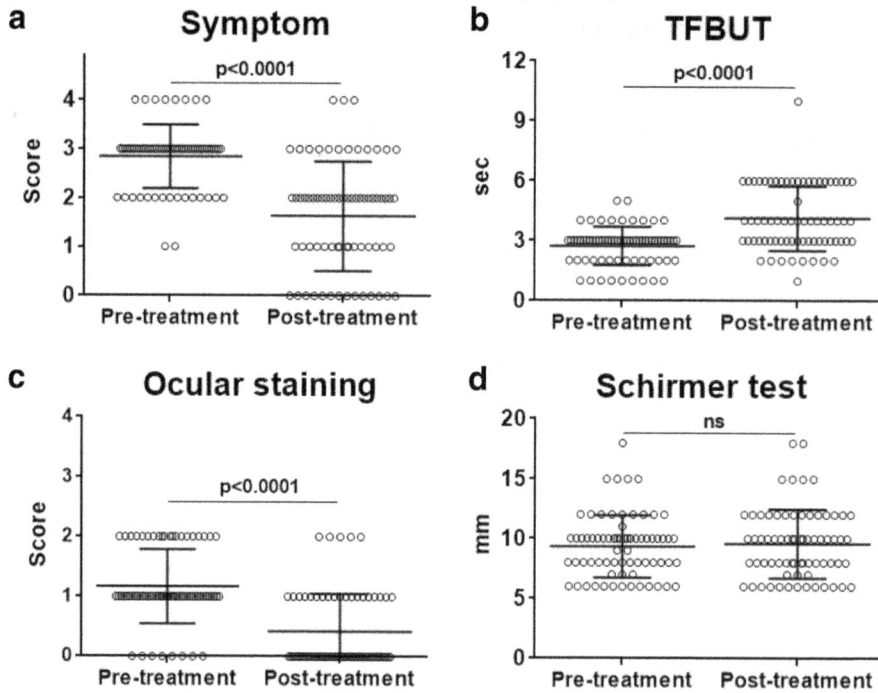

Fig. 1 Comparison of changes in dry eye parameters before and after 3% diquafosol ophthalmic solution administration. Changes in subjective dry eye symptom scores (**a**), tear film break-up time (TFBUT) (**b**), corneoconjunctival staining scores (**c**), and Schirmer I test values (**d**) before (pre-treatment) and after 4 weeks of 3% diquafosol ophthalmic solution administration (post-treatment)

of fluid and mucin secretion in conjunctival epithelial and goblet cells or promotion of membrane-binding mucin gene expression in corneal epithelial cells [13–16]. Therefore, diquafosol increases fluid secretion independent of lacrimal gland function and makes the ocular surface more hydrophilic, both of which lead to strengthening of the aqueous-mucin layer and stabilization of tear film in healthy subjects and DE patients [13–16].

Topical instillation of 3% diquafosol ophthalmic solution has been reported to be effective for both categories of DED: ADDE and EDE [14–20]. In particular, several studies recently reported that topical diquafosol is effective in alleviating symptoms and increasing TFBUT in patients with short TFBUT-type DE [10–12] which is characterized by a reduced TFBUT without much epithelial damage and

Table 3 The age of patients who showed improvement in dry eye symptoms and ocular signs after 4 weeks of topical 3% diquafosol ophthalmic solution administration

Changes after treatment	Age of patients (mean ± SD)		p value
	Improved	Not improved	
Subjective dry eye symptom	53.4 ± 27.5	63.3 ± 13.9	0.012
Tear film break-up time[a]	55.5 ± 13.8	56.5 ± 14.5	0.782
Ocular staining score	54.6 ± 13.9	57.8 ± 14.1	0.359

[a]An increase in tear film break-up time after treatment was defined as "Improved, and a decrease as "Worsened". The same values of tear film break-up time before and after treatment were defined as "No change

lacrimal gland dysfunction. In a study by Shimazaki-Den et al. [10], 39 eyes with DE symptoms and short TFBUT, but without epithelial damage and decreased Schirmer I values (≤ 5 mm), received 3% diquafosol ophthalmic solution 6 times a day. The subjective symptoms as assessed by a VAS (visual analog scale) score and TFBUT significantly improved from baseline at 1 and 3 months after treatment, whereas there was no significant change in Schirmer values. In another study by Jung et al. [11], 30 DED patients who had TFBUT < 5 s and basal tear secretion ≥5 mm on the Schirmer test were treated with 3% diquafosol 6 times a day in combination with 0.1% hyaluronic acid artificial tears. At 1 and 3 months, TFBUT was increased and DE symptoms decreased, although there were no differences in corneoconjunctival staining scores and Schirmer test results. In line with these studies, we here investigated clinical effects of 3% diquafosol in 70 patients with short TFBUT-type DE. Results demonstrate that topical application of 3% diquafosol for 1 month provided improvement of DE symptoms, TFBUT, and corneoconjunctival staining in 78.6%, 65.7%, and 62.8% of short TFBUT-type DE patients, respectively. Compared to before treatment, TFBUT was significantly increased after treatment, and DE symptoms and corneoconjunctival staining scores significantly decreased. Ocular adverse reactions were observed in 4.3% of patients, which is comparable to 6.3% in previous studies [17].

There are several novel findings in our study. One is that the age of patients who had symptomatic relief in response to diquafosol treatment was lower compared to patients who did not. Therefore, it is possible that diquafosol might serve as an effective treatment for short TFBUT-type DE related to environmental stresses such as VDT use or CL wear in young patients with normal lacrimal gland function [4–7]. Another is that the patients in our study had severe symptoms (the mean symptom score 2.84 on a scale of 0 to 4) relative to mild ocular surface damage (the mean staining score 1.17 on a scale of 0 to 4). All of them had normal lacrimal gland secretion (Schirmer I values > 5 mm), and the ocular surface inflammation was not clinically evident in most of patients. This type of DED corresponds to the level 1 and 2 DED according to the Korean Corneal Disease Study Group guidelines for the diagnosis of dry eye disease [21], and represents the most common type of DED in real world [2, 21]. Hence, our study suggests a possibility that 3% diquafosol ophthalmic solution might have a broader implication as a therapy for DED patients. In support for this, a multicenter, prospective, non-interventional observational study involving over 3000 "real-world" DED patients demonstrated that administration of 3% diquafosol ophthalmic solution was effective regardless of the severity of DED based on the ocular staining score, and a total of 76.0% of the enrolled patients responded that their condition had improved after 2 months of treatment [17]. Similarly, 3% diquafosol provided symptomatic relief in 78.6% of patients in our study.

Our study has several limitations. First, the treatment was not compared with a control treatment in parallel. Second, the therapeutic outcome and side effects were examined in the short-term (1 month after treatment). Third, it was performed in a small number of patients ($n = 70$), although our study involves the largest number of short TFBUT-type DE patients where the effects of diquafosol have been tested so far. In the future, a randomized controlled study in a larger number of patients with the longer follow-up period would be necessary to identify the DED type in which diquafosol is the most effective and to further broaden the disease indications for its use.

Conclusions

In conclusion, diquafosol tetrasodium 3% ophthalmic solution is effective in alleviating symptoms, stabilizing tear film, and decreasing ocular surface damage in patients with short TFBUT-type DE.

Abbreviations
ADDE: aqueous tear-deficient dry eye; CL: contact lens; DE: dry eye; DED: dry eye disease; EDE: evaporative dry eye; TFBUT: tear break-up time; VAS: visual analog scale; VDT: visual display terminal

Funding
This study was supported by Basic Science Research Program through the National Research Foundation of Korea (NRF) funded by the Ministry of Science, ICT and future Planning (2018R1A2B2004108).

Authors' contributions
YM analyzed the data and wrote the manuscript. JK analyzed the data and wrote the manuscript. JYO designed the study, analyzed and interpreted the patient data, and was a major contributor in writing the manuscript. All authors read and approved the final manuscript.

Competing interests
The authors declare that they have no competing interests.

Author details
[1]Department of Ophthalmology, Seoul National University Hospital, 101, Daehak-ro, Jongno-gu, Seoul 03080, South Korea. [2]Department of ophthalmology, Hanyang University College of Medicine Myongji Hospital, 14 Bungil 55, Hwasu-Ro, Deokyang-Gu, Goyang-si, Gyeonggi-do 14075, South Korea. [3]Laboratory of Ocular Regenerative Medicine and Immunology, Biomedical Research Institute, Seoul National University Hospital, 101 Daehak-ro, Jongno-gu, Seoul 03080, South Korea.

References
1. Craig JP, Nichols KK, Akpek EK, Caffery B, Dua HS, Joo CK, et al. TFOS DEWS II definition and classification report. Ocul Surf. 2017;15:26–83.
2. Tsubota K, Yokoi N, Shimazaki J, Watanabe H, Dogru M, Yamada M, et al. New perspectives on dry eye definition and diagnosis: a consensus report by the Asia dry eye society. Ocul Surf. 2017;15:65–76.
3. Shimazaki-Den S, Dogru M, Higa K, Shimazaki J. Symptoms, visual function, and mucin expression of eyes with tear film instability. Cornea. 2013;32:1211–8.
4. Uchino M, Yokoi N, Uchino Y, Dogru M, Kawashima M, Komuro A, et al. Prevalence of dry eye disease and its risk factors in visual display terminal users: the Osaka study. Am J Ophthalmol. 2013;156:759–66.
5. Yokoi N, Uchino M, Uchino Y, Dogru M, Kawashima M, Komuro A, et al. Importance of tear film instability in dry eye disease in office workers using visual display terminals: the Osaka study. Am J Ophthalmol. 2015;159:748–54.
6. Kojima T, Ibrahim OM, Wakamatsu T, Tsuyama A, Ogawa J, Matsumoto Y, et al. The impact of contact lens wear and visual display terminal work on ocular surface and tear functions in office workers. Am J Ophthalmol. 2011;152:933–40.
7. Yamamoto Y, Yokoi N, Higashihara H, Inagaki K, Sonomura Y, Komuro A, et al. Clinical characteristics of short tear film breakup time (BUT) -type dry eye. Nippon Ganka Gakkai Zasshi. 2012;116:1137–43.
8. Kawashima M, Yamada M, Suwaki K, Shigeyasu C, Uchino M, Hiratsuka Y, et al. A clinic-based survey of clinical characteristics and practice pattern of dry eye in Japan. Adv Ther. 2017;34:732–43.
9. Uchino M, Nishiwaki Y, Michikawa T, Shirakawa K, Kuwahara E, Yamada M, et al. Prevalence and risk factors of dry eye disease in Japan: Koumi study. Ophthalmology. 2011;118:2361–7.
10. Shimazaki-Den S, Iseda H, Dogru M, Shimazaki J. Effects of diquafosol sodium eye drops on tear film stability in short BUT type of dry eye. Cornea. 2013;32:1120–5.
11. Jung HH, Kang YS, Sung MS, Yoon KC. Clinical efficacy of topical 3% Diquafosol Tetrasodium in short tear film break-up time dry eye. J Korean Ophthalmol Soc. 2015;56:339–44.
12. Kaido M, Uchino M, Kojima T, Dogru M, Tsubota K. Effects of diquafosol tetrasodium administration on visual function in short break-up time dry eye. J Ocul Pharmacol Ther. 2013;29:595–603.
13. Nichols KK, Yerxa B, Kellerman DJ. Diquafosol tetrasodium: a novel dry eye therapy. Expert Opin Investig Drugs. 2004;13:47–54.
14. Lau OC, Samarawickrama C, Skalicky SE. P2Y2 receptor agonists for the treatment of dry eye disease: a review. Clin Ophthalmol. 2014;8:327–34.

15. Nakamura M, Imanaka T, Sakamoto A. Diquafosol ophthalmic solution for dry eye treatment. Adv Ther. 2012;29:579–89.
16. Koh S. Clinical utility of 3% diquafosol ophthalmic solution in the treatment of dry eyes. Clin Ophthalmol. 2015;9:865–72.
17. Yamaguchi M, Nishijima T, Shimazaki J, Takamura E, Yokoi N, Watanabe H, et al. Clinical usefulness of diquafosol for real-world dry eye patients: a prospective, open-label, non-interventional, observational study. Adv Ther. 2014;31:1169–81.
18. Tauber J, Davitt WF, Bokosky JE, Nichols KK, Yerxa BR, Schaberg AE, et al. Double-masked, placebo-controlled safety and efficacy trial of diquafosol tetrasodium (INS365) ophthalmic solution for the treatment of dry eye. Cornea. 2004;23:784–92.
19. Jeon HS, Hyon JY. The efficacy of Diquafosol ophthalmic solution in non-Sjögren and Sjögren syndrome dry eye patients unresponsive to artificial tear. J Ocul Pharmacol Ther. 2016;32:463–8.
20. Gong L, Sun X, Ma Z, Wang Q, Xu X, Chen X, et al. A randomised, parallel-group comparison study of diquafosol ophthalmic solution in patients with dry eye in China and Singapore. Br J Ophthalmol. 2015;99:903–8.
21. Hyon JY, Kim HM, Lee D, Chung ES, Song JS, Choi CY, et al. Korean guidelines for the diagnosis and management of dry eye: development and validation of clinical efficacy. Korean J Ophthalmol. 2014;28:197–206.

21

Implantable collamer lens surgery in patients with primary iris and/or ciliary body cysts

Zhen Li[*], Zhike Xu, Yaqin Wang, Qiang Liu and Bin Chen

Abstract

Background: The prevalence of primary iris and/or ciliary body cysts is common in myopia, though asymptomatic in nearly all cases. It's a very valuable thing to study the clinical safety and reliability of implantable collamer lens (ICL) surgery in patients with primary iris and/or ciliary body cysts.

Methods: A total of 108 patients (201 eyes) were included in this retrospective study. All eyes had been implanted with V4c implantable collamer lens (ICLV4c). According to the eyes with or without primary iris and/or ciliary body cysts, all eyes were divided into two groups. We observed preoperative and postoperative uncorrected distance visual acuity (UDVA), corrected distance visual acuity)(CDVA), intra-ocular pressure(IOP), anterior chamber volume(ACV), anterior chamber depth(ACD), trabecular-iris angle (TIA), angle opening distance at 500 μm (AOD500) ,vertical central distance between the corneal endothelium and the front surface of ICL(CE-ICL), and the central vault. The follow-up periods covered 12 months.

Results: Among all the 201 eyes, primary iris and/or ciliary body cysts were detected in 54 eyes (26.87%),but the prevalence was account to 36.11%(18males,21females).There were 30 eyes (55.56%) with unilateral single cyst, 12 eyes (22.22%) with unilateral double cysts, 12 eyes (22.22%) eyes with unilateral multiple and/or multi-quadrants cysts, the mean size of cysts was (0.714 ± 0.149)mm(range from 0.510 to 1.075 mm).30.4% of the cysts were located at iridociliary sulcus, 65.5% in pars plicata, and 4.1% in midzonal iris, which showed a characteristic distribution pattern, with cysts found predominantly in the inferior and temporal quadrants.The postoperative size and the number of cysts showed nearly no changes. The postoperative ACV, AOD500 and TIA showed a statistical reduction in both two groups ($P < 0.05$), but with no statistical significant between the two groups ($P > 0.05$), the parameters of postoperative IOP,CE-ICL and central vault also showed the same results as which. We did not observe serious complication and IOP elevating in the whole follow-up periods.

Conclusion: Primary iris and/or ciliary body cysts are not absolutely contraindication for ICL surgery. For some single cyst smaller than 1.075 mm or single quadrant cysts located at ciliary body are rare to lead some serious complications. But, for some multiple cysts, especially multi-quadrants cysts located at iridociliary sulcus, we still should remain cautions.

Keywords: Implantable collamer lens, Myopia, Phakic intraocular lens, Primary iris and ciliary body cyst, Ultrasound biomicroscope

* Correspondence: lizhen81131@163.com
Department of Ophthalmology, The People's Hospital of Leshan, 635
Wanghaoer Street, Leshan, Sichuan Province 614000, People's Republic of
China

Background

The implantable collamer Lens (ICL) (STAAR Surgical Co.), which have been reported to perform well for the correction of moderate to high myopia [1–4]. But the prevalence of primary iris and/or ciliary body cysts in myopia is common, especially in young adult or middle-aged women [5]. In the last years, primary iris and /or ciliary body cysts were hardly detected by using common ophthalmic examinations. With the development of advanced medical technique, UBM is an important investigation which could effectively excludes the differential diagnosis of some ring melanoma of the iris and multiple separate cysts of the iris pigment epithelium [6]. Primary iris and/or ciliary body cysts are usually located inferotemporally in the anterior segment, most commonly in the iridociliary sulcus [7].Though asymptomatic in nearly all cases, they may rarely enlarge or cause secondary glaucoma, corneal decompensation [8]. Because, there were no relative reports about the safety and reliability of ICL implantation in patients with iris and/or ciliary body cysts. Our research was aimed to evaluate the clinical safety and reliability of ICL surgery in patients with primary iris and/or ciliary body cysts.

Methods

Patient and public involvement

Our study was a retrospective analysis. A total of 108 patients (201 eyes) were included in this study. All eyes were implanted with the myopic ICLV4c (ICMV4C model) by an experienced doctor at the Department of ophthalmology, The People's Hospital of Leshan, Sichuan Province, China, from July 2015 to December 2016. Group1 included 54 eyes with primary iris and/or ciliary body cysts. Group2 included 147 eyes without cysts. Before our analysis, all patients and /or public were not involved in the design of this study. This project was approved by the science and technology foundation of Sichuan Provincial Health and Family Planning Commission (NO.150065), which met the demand of Declaration of Helsinki. Informed consents were obtained from all subjects.

Data collection

Inclusion criteria for this study included patients age between 18 and 45 years, myopia between --2.50 and –21.00DS, astigmatism between 0 and – 6.00 DC, anterior chamber depth (ACD) of 2.80 mm or more, and an endothelial cell density greater than 2000 cells/mm^2. Patients were also required to have a reasonable expectation of surgical outcomes, no preexisting ocular pathology, no keratoconus, cataract or glaucoma, and no serious systemic diseases [9]. Preoperatively, all the patients underwent a complete ophthalmic examination,which included uncorrected distance visual acuity

(UDVA), corrected distance visual acuity(CDVA), slit lamp biomicroscopy, indirect ophthalmoscopy, corneal thickness (CT), anterior chamber volume (ACV) (Pentacam, Oculus,Germany), intra-ocular pressure (IOP), the horizontal white-to-white distance, endothelial cell density, anterior chamber depth (ACD),trabecular-iris angle (TIA) and angle opening distance at 500 μm (AOD500). ACD was measured from the endothelial surface of cornea to the anterior surface of lens. TIA was measured with the apex in the iris recess and the arms of the angle passing through a point on the trabecular meshwork from the scleral spur and the point on the iris perpendicularly opposite.AOD500 was the distance between the posterior cornea surface and the anterior iris surface measured on a line perpendicular to the trabecular meshwork at 500 mm from the scleral spur [10]. Gonioscopy showed an open anlge all over in both eyes. The follow-up periods covered 12 months. By the end of the 1st,the 3rd,the 6th and the 12th month postoperatively, we observed the vertical central distance between the corneal endothelium and the front surface of ICL (CE-ICL), central vault, IOP, AOD500, TIA,ACV, endothelial cell density,UDVA and CDVA. AOD500 and TIA were measured by UBM, ACV by Pentcam. Endothelial cell density was determined using a noncontact specular microscope by one single operator (J.Y.) (SP-8800, Konan, Nishinomiya, Japan).All image acquisitions were operated by the same physician. The central vault was defined as the distance between the back surface of the ICL and the anterior crystalline lens pole. The UDVA and CDVA were checked using Snellen charts and converted to the logMAR scale for statistical analysis.

Ultrasound biomicroscopy

ACD, TIA,CE-ICL,AOD500,central vault were performed using a high-resolution UBM (SW-3200, SUOER, China) with a 50–100 MHz transducer-probe. All procedures were performed by the same experienced examiner in constant ambient lighting conditions. Any cysts detected in UBM were recorded for the size (the horizontal and vertical diameters in radial position), location, clock position, corresponding AOD500 and TIA. The parameters of AOD500 and TIA in 3, 6, 9, 12'o clock were separately recorded. By the end of the 6th month postoperatively, the mean value of TIA and AOD500 in 3, 6, 9, 12'o clock was separately considered to statistical analysis. Anterior chamber angle was considered to be closed on UBM image if any contact between the iris and angle wall anterior to the scleral spur. The anterior chamber angle corresponding to the cysts, which is defined as the anterior chamber angle with cyst in the largest vertical diameter on UBM image, was further assessed by AOD500 and TIA (Fig. 1). According to the distribution of cysts, single quadrant cysts were defined as a distribution of the cysts

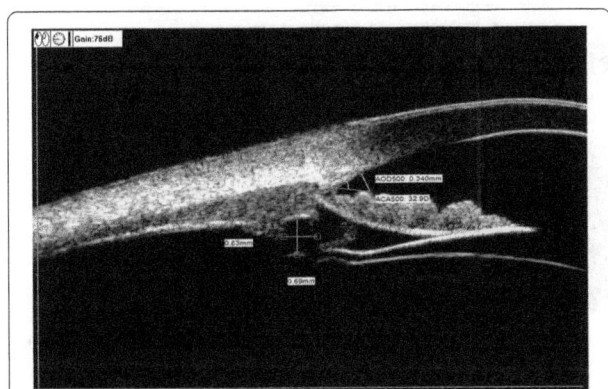

Fig. 1 Postoperative parameters of TIA and AOD500 corresponding to the cysts on the UBM image

equal to or less than one quadrant, multi-quadrant cysts were defined as cysts in more than one quadrant. According to the number of cysts, single cyst was defined as only one cyst found within the iris and/or ciliary body, double cysts were defined as 2 cysts, and multiple cysts were defined as equal to or more than 3 cysts [11].

ICL surgical procedure

After topical anaesthesia (0.4% oxybuprocaine hydrochloride, Santen, Japan) and injection f a viscoelastic surgical agent (1.7% Sodium hyaluronate; Bausch & Lomb, China) into the anterior chamber, an ICLV4c was inserted via a 3.0 mm temporal clear corneal incision with the use of an injector cartridge (STAAR Surgical). After the ICL was placed in the posterior chamber, the surgeon then completely removed the viscoelastic surgical agent from the eye using a balanced salt solution. All surgeries were uneventful and no intra-operative complications were observed. Following surgery, a combination antibacterial and steroidal medication (0.1% Tobramycin dexamethasone,

Alcon, China) was prescribed four times daily for 2 weeks.

Statistical analysis

Statistical analysis was performed by using SPSS 20.0. Parametric and nonparametric tests were used to compare continuous variables, according to data distribution. For nonparametric data, Kolmogorov-Smirnov test was applied for all variables and resulted in nonsignificant outcomes indicating the normality of data distribution. The Mann–Whitney U test was used to analyze the differences between the two groups. Differences in mean values of preoperative and postoperative ocluar biometric parameters within one group were examined using a paired Student's t-test. P value less than 0.05 was considered significant statistically.

Results

A total of 108 patients (201 eyes) were included in this retrospective study. Preoperative parameters showed no statistical difference between the two groups in the terms of biometric data, UDVA, CDVA, IOP, ACD, ACV, AOD500, TIA and CT (Table 1). There were no intra-operative and postoperative ocular or systemic complications.

Primary iris and ciliary body cysts

Among all the 201 eyes, primary iris and/or ciliary body cysts were detected in 54 eyes (26.87%), but the prevalence of cysts in patients was account to 36.11% (18males,21females). Among all the eyes with cysts, there were 30 eyes (55.56%) with unilateral single cyst, 12 eyes (22.22%) with unilateral double cysts, 12 eyes (22.22%) eyes with unilateral multiple and/or multi-quadrants cysts, the mean size of cysts was (0.714 ± 0.149)mm(range from 0.510 to 1.075 mm).30.4% of the cysts were located at iridociliary sulcus, 65.5% at pars plicata, and 4.1% at midzonal ris,

Table 1 Preoperative ocular parameters in two groups (Mean ± _ Standard Deviation)

Parameters	Groups			
	Group1(Mean ± SD)	Group 2(Mean ± SD)	t	P
UDVA	0.04 ± 0.03	0.03 ± 0.03	1.460	0.149
CDVA	0.91 ± 0.18	0.78 ± 0.25	1.948	0.056
Manifest refractive sphere(D)	12.76 ± 4.00	13.71 ± 5.01	−0.723	0.427
Manifest refractive cylinder(D)	1.78 ± 1.13	1.44 ± 0.92	1.235	0.221
IOP	15.33 ± 3.76	16.14 ± 3.13	−0.889	0.377
ACD	3.25 ± 0.19	3.16 ± 0.24	1.422	0.160
CT	528.61 ± 37.98	526.06 ± 28.31	0.297	0.797
ACV	216.00 ± 30.07	199.90 ± 30.57	1.938	0.057
AOD500	0.617 ± 0.222	0.583 ± 0.185	0.639	0.525
TIA	47.92 ± 9.79	47.40 ± 9.43	0.199	0.843

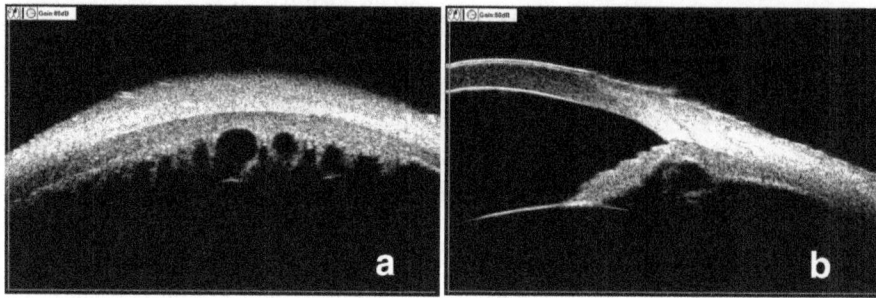

Fig. 2 Preoperative vertical and horizontal scanning images of multiple cysts. **a**. Preoperative vertical scanning image of multiple cysts in 3'o clock in left eye. **b**. Preoperative horizontal scanning image of multiple cysts in 3'o clock in left eye

which showed a characteristic distribution pattern, where cysts found predominantly in the inferior and temporal quadrants. Postoperatively, the size and the number of cysts showed nearly no changes. Figure 2a and b showed a 31-year-old patient in her left eye with multiple and multi-quadrant cysts.

Change of anterior chamber parameters

We observed the change of anterior chamber according to the parameters, which included the ACV, AOD500 and TIA. Table 2 showed the preoperative mean AOD500, TIA corresponding to the cysts and the mean value of AOD500, TIA in four clocks. Statistical analysis showed no statistical significant ($P > 0.05$). The range of AOD500 was 0.183 mm to 1.129 mm corresponding to the location of cysts, while the degree of TIA was 20.20° to 64.70°. Table 3 showed the preoperative and postoperative parameters of AOD500 and TIA in 3, 6, 9, 12'o clock. By the end of 6th month postoperatively, all the parameters of AOD500 and TIA in 3, 6, 9, 12'o clock were proved to be significant reduced in both two groups ($P < 0.05$). But, the preoperative and postoperative parameters of AOD500 and TIA in 3, 6, 9, 12'o clock showed no statistical significant between the two groups ($P > 0.05$).The postoperative parameters of ACV also showed the same reduction as AOD and TIA in both two groups ($P < 0.05$), but with no statistical significant between the two groups ($P > .005$).

Visual outcomes

The postoperative UDVA was proved to be significantly improved for both two groups ($p < 0.05$), but, which showed

no statistical significant between the two groups in follow-up periods ($P > 0.05$).

IOP, vault and CE-ICL

Table 4 showed the change of IOP, central vault and CE-ICL, which showed no statistical significant between the two groups in follow-up periods ($P > 0.05$).

Discussion

Compared with custom corneal laser refractive surgery or clear lens extraction surgery, the ICL surgery has been proved to have many potential advantages, including the possibility of correction of high refractive errors, maintaining the integrity of the corneal structure and accommodation of the lens, and the reversibility [3, 4]. In our study, all cases in both two groups finally gained good UDVA and also showed no serious complications, which means primary iris and/or ciliary body cysts had no direct impact on the visual outcome in ICL surgery. The diagnosis of primary iris and/or ciliary body cysts was made according to the patients' history and clinical manifestation, after excluding other possible etiological factors that can cause secondary cysts. Most of primary iris and/or ciliary body cysts are located at the iridociliary sulcus and/or pars plicata, which mainly arise from the iris pigment epithelium [8]. In our study, we still found that almost all cysts were located at the iridociliary sulcus or pars plicata, and were predominantly distributed in the inferior and temporal quadrants. These results were well according with the finding of Kunimatsu [6]. The prevalence of primary cysts was amount to 36.11%, which was higher than 34.4% found by Wang

Table 2 Comparison of the preoperative TIA and AOD500 corresponding to the cysts (Mean ± _ Standard Deviation)

	Location			
	Corresponding to the cysts (Mean ± SD)	mean value of 4 clocks (Mean ± SD)	t	P
AOD500	0.573 ± 0.202	0.617 ± 0.222	0.719	0.476
TIA	47.17 ± 10.75	47.92 ± 9.79	0.818	0.807

Table 3 Comparing the parameters of AOD500 and TIA in 3,6,9,12'o clock

Location Group and P-value		TIA(°)			AOD500(mm)		
		Pre-operation	post-operation(6th month)	P	Pre-operation	post-operation (6th month)	P
3'o clock	Group1	45.40 ± 8.29	22.67 ± 6.15	0.000	0.51 ± 0.14	0.21 ± 0.06	0.000
	Group2	47.37 ± 8.29	27.56 ± 8.50	0.000	0.53 ± 0.13	0.26 ± 0.09	0.000
	P-value	0.560	0.368		0.750	0.314	
6'o clock	Gropu1	40.77 ± 12.98	24.11 ± 4.27	0.000	0.46 ± 0.20	0.21 ± 0.04	0.001
	Group2	52.71 ± 7.87	21.60 ± 2.97	0.013	0.68 ± 0.23	0.19 ± 0.03	0.009
	P-value	0.090	0.368		0.101	0.633	
9'o clock	Group1	44.96 ± 9.00	26.30 ± 7.11	0.001	0.53 ± 0.19	0.25 ± 0.09	0.001
	Group2	48.03 ± 4.53	25.54 ± 5.72	0.000	0.56 ± 0.09	0.26 ± 0.06	0.001
	P-value	0.314	1.000		0.315	0.832	
12'o clock	Group1	42.96 ± 9.15	20.84 ± 5.80	0.000	0.48 ± 0.19	0.19 ± 0.05	0.000
	Group2	45.16 ± 4.41	19.67 ± 4.53	0.000	0.52 ± 0.08	0.19 ± 0.06	0.002
	P-value	0.289	0.711		0.20	0.791	

et al. [12]. It was reported that iris-ciliary cysts were the main cause of glaucoma and closure glaucoma [13–15] .If the patients with cysts had been implanted with ICL, the potential risk would include: (1) cysts stimulated ciliary body, causing an increase in aqueous fluid;(2) mucus and other materials produced by cysts deposited trabecular meshwork, thus preventing aqueous fluid from flowing out; (3) If the haptics of ICL just were located at the position of cysts, which might be more likely to push the root of iris forwarding and lead the anterior chamber

Table 4 Postoperative parameters of IOP, Vault and CE-ICL for the two groups

Parameters	Time	Groups		
		Group 1(Mean ± SD)	Group2(Mean ± SD)	1P
IOP(mmHg)	1mo	17.11 ± 2.95	16.20 ± 3.25	0.295
	3mo	16.83 ± 2.04	17.27 ± 2.62	0.578
	6mo	16.33 ± 2.74	16.71 ± 2.64	0.560
	12mo	16.44 ± 1.98	16.78 ± 2.35	0.580
2 P	P > 0.05			
Vault(mm)	1mo	0.62 ± 0.26	0.50 ± 0.27	0.157
	3mo	0.62 ± 0.25	0.52 ± 0.24	0.197
	6mo	0.62 ± 0.25	0.51 ± 0.23	0.111
	12mo	0.61 ± 0.23	0.51 ± 0.22	0.109
2P	P > 0.05			
CE-ICL (mm)	1mo	2.23 ± 0.32	2.37 ± 0.37	0.132
	3mo	2.25 ± 0.27	2.35 ± 0.33	0.243
	6mo	2.25 ± 0.26	2.34 ± 0.33	0.264
	12mo	2.26 ± 0.24	2.35 ± 0.33	0.229
2P	P > 0.05			

angle becoming narrowed or closed up;(4) The haptics of ICL might cause the broken of cyst capsule, the fluid of cysts might cause serious inflammation (Fig. 3a, b). But, in the whole follow-up periods, we did not find an elevating of IOP in the eyes with cysts. The size of cysts also showed no changes. According to the study of Wang et al. [11], the cysts larger than 0.8 mm or located at iridociliary sulcus were inclined to narrow or close the corresponding angles. When compared with the eyes without cysts, the eyes with multiple and/or multi-quadrants cysts would be more likely to narrow or close the whole anterior chamber angle. But, the eyes only with unilateral single or double cysts did not show the same result. In our study, all the postoperative parameters of AOD500, ACV and TIA in 3, 6, 9, 12'o clock were proved to be significant reduced in both two groups. But, the difference between the two groups showed no statistical significant. The result also showed that the unilateral single cyst or single quadrant cysts would have no significant effect on narrowing or closing anterior chamber angle in ICL surgery. As Zhu's [16] study, he found significant correlation between high intraocular pressure and the presence of iris-ciliary cysts, particularly the quantity and the size of the cysts. We sincerely suggest that ophthalmologists should monitor the changes of IOP and anterior chamber angle for extended follow-up periods, once the larger primary iris-ciliary cysts or multiple cysts, especially multi-quadrants cysts located at iridociliary sulcus were detected. Central vault is of crucial value for estimating the safety of ICL surgery. Excessive vault is one of risk factors to induce secondary glaucoma, and insufficient vault is responsible for the formation of anterior subcapsular cataract [17, 18]. Previous studies had defined an excellent vault was 250 to 750 μm [19]. In our study, we found that the postoperative mean

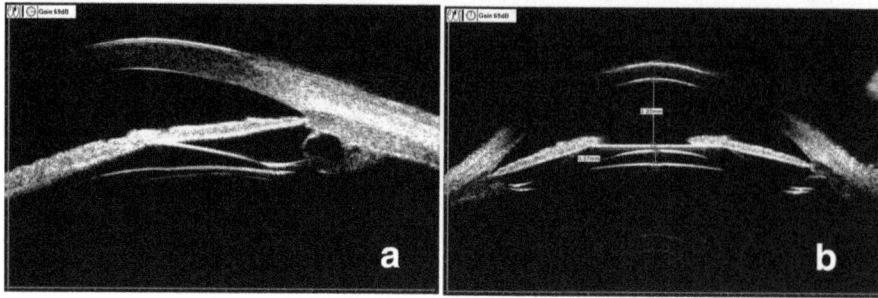

Fig. 3 Postoperative horizontal scanning image of multiple cysts in 3'o clock in left eye. **a**. The haptics of ICL would induce the broken of cyst capsule. **b**. The haptics of ICL in the location of cysts in ciliary sulcus, which would be likely to push the root of iris forwarding and induce the anterior chamber angle narrow or close up

vault and CE-ICL had no statistical significant between two groups. As we all known that the changes of central vault are mainly according to the difference between the size of ICL and sulcus-to-sulcus (STS) diameter, which would explain why primary iris and/or ciliary body cysts had no direct impact on the change of central vault. In our study, we found the postoperative anterior chamber angle was closed in 3'o clock positions in one eye without cysts. Form the images of UBM (Fig. 4), we observed that the central vault was more than 1.25 mm, the anterior chamber angle was closed at the location corresponding to the ICL haptic. Excessive vaults would induce secondary glaucoma, owe to persistent angle closure, pupil blocking, or pigmentary dispersion [20–24].For all eyes, we did not find an elevating IOP in follow-up periods. We considered, whether the secondary angle closure glaucoma would be happen, which was decided by the range of closed anterior chamber angle. If only one clock position or less than one quarter anterior chamber angle was closed, the secondary glaucoma would not be happen.

Besides, with a hole in the central of the lens, which reduce the risk of papillary block.

Conclusion

In conclusion, primary iris and/or ciliary body are not absolutely contraindication for ICL surgery. For some single cyst smaller than 1.075 mm or single quadrant cysts located at ciliary body are rare to lead some serious complications. But, for some multiple cysts, especially multi-quadrants cysts located at iridociliary sulcus, we still should remain cautions. In the future study, we would collect more samples and monitor longer follow-up periods to prove the safety and reliability of ICL surgery in patients with primary iris and/or ciliary body cysts.

Abbreviations
ACD: Anterior chamber depth; ACV: Anterior chamber volume; AOD500: Angle opening distance at 500 μm; BCVA: Best corrected visual acuity; CDVA: Corrected distance visual acuity; CE-ICL: Vertical central distance between the corneal endothelium and the front surface of ICL; CT: Corneal thickness; D: Dioptometer; ICL: Implantable collamer lens; IOP: Intraocular pressure; TIA: Trabecular-iris angle

Acknowledgements
The authors thank Yu Han, The People's Hospital of Leshan, for his surgical technical guidance.

Funding
This study was supported by the science and technology foundation of Sichuan provincial health and family planning commission (NO:150065). This study was also partially supported by the Innovation Project of Leshan people's hospital. The funding body had no role in the design or conduct of this study. The funding organizations had no role in the study design, conduct of this research, data analysis, decision to publish, or preparation of the manuscript.

Authors' contributions
ZL and ZKX involved in design and conduct of the study and preparation of manuscript; YQW and QL participated in the acquisition of the data and equipment technical support; ZL and BC participated in management, analysis, and interpretation of the data; All authors review and approval of the final manuscript.

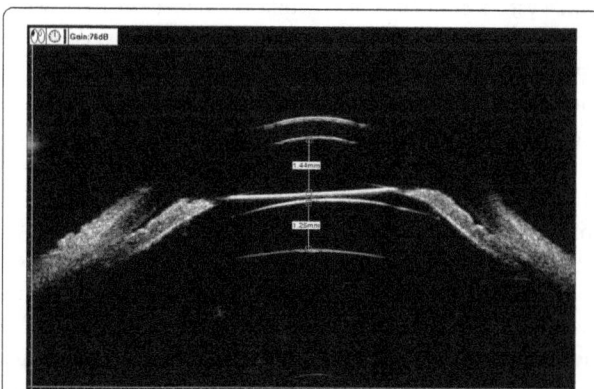

Fig. 4 Excessive vault is a high risk factor to induce glaucoma. In this eye, the central vault was more than 1.25 mm, and the anterior chamber angle was closed in the location of ICL haptics

Competing interests
The authors declare that they have no competing interests.

References

1. Alfonso JF, Baamonde B, Fernández-Vega L, et al. Posterior chamber collagen copolymer phakic intraocular lenses to correct myopia: five-year follow-up. J Cataract Refract Surg. 2011;37:873–80.

2. Kamiya K, Shimizu K, Igarashi A, et al. Four-year follow-up of posterior chamber phakic intraocular lens implantation for moderate to high myopia. Arch Ophthalmol. 2009;127:845–50.

3. Pérez-Vives C, Domínguez-Vicent A, Ferrer-Blasco T, et al. Optical quality of the Visian implantable Collamer Lens for different refractive powers. Graefes Arch Clin Exp Ophthalmol. 2013;251:1423–9.

4. Schallhorn S, Tanzer D, Sanders DR, et al. Randomized prospective comparison of visian toric implantable collamer lens and conventional photorefractive keratectomy for moderate to high myopic astigmatism. J Refract Surg. 2007;23:853–67.

5. Shields JA, Shields CL. Cysts of the Iris pigment epithelium. What is new and interesting? The 2016 Jose Rizal international medal lecture. Asia-Pac. J Ophthalmol. 2017;1:64–9.

6. Kunimatsu S, Araie M, Ohara K, et al. Ultrasound biomicroscopy of ciliary body cysts. Am J Ophthalmol. 1999;127:48–55.

7. Rotsos T, Diagourtas A, Symeonidis C, et al. Phacoemulsification in a patient with small pupil and a large iris cyst. Eur J Ophthalmol. 2012;22(2):278–9.

8. Kanski JJ. Kanski's clinical ophthalmology: a systematic approach, 8th ed. Elsevier Butterworth-266 Heinmann publications; 2015. p. 480–2.

9. Sanders DR, et al. U.S. Food and Drug Administration clinical trial of the implantable contact Lens for moderate to high myopia. Ophthalmology. 2003;110:255–66.

10. Shukla S, Damji KF, Harasymowycz P, et al. Clinical features distinguishing angle closure from pseudoplateau versus plateau iris. Br J Ophthalmol. 2008; 92:340–4.

11. Wang BH, Yao YF. Effect of primary iris and ciliary body cyst on anterior chamber angle in patients with shallow anterior chamber. J Zhejiang Univ-Sci B (Biomed & Biotechnol). 2012;13(9):723–30.

12. Wang BH, Nie X, Zhou CX, et al. Primary Iris-eulacy body cyst and its relevance with the change of anterior chamber angle. Chin J Ophthalmol. 2008;44:993–7.

13. Steigerwalt JR, Vingolo EM, Plateroti P, et al. The effect of latanoprost and influence of changes in body position on patients with glaucoma and ocular hypertension. Eur Rev Med Pharmacol Sci. 2012;16:1723–8.

14. Kaushik S, Ichhpujani P, Kaur S, et al. Optic disk pit and Iridociliary cyst precipitating angle closure Glaucoma. J Current Glau Prac. 2014;8:33–5.

15. Seki M, Fukuchi T, Yoshino T, et al. Secondary Glaucoma associated with bilateral complete ring cysts of the ciliary body. J Glaucoma. 2014; 23:477–81.

16. Zhu R, Cheng L, Wang D-M. Correlation between presence of primary irisand cilliary body cysts and intraocular pressure. Eur Rev Med Pharmacol Sci. 2017;21:3985–9.

17. Fernandes P, Gonzalez-Meijome JM, Madrid-Costa D, et al. Implantable collamer posterior chamber intraocular lenses: a review ofpotential complications. J Refract Surg. 2011;27:765–76.

18. Shi M, Kong J, Li X, et al. Observing implantable collamer lens dislocation by panoramic ultrasound biomicroscopy. Eye. 2015;29:499–504.

19. Kamiya K, Shimizu K, Komatsu M. Factors affecting vaulting after implantable collamer lens implantation. J Cataract Refract Surg. 2009;25:259–64.

20. Smallman DS, Probst L, Rafuse PE. Pupillary block glaucoma secondary to posterior chamber phakic intraocular lens implantation for high myopia. J Cataract Refract Surg. 2004;30:905–7.

21. Vetter JM, Tehrani M, Dick HB. Surgical management of acute angle-closure glaucoma after toric implantable contact lens implantation. J Cataract Refract Surg. 2006;32:1065–7.

22. Bylsma SS, Zalta AH, Foley E, et al. Phakic posterior chamber intraocular lens pupillary block. J Cataract Refract Surg. 2002;28:2222–8.

23. Chung TY, Park SC, Lee MO, et al. Changes in iridocorneal angle structure and trabecular pigmentation with STAAR implantable Collamer lens during 2 years. J Refract Surg. 2009;25:251–8.

24. Ju Y, Gao XW, Ren B. Posterior chamber phakic intraocular lens implantation for high myopia. Int J Ophthalmol. 2013;116:1523–6.

22

Effect of amblyopia treatment on choroidal thickness in hypermetropic anisometropic amblyopia using swept-source optical coherence tomography

Syunsuke Araki[1], Atsushi Miki[1,2*], Katsutoshi Goto[1], Tsutomu Yamashita[1,2], Go Takizawa[1], Kazuko Haruishi[1], Tsuyoshi Yoneda[1,2], Yoshiaki Ieki[1], Junichi Kiryu[1], Goro Maehara[3] and Kiyoshi Yaoeda[4]

Abstract

Background: Recent studies using optical coherence tomography (OCT) have indicated that choroidal thickness (CT) in the anisometropic amblyopic eye is thicker than that of the fellow and normal control eyes. However, it has not yet been established as to how amblyopia affects the choroid thickening. The purpose of the present study was to investigate the effect of amblyopia treatment on macular CT in eyes with anisometropic amblyopia using swept-source OCT.

Methods: Thirteen patients (mean age: 6.2 ± 2.4 years) with hypermetropic anisometropic amblyopia were included in this study. Visual acuity (VA), axial length (AL), and CT were measured at the enrollment visit and at the final visit, after at least 6 months of treatment. CT measurements were corrected for magnification error and were automatically analyzed using built-in software and divided into three macular regions (subfoveal choroidal thickness (SFCT), center 1 mm, and center 6 mm). A one-way analysis of covariance using AL as a covariate was performed to determine whether CT in amblyopic eyes changed after amblyopia treatment.

Results: The average observation period was 22.2 ± 11.0 months. After treatment, VA (logMAR) improvement in the amblyopic eyes was 0.41 ± 0.19 ($p < 0.001$). SFCT, center 1 mm CT, and center 6 mm CT were significantly thicker in the amblyopic eyes compared with the fellow eyes both before and after treatment ($p < 0.05$ for all comparisons). There were no significant changes in SFCT, center 1 mm CT, or center 6 mm CT before and after treatment in the amblyopic ($p = 0.25, 0.21,$ and $0.84,$ respectively) and fellow ($p = 0.75, 0.84,$ and $0.91,$ respectively) eyes. The correlation between changes in logMAR versus changes in CT after treatment was not significant.

Conclusions: Although VA in amblyopic eyes was significantly improved after treatment, the choroid thickening of anisometropic amblyopic eyes persisted, and there was no significant change found in the CT after the treatment. Our findings suggest that thickening of the CT in amblyopia is not directly related to visual dysfunction.

Keywords: Amblyopia, Choroid, Treatment, Optical coherence tomography

* Correspondence: amiki@tc5.so-net.ne.jp
[1]Department of Ophthalmology, Kawasaki Medical School, 577 Matsushima, Kurashiki, Okayama 701-0192, Japan
[2]Department of Sensory Science, Faculty of Health Science and Technology, Kawasaki University of Medical Welfare, 288 Matsushima, Kurashiki, Okayama 701-0193, Japan
Full list of author information is available at the end of the article

Background

Amblyopia is defined as a disorder in which there is dysfunction in processing visual information such as reduced recognition visual acuity (VA) [1]. The pathogenesis of amblyopia has been thought to be based on morphological and functional abnormalities in the visual cortex and lateral geniculate nucleus [2–5]. In contrast, it is unclear whether or not dysfunction or structural abnormality of the retina is present in amblyopia [6].

Recent studies using optical coherence tomography (OCT) have indicated that retinal or choroidal thickness (CT) in amblyopic eyes is thicker than in fellow and normal control eyes [7, 8]. However, since amblyopic eyes are often smaller than fellow eyes [9], it is almost impossible to find control subjects, as these small eyes are almost always hyperopic and normally amblyopic. Therefore, a consensus as to whether the retina or choroid thickening in amblyopic eyes is affected by the "pathologic condition of amblyopia" or a "difference in the ocular size" has yet to be established. In our previous study [10], we found there was no significant difference in the macular inner retinal thickness in unilateral amblyopia patients. In addition, although we found significant differences in CT in patients with hypermetropic anisometropic amblyopia, there was no significant difference found for strabismic amblyopia. The results of our previous study do not support the hypothesis that the choroid thickening is simply due to differences in ocular size, as we analyzed the choroidal thickness after adjusting for the axial length (AL). There must be another contributing factor, but it remains unclear as to how amblyopia is able to affect the choroid thickening.

A few recent studies researched the effect of amblyopia treatment on CT in order to investigate the relationship between amblyopia and choroid [11–14]. However, to the best of our knowledge, there have been no studies in which a swept-source OCT (SS-OCT) has been used to compare the CT before and after treatment. Furthermore, as SS-OCT uses a long-wavelength light source of 1 μm, utilizing this technique to examine the choroid can provide superior imaging as compared to spectral-domain OCT (SD-OCT). Thus, the purpose of the present study was to investigate the effect of amblyopia treatment on the macular CT in anisometropic amblyopia eyes using the SS-OCT technique.

Methods

All of the investigative procedures used respect the Declaration of Helsinki and approval from the Institutional Review Board Committee of Kawasaki Medical School (registration number: 2458–1) was obtained. This study was designed as an observational case series and conducted from November 2013 to June 2017 in the Department of Ophthalmology at Kawasaki Medical School Hospital. Informed consent for the examinations was obtained from one of the parents of each patient.

Subjects

This study enrolled 16 patients aged 4 to 12 years. All patients were diagnosed with hypermetropic anisometropic amblyopia, and underwent ophthalmologic examinations at the first visit including best-corrected VA (BCVA), cycloplegic refraction using an autorefractor (RKT-7700, NIDEK Co., Ltd., Gamagori, Japan), intraocular pressure, AL (IOL Master®, Carl Zeiss Meditec AG, Jena, Germany), cover test, extraocular movements, slit-lamp, funduscopy, and SS-OCT (DRI OCT-1 Atlantis®, Topcon Corporation, Tokyo, Japan).

The exclusion criteria were as follows: presence of BCVA better than 0.0 logMAR within two months after full refractive correction, history of amblyopia treatment, ocular diseases, history of intraocular surgery, presence of systemic diseases that may have had an influence on the eye, and an SS-OCT image in which the auto-segmentation was difficult to obtain due to signal attenuation.

Anisometropia was defined as an interocular difference in refraction (spherical equivalent) of more than 2.0 diopters (D). Hypermetropic anisometropic amblyopia was defined as the presence of a BCVA worse than 0.1 logMAR in the eye which had more diopters after full refractive correction.

Initially all patients received the full refractive correction. BCVA was measured at least every 1 to 2 months. After no further VA improvement, patients underwent additional patching treatment (2 to 6 h/day) [15]. Patching treatment was reduced or stopped once the patient achieved the maximum VA. BCVA, AL, and CT were measured at the enrollment visit and at the final visit after treatments of at least 6 months.

CT measurements

CT measurements were performed using SS-OCT. SS-OCT parameters included a 1050 nm wavelength light source, depth resolution of 8.0 μm, and a scan speed of 100,000 A-scans/second. Data analysis was performed using the DRI OCT-1 Atlantis® software program version 9.30.

The scanning protocol used was the 3D macula with a scan density of 512×256 and an area of 12×9 mm². After automatically analyzing CT using the built-in tools, the area was divided into three macular regions: subfoveal choroidal thickness (SFCT), radii of 0.5 mm (center 1 mm), and radii of 3.0 mm (center 6 mm) (Fig. 1). Thickness data was corrected for magnification errors through the use of the individual AL, spherical refraction, cylinder refraction, and corneal radius. All SS-OCT examinations were performed by an experienced technician (S.A.) between 9:00 AM and 12:00 PM in order to avoid the inclusion of any diurnal variations in the CT [16].

Statistical analyses

All statistical analyses were performed using the Bell Curve for Excel version 2.0 software program (Social

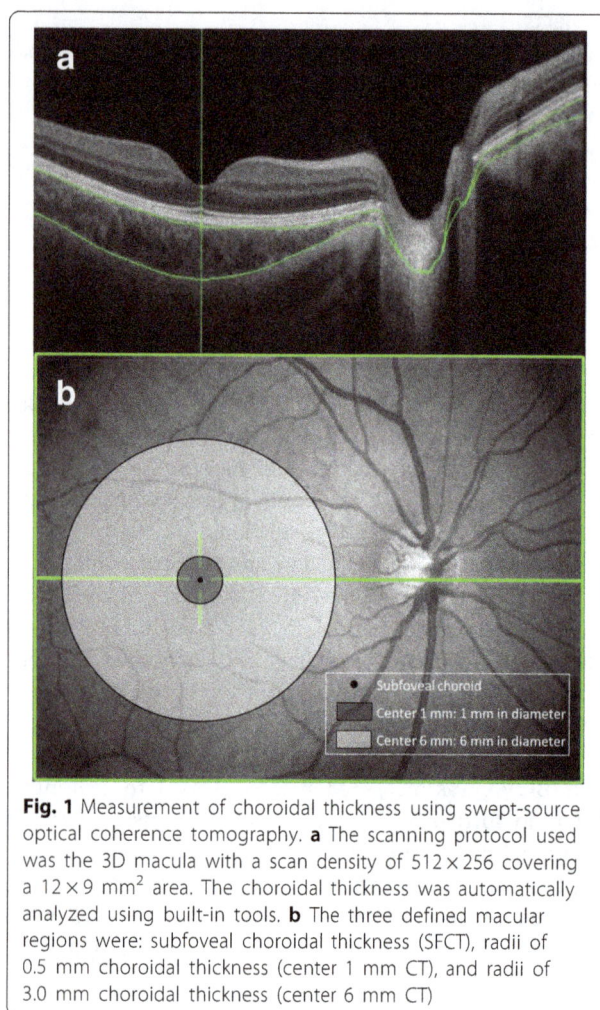

Fig. 1 Measurement of choroidal thickness using swept-source optical coherence tomography. **a** The scanning protocol used was the 3D macula with a scan density of 512×256 covering a 12×9 mm^2 area. The choroidal thickness was automatically analyzed using built-in tools. **b** The three defined macular regions were: subfoveal choroidal thickness (SFCT), radii of 0.5 mm choroidal thickness (center 1 mm CT), and radii of 3.0 mm choroidal thickness (center 6 mm CT)

Survey Research Information Co., Ltd., Tokyo, Japan). Data are presented as the means ± standard deviations. A paired t-test, two sample t-test, and a one-way analysis of covariance (ANCOVA), which was controlled using AL, were used to evaluate the differences between the amblyopic and fellow eyes. CT differences before and after treatment were compared by ANCOVA, which was controlled using AL. Pearson's correlation coefficient was used to evaluate correlations in logMAR changes versus CT changes after amblyopia treatment. A *p*-value of less than 0.05 was considered to be statistically significant.

Results

Demographic data

Initially, 16 Japanese patients with hypermetropic anisometropic amblyopia were enrolled in this study. In three patients the auto-segmentation of the choroid from the sclera was incorrect and SS-OCT image quality was poor, so they were excluded from the study. Therefore, our current study analyzed a total of 13 patients. Table 1 shows the

demographic and clinical data of the patients. The mean age of the patients at the enrollment visit was 6.2 ± 2.4 years (range: 4.0 to 11.3 years). The average observation period was 22.2 ± 11.0 months (range: 7 to 36 months). As for the details of the treatment, refractive correction only was performed in four patients, while combined refractive correction and patching was administered in nine patients. The logMAR in amblyopic eyes at the time of enrollment was 0.44 ± 0.27 (range: 1.00 to 0.10), while it was 0.03 ± 0.15 (range: 0.22 to -0.18) after the treatment. After amblyopia treatment, the logMAR improvement in the amblyopic eyes was 0.41 ± 0.19 ($p < 0.001$). Refraction in the amblyopic eyes was more hyperopic as compared to that for the fellow eyes both before and after the treatment ($p < 0.001$ for both comparisons). The AL in the amblyopic eyes was significantly shorter than that found in the fellow eyes both before and after treatment ($p < 0.001$ for both comparisons). There was a significant extension of the AL in both eyes at the final versus the enrollment visit (amblyopic eyes: 0.33 ± 0.14 mm, $p < 0.001$; fellow eyes: 0.21 ± 0.15 mm, $p < 0.001$).

CT

Table 2 shows the CT before and after the treatment. SFCT, center 1 mm CT, and center 6 mm CT in the amblyopic eyes were significantly thicker than that in the fellow eyes both before and after the treatment ($p < 0.05$ for all comparisons). There was no significant change in SFCT, center 1 mm CT, and center 6 mm CT seen in either the amblyopic or fellow eye after the treatment.

Figure 2 shows that there are not significant correlations between logMAR changes and CT changes in the amblyopic eyes after treatment [SFCT (Fig. 2a): $r = -0.09$, $p = 0.77$, center 1 mm CT (Fig. 2b): $r = 0.04$, $p = 0.90$, or center 6 mm CT (Fig. 2c): $r = -0.21$, $p = 0.49$].

Discussion

Our current study demonstrates that macular CT in the eyes with hypermetropic anisometropic amblyopia, as measured by SS-OCT, was significantly thicker than that in the fellow eyes, similar to that reported by our previous study [10]. In addition, although the treatment significantly improved the VA in the amblyopic eyes, the choroidal thickening of the amblyopic eyes persisted, and there was no significant change found in CT after the amblyopia treatment.

To the best of our knowledge, there have been four previous studies that evaluated CTs before and after amblyopia treatment [11–14]. Öner et al. [11] found no significant differences between the pre- and post-treatment SFCT in the amblyopic and fellow eyes, although they did report that SFCT was larger in the amblyopic versus the fellow eyes before and after treatment. Our results were in agreement with their previous findings. In contrast, Bayhan et al. [12] reported that there was a significant decrease in CT after

Table 1 Demographic and clinical data of the patients before and after treatment

	Before treatment			After treatment		
	AE (n = 13)	FE (n = 13)	p-value[†]	AE (n = 13)	FE (n = 13)	p-value[†]
Age	6.2 ± 2.4		–	8.1 ± 2.3		–
Sex (Male: Female)	2: 11		–	–		–
Visual acuity (logMAR)	0.44 ± 0.27	− 0.12 ± 0.07	$p < 0.001^*$	0.03 ± 0.15	− 0.16 ± 0.05	$p < 0.001^*$
Refraction (diopters)	5.58 ± 1.23	2.27 ± 1.43	$p < 0.001^*$	5.50 ± 1.39	2.29 ± 1.99	$p < 0.001^*$
Axial length (mm)	20.97 ± 0.88	22.11 ± 1.22	$p < 0.001^*$	21.31 ± 0.91	22.32 ± 1.25	$p < 0.001^*$

AE, amblyopic eyes, FE fellow eyes
Values are shown as mean ± standard deviation
[†]Two sample t-test; * $p < 0.01$

treatment in amblyopic eyes. In addition, Hashimoto et al. [13] reported that treatment in two anisohypermetropic amblyopia patients resulted in a gradual increase in choroidal blood flow of the macular regions along with an improvement in VA and a decrease in CT. On the other hand, Nishi et al. [14] found that SFCT in eyes with thicker choroid tended to decrease while eyes with a thinner choroid tended to increase in both the amblyopic and fellow eyes after treatment. As the results appear to differ from study to study, there is not yet a consensus regarding CT changes after amblyopia treatment.

There were some differences noted between our current study and the above previous reports. First, the previous studies used a manual analysis to compile CT measurements obtained by SD-OCT [11–14]. However, in our current study, we used SS-OCT, which performs an automatic analysis using a 3D scan. Since our automatic analysis should have evaluated CT more objectively than the manual analysis, differences between the types of analysis used may have led to the disagreement between the results of the previous studies and our current study. Second, the duration of the treatment varied across studies. The studies by Öner et al. and Bayhan et al. evaluated CT at 6 months after starting the treatment [11, 12]. In contrast, we observed the patients after the treatment for a longer term, ranging from 7 to 36 months (mean; 22.2 ± 11.0 months). The difference in the length of the observation period could have had an influence on the degree of the VA improvement. In fact,

the improvement of VA in the amblyopic eyes after treatment in our study (logMAR; 0.44 ± 0.27 to 0.03 ± 0.15) was greater than that found by Öner et al. (logMAR; 0.35 ± 0.3 to 0.16 ± 0.2) [11] and Bayhan et al. (Snellen; 0.32 ± 0.2 to 0.74 ± 0.3) [12]. Nevertheless, we did not find any significant change in CT after treatment. Furthermore, our current study also did not find any significant correlation between logMAR changes and CT changes after amblyopia treatment. Nishi et al. [14] showed that the changes in CT were found not only in the amblyopic eye but also in the fellow eye one year after optical correction. Therefore, we believe that the improvement of VA that occurs after the amblyopia treatment does not have a significant effect on CT.

It has been previously reported that an increased macular choroidal thickness correlates with hypermetropia, so in consequence it correlates with a short AL [17, 18]. However, other studies, including our study, show that CT of hypermetropic anisometropic amblyopic eyes is thick, even when the difference in the AL or refractive error between amblyopic and fellow eyes is taken into account in the statistical analysis [10, 12, 19]. Furthermore, other investigations have reported changes in the profile of CT [20], in the choroidal structure [21], and in the choroidal blood flow [13] exist in hypermetropic anisometropic amblyopic eyes. Based on these findings, we assume that there are some structural changes that do occur in the choroid of hypermetropic anisometropic amblyopic eyes. In normal human eyes, it has been

Table 2 CT comparisons before and after treatment in the amblyopic and fellow eyes

	Before treatment		After treatment		p-value[‡]			
	AE (n = 13)	FE (n = 13)	AE (n = 13)	FE (n = 13)	Before: AE vs. FE	After: AE vs. FE	AE: before vs. after	FE: before vs. after
SFCT (μm)	353.7 ± 86.6	281.1 ± 56.2	336.3 ± 67.9	286.4 ± 57.9	0.013*	0.042*	0.25	0.75
Center 1 mm CT (μm)	352.8 ± 80.1	283.2 ± 54.1	334.6 ± 63.4	285.0 ± 57.3	0.015*	0.043*	0.21	0.84
Center 6 mm CT (μm)	295.1 ± 43.5	259.9 ± 50.7	288.5 ± 36.1	258.8 ± 44.8	0.043*	0.036*	0.84	0.91

AE amblyopic eyes, FE fellow eyes, SFCT subfoveal choroidal thickness, CT choroidal thickness
Values are shown as mean ± standard deviation
[‡]ANCOVA using axial length as a covariate; * $p < 0.05$

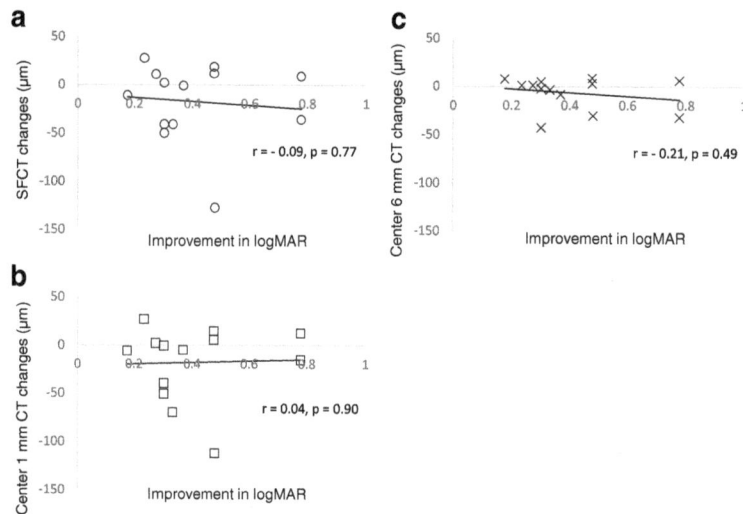

Fig. 2 Correlations between logMAR changes versus choroidal thickness changes after treatment in the amblyopic eyes. **a** Scatter plot of improvement in logMAR versus subfoveal choroidal thickness (SFCT) changes. **b** Scatter plot of improvement in logMAR versus center 1 mm choroidal thickness (CT) changes. **c** Scatter plot of improvement in logMAR versus center 6 mm CT changes. The correlations between improvement in logMAR and changes in the SFCT, center 1 mm CT, and center 6 mm CT were not significant

reported that SFCT decreases during accommodation [22]. Also, Chakraborty et al. reported that the presence or absence of hyperopic defocus affects the amplitude of the diurnal change in CT [23]. Therefore, these findings suggest that CT might be closely related to the accommodative function and/or hyperopic defocus. On the other hand, it has been reported that amblyopic eyes have accommodative dysfunction compared to fellow eyes for which refractive correction is unnecessary [24]. Therefore, it can be hypothesized that the difference in CT between hypermetropic anisometropic amblyopic eyes and fellow eyes is not entirely due to a short AL, as the accommodative dysfunction and/or hyperopic defocus imposes a secondary effect on the morphology of the choroid in amblyopia. A future study that evaluates the relationship between the accommodative function and CT in amblyopic eyes will need to be undertaken.

The limitation of our present study was the small number of patients examined. A further study that includes a larger number of patients will need to be undertaken in order to definitively confirm the results.

Conclusion

In conclusion, we found that even though there was a significant improvement of the VA in amblyopic eyes after treatment, the choroidal thickening of amblyopic eyes persisted, and there was no significant correlation between logMAR changes and CT changes after treatment. Therefore, our findings suggest that thickening of CT in amblyopia is not directly related to visual dysfunction.

Abbreviations
AE: Amblyopic eyes; AL: Axial length; ANCOVA: A one-way analysis of covariance; BCVA: Best-corrected visual acuity; CT: Choroidal thickness; FE: Fellow eyes; logMAR: Logarithm of the minimum angle of resolution; OCT: Optical coherence tomography; SD-OCT: Spectral-domain optical coherence tomography; SFCT: Subfoveal choroidal thickness; SS-OCT: Swept-source optical coherence tomography; VA: Visual acuity

Funding
The Japan Society for the Promotion of Science (JPSP) provided financial support in the form of KAKENHI Grants-in-Aid (Grant Number: 17 K04506, Grant Recipient: Goro Maehara).

Authors' contributions
SA and AM designed the study, collected and interpreted the data, drafted the manuscript, and reviewed the literature. TY (Yamashita), KG, GT, KH, and TY (Yoneda) participated in the collection and interpretation of the data. SA and KY performed statistical analysis. YI, JK, and GM interpreted the data and critically reviewed the manuscript. All authors read and approved the final manuscript.

Competing interests
The authors declare that they have no competing interests.

Author details
[1]Department of Ophthalmology, Kawasaki Medical School, 577 Matsushima, Kurashiki, Okayama 701-0192, Japan. [2]Department of Sensory Science, Faculty of Health Science and Technology, Kawasaki University of Medical Welfare, 288 Matsushima, Kurashiki, Okayama 701-0193, Japan. [3]Department of Human Sciences, Kanagawa University, 3-27-1 Rokkakubashi, Yokohama, Kanagawa 221-8686, Japan. [4]Yaoeda Eye Clinic, 2-1649-1 Naga-Chou, Nagaoka, Niigata 940-0053, Japan.

References
1. Holmes JM, Clarke MP. Amblyopia. Lancet. 2006;367(9519):1343–51.
2. Hubel DH, Wiesel TN. Binocular interaction in striate cortex of kittens reared with artificial squint. J Neurophysiol. 1965;28:1041–59.

3. von Noorden GK. Histological studies of the visual system in monkeys with experimental amblyopia. Investig Ophthalmol. 1973;12:727–38.

4. Miki A, Liu GT, Goldsmith ZG, Liu CS, Haselgrove JC. Decreased activation of the lateral geniculate nucleus in a patient with anisometropic amblyopia demonstrated by functional magnetic resonance imaging. Ophthalmologica. 2003;217:365–9.

5. Hess RF, Thompson B, Gole G, Mullen KT. Deficient responses from the lateral geniculate nucleus in humans with amblyopia. Eur J Neurosci. 2009; 29:1064–70.

6. Hess RF. Amblyopia: site unseen. Clin Exp Optom. 2001;84:321–36.

7. Li J, Ji P, Yu M. Meta-analysis of retinal changes in unilateral amblyopia using optical coherence tomography. Eur J Ophthalmol. 2015;25:400–9.

8. Liu Y, Dong Y, Zhao K. Meta-analysis of choroidal thickness changes in unilateral amblyopia. J Ophthalmol. 2017;2017:2915261. https://doi.org/10.1155/2017/2915261.

9. Lempert P. The axial length/disc area ratio in anisometropic hyperopic amblyopia: a hypothesis for decreased unilateral vision associated with hyperopic anisometropia. Ophthalmology. 2004;111(2):304–8.

10. Araki S, Miki A, Goto K, Yamashita T, Takizawa G, Haruishi K, et al. Macular retinal and choroidal thickness in unilateral amblyopia using swept-source optical coherence tomography. BMC Ophthalmol. 2017; 17(1):167. https://doi.org/10.1186/s12886-017-0559-3.

11. Öner V, Bulut A. Does the treatment of amblyopia normalise subfoveal choroidal thickness in amblyopic children? Clin Exp Optom. 2016;100(2): 184–8.

12. Aslan Bayhan S, Bayhan HA. Effect of amblyopia treatment on choroidal thickness in children with hyperopic Anisometropic amblyopia. Curr Eye Res. 2017;42(9):1254–9.

13. Hashimoto R, Kawamura J, Hirota A, Oyamada M, Sakai A, Maeno T. Changes in choroidal blood flow and choroidal thickness after treatment in two cases of pediatric anisohypermetropic amblyopia. American Journal of Ophthalmology Case Reports. 2017;8:39–43.

14. Nishi T, Ueda T, Mizusawa Y, Semba K, Shinomiya K, Mitamura Y, et al. Effect of optical correction on subfoveal choroidal thickness in children with anisohypermetropic amblyopia. PLoS One. 2017;12(12):e0189735.

15. Pediatric Eye Disease Investigator Group. A randomized trial of increasing patching for amblyopia. Ophthalmology. 2013;120:2270–7.

16. Gabriel M, Esmaeelpour M, Shams-Mafi F, Hermann B, Zabihian B, Drexler W, et al. Mapping diurnal changes in choroidal, Haller's and Sattler's layer thickness using 3-dimensional 1060-nm optical coherence tomography. Graefes Arch Clin Exp Ophthalmol. 2017;255:1957–63.

17. Ikuno Y, Kawaguchi K, Nouchi T, Yasuno Y. Choroidal thickness in healthy Japanese subjects. Invest Ophthalmol Vis Sci. 2010;51:2173–6.

18. Kaderli A, Acar MA, Ünlü N, Üney GÖ, Örnek F. The correlation of hyperopia and choroidal thickness, vessel diameter and area. Int Ophthalmol. 2018;38: 645–53.

19. Xu J, Zheng J, Yu S, Sun Z, Zheng W, Qu P, et al. Macular choroidal thickness in unilateral amblyopic children. Invest Ophthalmol Vis Sci. 2014; 55:7361–8.

20. Nishi T, Ueda T, Hasegawa T, Miyata K, Ogata N. Choroidal thickness in children with hyperopic anisometropic amblyopia. Br J Ophthalmol. 2014;98: 228–32.

21. Nishi T, Ueda T, Mizusawa Y, Shinomiya K, Semba K, Mitamura Y, et al. Choroidal structure in children with anisohypermetropic amblyopia determined by binarization of optical coherence tomographic images. PLoS One. 2016;11:e0164672.

22. Woodman-Pieterse EC, Read SA, Collins MJ, Alonso-Caneiro D. Regional changes in choroidal thickness associated with accommodation. Invest Ophthalmol Vis Sci. 2015;56:6414–22.

23. Chakraborty R, Read SA, Collins MJ. Hyperopic defocus and diurnal changes in human choroid and axial length. Optom Vis Sci. 2013;90:1187–98.

24. Toor S, Horwood AM, Riddell P. Asymmetrical accommodation in hyperopic anisometropic amblyopia. Br J Ophthalmol. 2018;102:772–8.

23

Corneal higher-order aberrations of the anterior surface, posterior surface, and total cornea after small incision lenticule extraction (SMILE): high myopia versus mild to moderate myopia

Hong-Ying Jin[*], Ting Wan, Xiao-Ning Yu, Fang Wu and Ke Yao

Abstract

Background: To investigate corneal higher-order aberrations (HOAs) of the anterior surface, posterior surface, and total cornea after small incision lenticule extraction (SMILE) in high myopic and mild to moderate myopic patients.

Methods: This retrospective study included 197 eyes (101 patients) undergoing SMILE surgery. According to the preoperative spherical equivalent (SE), treated eyes were divided into two groups: a high myopic group (more than − 6.0 D, Group H) and a mild to moderate myopic group (less than − 6.0 D, Group M). Corneal HOAs of the anterior surface, posterior surface, and total cornea were measured using a Scheimpflug camera preoperatively and 3 months postoperatively. Pearson's correlation analysis was conducted to determine relationships between corneal aberrations and the SE.

Results: There were no significant differences in third-order to eight-order aberrations (RMS HOAs) of the anterior surface, posterior surface, and total corneal between the two groups before SMILE surgery. However, after SMILE, anterior and total corneal HOAs, especially vertical coma and spherical aberrations, significantly increased in both groups ($p < 0.0167$), whereas posterior corneal HOAs remained relatively stable ($p > 0.0167$). The induction of HOAs was significantly greater in Group H than Group M postoperatively ($p < 0.0167$). Changes in anterior surface and total corneal HOAs, especially vertical coma and spherical aberrations, were related to the SE ($p < 0.05$).

Conclusions: Anterior and total corneal HOAs, particularly vertical coma and spherical aberrations, significantly increased after SMILE in both groups, whereas posterior corneal HOAs remained stable. Aberration changes were related to SE.

Keywords: SMILE, Higher-order aberrations, Posterior cornea

* Correspondence: hongyingj@zju.edu.cn
Eye Center, 2nd Affiliated Hospital, School of Medicine, Zhejiang University, Hangzhou 310009, China

Background

Visual acuity is the most commonly used parameter for assessments of overall visual function in the clinical setting. However, under dim light conditions or low contrast sensitivity conditions, visual acuity does not truly reflect a patient's subjective vision function [1], especially after corneal refractive surgeries. Higher-order aberrations (HOAs) increase after successful refractive surgery and influence the vision quality of patients. Measurements of changes in wavefront aberrations are used to evaluate the impact of refractive surgery on vision quality [1]. Previous studies indicated that posterior corneal HOAs influenced corneal biomechanical responses and provided valuable information in determining the cause of poor vision quality after corneal refractive surgery [2, 3].

Small incision lenticule extraction (SMILE) surgery is a newly developed corneal refractive technique, which is less invasive than LASIK (Laser-assisted in situ keratomileusis) and FS-LASIK (femtosecond laser-assisted LASIK), with only a small incision required [4, 5]. Recent studies suggested that the SMILE procedure provided excellent clinical outcomes, considering its safety, efficacy, predictability, and postoperative ocular surface health [6–8]. Therefore, SMILE is considered to be a good choice for refractive surgery. Previous studies of changes of corneal HOAs after the SMILE procedure focused mainly on anterior corneal HOAs or total corneal HOAs [8–11]. Only a few studies have compared anterior, posterior, and total corneal HOAs following different refractive surgery procedures [2, 3, 12]. The potential effect of the SMILE procedure on posterior corneal HOAs is not well understood. In this study, we compared HOAs of the anterior surface, posterior surface, and total cornea after SMILE surgery for high myopia and mild to moderate myopia.

Material and methods

Subjects

This is a retrospective study, which recruited 197 eyes (101 patients). All patients aged between 18 and 47 years underwent SMILE surgery at the Department of Ophthalmology, Second Affiliated Hospital, College of Medicine, Zhejiang University from December 2016 to May 2017 were included in this study. This research followed the tenets of the Declaration of Helsinki was approved by the Institutional review board (No: 2017–017). Informed written consent was obtained from the all subjects. The inclusion criteria were aged ≥18 years, myopic spherical correction < − 10.00 diopters, no ocular or systemic diseases, and stable refraction for at least one year. The exclusion criteria were the presence of active ocular disease or a history of ocular surgery and trauma. Patients were instructed to stop wearing soft contact lenses for at least 1 week prior to the surgery. The cases were divided into two groups according to the degree of preoperative spherical equivalent (SE): a high myopic group (more than − 6.0 D,Group H) and a mild to moderate myopic group (less than − 6.0 D, Group M).

Surgical technique

All surgeries were performed by the same experienced surgeon (H.Y.J.). A VisuMax femtosecond laser system (Carl Zeiss Meditec AG, Jena, Germany) was used for surgical refractive corrections in all patients, with a repetition rate of 500 kHz and pulse energy of 155 nJ. The stroma cap was set at thickness of 120 μm, diameter of 7.5–7.6 mm. Prior to the initiation of suction, the patients were instructed to fixate on a target light. Four cleavage planes were created, including anterior and posterior surfaces of the refractive lenticule and vertical edge of the refractive lenticule. A single side-cut incision (width of 2 mm) was made at an angle of 120°. The lenticule was removed using a forceps. The target refraction was emmetropia. After surgery, all the patients received a topical antibiotic for 7 days and a topical steroid for 2 weeks. Artificial tears were used for more than 4 weeks.

Measurement of corneal aberrations

Corneal aberrations of the anterior surface, posterior surface, and total cornea were measured by a rotating Scheimpflug Camera (Pentacam HR; Oculus, Wetzlar, Germany). The Pentacam HR is a noninvasive and reproducible diagnostic method. The measurements were made in a dark room. To minimize the potential effect of tear film on corneal imaging, the patients were instructed to remain fixated on a target light immediately after blinking. The Pentacam HR camera then started rotating and scanning the cornea. Only measurements marked as "OK" quality were considered valid. Corneal aberrations of the anterior surface, posterior surface, and total cornea were analyzed over a 6.0-mm central diameter preoperatively, 1 and 3 months postoperatively. Root mean square (RMS) values of higher-order aberrations (HOAs) (third-order to eight-order), including coma, trefoil, quadrafoil, and secondary astigmatism, were calculated.

Statistical analysis

Statistical analyses were performed using SPSS software, ver. 18 (SPSS, Chicago, IL, USA). The Kolmogorov–Smirnov test was used to test for normality. An independent-sample t test was conducted for comparisons between Group H and Group M. A paired-sample t test was performed for preoperative and postoperative comparisons. The Bonferroni correction for multiple testing was used to reduce the rate of type I error. In addition, Pearson's correlation analysis was performed to determine relationships between the preoperative spherical equivalent (SE) and corneal aberrations. All values are given as the mean ± standard deviation. $P < 0.05$ was considered statistically significant, otherwise indicated.

Results

All 101 patients attended the 1-month, and 3-month follow-up examinations. Group H and Group M comprised 65 and 132 eyes, respectively. Preoperative characteristics of both groups are listed in Table 1. There were no statistically significant differences between the two groups as regards the patient's age, preoperative SE, spherical diopter, cylindrical diopter, central corneal thickness(CCT), intraocular pressure(IOP), and mean corneal power, making it possible to compare corneal HOAs without confounders ($p > 0.05$).

Comparison of surgically induced third-order to eight-order aberrations (RMS HOAs) after SMILE in group H and group M

As shown by RMS values, third-order to eight-order aberrations of the anterior corneal surface (RMS-HOA-CF) and total cornea (RMS-HOA-cornea) significantly increased after SMILE surgery in Group H and Group M ($p < 0.0167$) (Fig. 1a and c). According to RMS values, posterior corneal HOAs (RMS-HOA-CB) slightly increased, but remained relatively stable in both groups ($p > 0.0167$) (Fig. 1b).

Comparison of preoperative HOAs versus surgically induced HOAs (third-order to eight-order, RMS HOAs) between group H and group M

As shown by RMS values, there were no significant differences in HOAs between Group H and Group M preoperatively ($p > 0.0167$). However, there were significant differences in HOAs in anterior cornea and total cornea between the two groups 1 and 3 months after surgery ($p < 0.0167$). There was no significant difference in HOAs

of posterior cornea surface between the two groups after the surgery ($p > 0.0167$) (Table 2).

Comparison of surgically induced anterior corneal surface HOAs in group H and group M

There were no significant differences in coma and spherical aberrations of the anterior surface between the two groups preoperatively ($p > 0.0167$). However, there was a significant increase in vertical coma ($Z^{3,-1}$) and spherical aberrations ($Z^{4,\,0}$) in the two groups 1 and 3 months postoperatively ($p < 0.0167$). More coma and spherical aberrations of the anterior corneal surface were induced in Group H than Group M postoperatively ($p < 0.0167$) (Fig. 2).

Comparison of surgically induced posterior corneal surface HOAs in group H and group M

There was no significant difference in spherical aberrations ($Z^{4,\,0}$) of the posterior cornea between the two groups preoperatively or postoperatively ($p > 0.0167$). There was also no significant increased in spherical aberration in the two groups after smile surgery ($p > 0.0167$). There was no significant differences between-group in coma aberrations preoperatively ($p > 0.0167$). However, there were significant changes in vertical coma ($z^{3,-1}$) and vertical trefoil ($Z^{3,\,-3}$) after SMILE surgery in the two groups ($p < 0.167$). In addition, there was significant difference in vertical coma between the two groups after surgery ($p < 0.167$) (Fig. 3).

Comparison of surgically induced total corneal HOAs in group H and group M

There were no significant differences in total corneal HOAs (coma and spherical aberrations) between the two groups preoperatively ($p > 0.0167$). In contrast, there were significant differences in vertical coma ($z^{3,-1}$) and

Table 1 Demographic and preoperative patient information (mean ± SD)

Parameter	Group H	Group M	t	p
Eye (n)	65	132		
Sex (M/F)	31/34	77/56		
Age (y)	24.46 ± 7.34 (18 to 47)	23.84 ± 5.92 (18 to 47)	0.64	0.52
IOP (mmHg)	15.80 ± 2.12 (11 to 23)	15.48 ± 2.36 (10 to 23)	0.93	0.36
CCT (µm)	552.58 ± 25.61 (502 to 616)	541.52 ± 28.03 (482 to 627)	1.66	0.10
Mean corneal power (D)	43.16 ± 1.42 (40.60 to 46.55)	43.24 ± 1.25 (41.25 to 45.95)	−0.42	0.67
SE (D)	−7.32 ± 0.99 (−6.00 to −9.88)	−4.45 ± 1.01 (− 1.13 to − 5.88)	− 18.85	0.00*
Sphere (D)	−6.94 ± 1.00 (− 5.00 to − 9.75)	−4.13 ± 1.00 (−0.75 to −5.75)	− 18.60	0.00
Cylinder (D)	−0.76 ± 0.68 (0 to − 3.00)	−0.64 ± 0.50 (0 to − 2.75)	−1.35	0.18
Lenticule thickness (µm)	128.48 ± 10.27 (109 to148)	92.23 ± 15.53 (50 to 120)	19.51	0.00*
Lenticule diameter (mm)	6.52 ± 0.14 (6.1 to 6.6)	6.58 ± 0.05 (6.1 to 6.6)	−5.84	0.00*

SD standard deviation, D diopters, SE spherical equivalent, CCT central corneal thickness, IOP intraocular pressure, Group H high myopia group, Group M mild to moderate myopia group.*p < 0.05

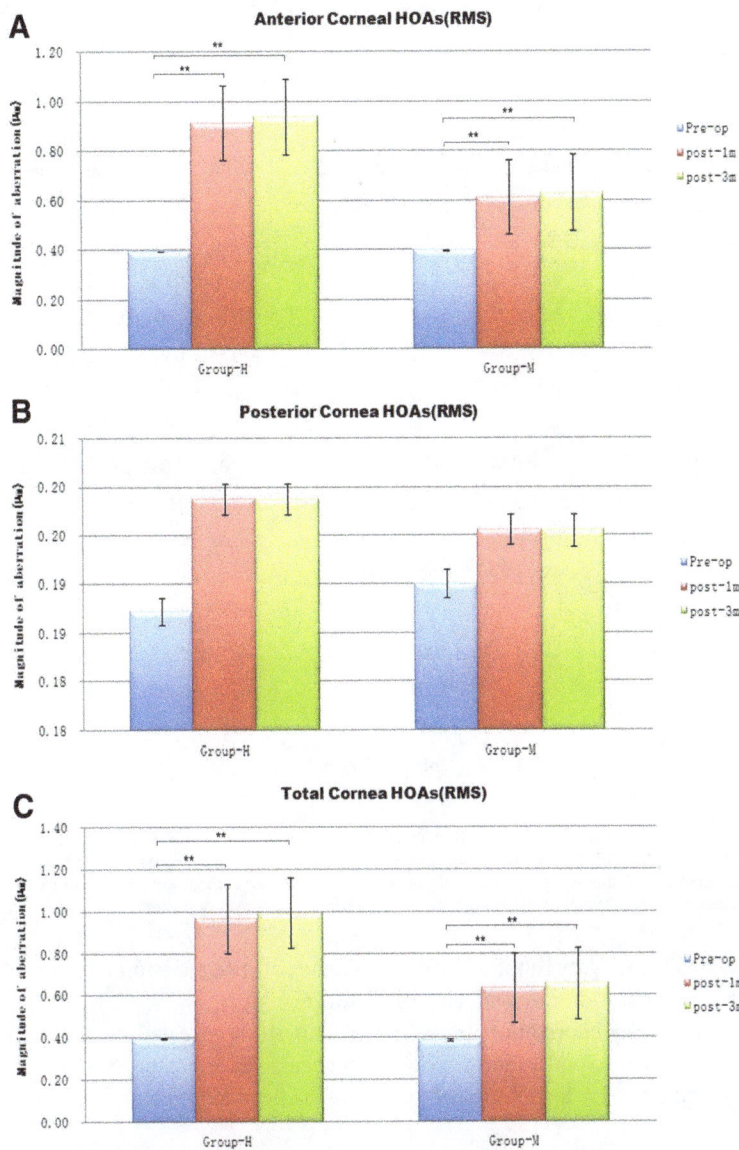

Fig. 1 Third-order to eight-order higher-order aberrations (RMS HOAs) of the cornea preoperatively and 1 and 3 months postoperatively in Group H and Group M. **a** Anterior corneal surface (RMS-HOA-CF, root mean square –HOA- cornea front); **b** Posterior corneal surface (RMS-HOA-CB, root mean square-HOA- cornea back); **c** Total cornea (RMS-HOA-cornea, root mean square- HOA- cornea). *$p < 0.0167$ (the modified Bonferroni correction, 0.05/3 tests)

spherical aberrations ($Z^{4,\ 0}$) between the two groups 1 and 3 months postoperatively ($p < 0.0167$). More total corneal coma and spherical aberrations were induced in Group H than Group M postoperatively ($p < 0.0167$) (Fig. 4).

Correlations between the preoperative SE and surgically induced corneal HOAs

Correlations between the preoperative SE and surgically induced corneal HOAs are shown in Table 3. The SE was significantly correlated with the induction of HOAs (third-order to eight-order, RMS HOAs) of the anterior

surface and total cornea, especially vertical coma and spherical aberrations after SMILE surgery ($p < 0.05$) (Table 3).

Discussion

This study is the first to compare corneal HOAs of the anterior surface, posterior surface, and total cornea in high and mild to moderate myopic eyes after SMILE surgery. The results indicated that HOAs of the anterior cornea surface and total cornea significantly increased after SMILE surgery in both groups. However, HOAs of the posterior corneal surface remained relatively

Table 2 Comparison of higher-order aberrations (HOAs) between the two groups preoperatively and postoperatively 1 and 3 months (mean ± SD)

Time	Preop.			Postop. 1 month			Postop. 3 months		
Group	Group H (n = 65)	Group M (n = 132)	p	Group H (n = 65)	Group M (n = 132)	p	Group H (n = 65)	Group M (n = 132)	P
RMS HOA (CF)	0.39 ± 0.08	0.40 ± 0.11	0.754	0.91 ± 0.28	0.61 ± 0.18	0.000*	0.94 ± 0.26	0.63 ± 0.19	0.000#
RMS HOA (CB)	0.19 ± 0.03	0.19 ± 0.03	0.546	0.20 ± 0.03	0.20 ± 0.03	0.219	0.19 ± 0.03	0.20 ± 0.03	0.640
RMS HOA (cornea)	0.40 ± 0.09	0.39 ± 0.12	0.710	0.97 ± 0.30	0.64 ± 0.19	0.000	0.99 ± 0.28	0.66 ± 0.20	0.000#
Oblique trefoil $Z^{3,3}$ (CF)	0.00 ± 0.07	−0.01 ± 0.09	0.294	0.01 ± 0.10	−0.01 ± 0.09	0.486	0.03 ± 0.11	0.01 ± 0.11	0.376
Horizontal coma $Z^{3,1}$ (CF)	−0.01 ± 0.15	−0.03 ± 0.15	0.304	0.01 ± 0.37	−0.04 ± 0.25	0.434	−0.03 ± 0.38	−0.05 ± 0.26	0.996
Vertical coma $Z^{3,-1}$ (CF)	−0.03 ± 0.19	0.01 ± 0.18	0.276	−0.60 ± 0.31	−0.34 ± 0.23	0.000*	−0.62 ± 0.29	−0.32 ± 0.26	0.000#
Vertical trefoil $Z^{3,-3}$ (CF)	−0.04 ± 0.10	−0.05 ± 0.11	0.666	−0.03 ± 0.13	−0.02 ± 0.11	0.988	−0.04 ± 0.12	−0.03 ± 0.13	0.661
Spherical aberration $Z^{4,0}$ (CF)	0.24 ± 0.07	0.26 ± 0.07	0.188	0.44 ± 0.14	0.31 ± 0.11	0.000*	0.45 ± 0.13	0.30 ± 0.11	0.000#
Oblique trefoil $Z^{3,3}$ (CB)	−0.01 ± 0.05	0.00 ± 0.04	0.619	0.00 ± 0.05	−0.01 ± 0.04	0.490	−0.01 ± 0.04	−0.01 ± 0.05	0.895
Horizontal coma $Z^{3,1}$ (CB)	0.00 ± 0.02	0.00 ± 0.02	0.408	−0.01 ± 0.03	0.00 ± 0.03	0.180	−0.01 ± 0.03	0.00 ± 0.03	0.461
Vertical coma $Z^{3,-1}$ (CB)	−0.02 ± 0.03	−0.03 ± 0.04	0.025	0.01 ± 0.04	−0.01 ± 0.04	0.000*	0.01 ± 0.03	−0.01 ± 0.04	0.000#
Vertical trefoil $Z^{3,-3}$ (CB)	−0.02 ± 0.05	−0.02 ± 0.05	0.220	−0.05 ± 0.05	−0.04 ± 0.06	0.249	−0.04 ± 0.05	−0.04 ± 0.05	0.470
Spherical aberration $Z^{4,0}$ (CB)	−0.15 ± 0.03	−0.16 ± 0.03	0.306	−0.16 ± 0.03	−0.16 ± 0.03	0.821	−0.16 ± 0.03	−0.16 ± 0.03	0.857
Oblique trefoil $Z^{3,3}$ (cornea)	0.00 ± 0.09	−0.02 ± 0.10	0.506	0.01 ± 0.11	−0.01 ± 0.09	0.250	0.02 ± 0.12	0.00 ± 0.12	0.339
Horizontal coma $Z^{3,1}$ (cornea)	−0.01 ± 0.15	−0.03 ± 0.15	0.307	0.00 ± 0.39	−0.05 ± 0.26	0.457	−0.04 ± 0.40	−0.06 ± 0.27	0.964
Vertical coma $Z^{3,-1}$ (Cornea)	−0.04 ± 0.20	−0.01 ± 0.18	0.351	−0.66 ± 0.23	−0.39 ± 0.23	0.000*	−0.68 ± 0.31	−0.36 ± 0.27	0.000#
Vertical trefoil $Z^{3,-3}$ (cornea)	−0.07 ± 0.12	−0.07 ± 0.12	0.864	−0.08 ± 0.14	−0.06 ± 0.12	0.600	−0.08 ± 0.14	−0.07 ± 0.14	0.454
Spherical aberration $Z^{4,0}$ (cornea)	0.19 ± 0.08	0.20 ± 0.07	0.398	0.41 ± 0.16	0.26 ± 0.12	0.000*	0.42 ± 0.14	0.26 ± 0.13	0.000#

*Significant difference in HOAs 1 months postoperatively ($p < 0.0167$) (the modified Bonferroni correction, 0.05/3 tests) between Group-H and Group-M; #Significant difference in HOAs 3 months postoperatively ($p < 0.0167$) (the modified Bonferroni correction, 0.05/3 tests) between Group-H and Group-M. HOAs higher-order aberrations, RMS root mean square, RMS-HOA-CF: third-order to eight-order aberrations of anterior corneal surface (cornea front, CF); RMS-HOA-cornea: third-order to eight-order aberrations of total corneal surface; RMS-HOA-CB: third-order to eight-order aberrations of posterior corneal surface (cornea back, CB)

stable. These results are consistent with those of other studies, which indicated that posterior corneal HOAs could complement corneal topography information, provide insight into the corneal biomechanical response, and provide valuable information that could be used to determine the cause of poor vision quality after corneal refractive surgery [2, 3].

This study revealed no significant differences in anterior cornea surface, posterior cornea surface and total corneal HOAs between high and mild to moderate myopic groups

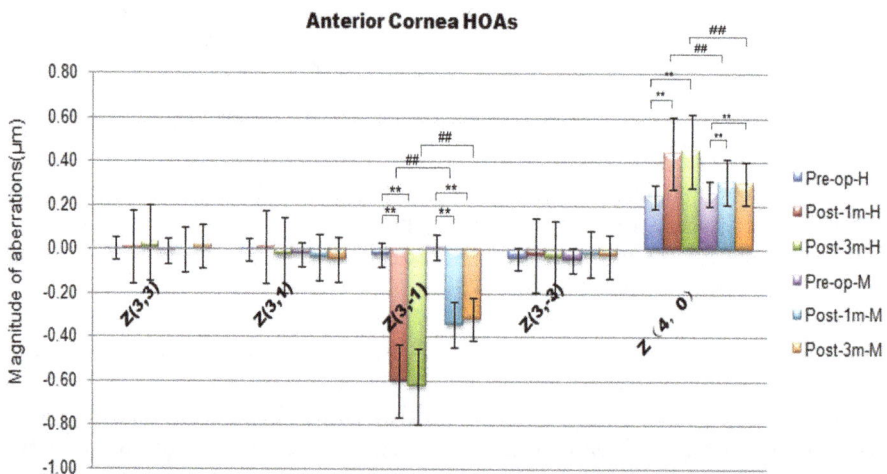

Fig. 2 Higher-order aberrations (HOAs) of the anterior cornea surface before and after SMILE surgery in Group H and group M. *p, #p < 0.0167 (the modified Bonferroni correction, 0.05/3 tests)

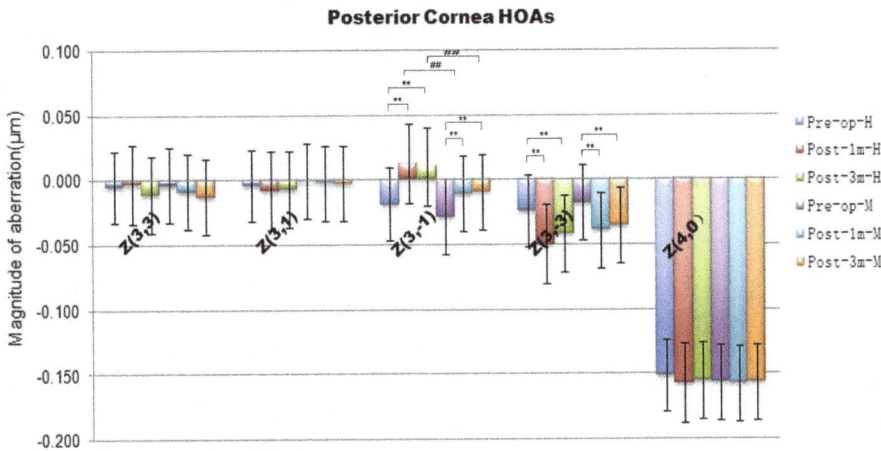

Fig. 3 Higher-order aberrations (HOAs) of the posterior cornea surface before and after SMILE surgery in Group H and group M. *p, #$p < 0.0167$ (the modified Bonferroni correction, 0.05/3 tests)

before SMILE surgery. However, significant between-group differences in anterior cornea surface HOAs and total corneal HOAs were detected postoperatively. In terms of SMILE-induced HOAs, there were significantly more HOAs in the high myopic group than mild to moderate group postoperatively, whereas HOAs of the posterior cornea remained almost unchanged postoperatively in both groups. The lack of significant changes in the posterior corneal surface is in agreement with that of previous studies, which examined the posterior corneal surface after PRK (Photo Refractive Keratectomy), FS-LASIK, and SMILE using Pentacam [3, 12, 13]. Wu et al. compared HOAs after SMILE, FS-LASIK, and FLEx (Femtosecond Lenticule Extraction) surgeries [3]. They reported a value of 0.19 ± 0.03 μm for third-order to eight-order aberrations of the posterior corneal surface in each surgical group postoperatively. They found that these HOAs not

only remained stable postoperatively but were similar to values for HOAs obtained prior to surgery. In the present study, the number of third-order to eight-order aberrations of the posterior corneal surface in each group preoperatively and postoperatively was similar to that found by Wu [3]. Gyldenkerne et al. reported that the posterior corneal surface showed almost no change after FS-LASIK and SMILE procedures, which was consistent with our study [13]. Juhasz et al. analyzed changes in anterior and posterior corneal surface HOAs after PRK [12]. They found that PRK-induced HOAs increased significantly more than 76.78 μm ablation depths. And the HOAs on the anterior corneal surface increased total corneal aberrations. However, posterior corneal surface HOAs remained relatively stable after surgery. They also pointed out that aberrations of the anterior corneal surface were statistically significantly higher than that of the total cornea,

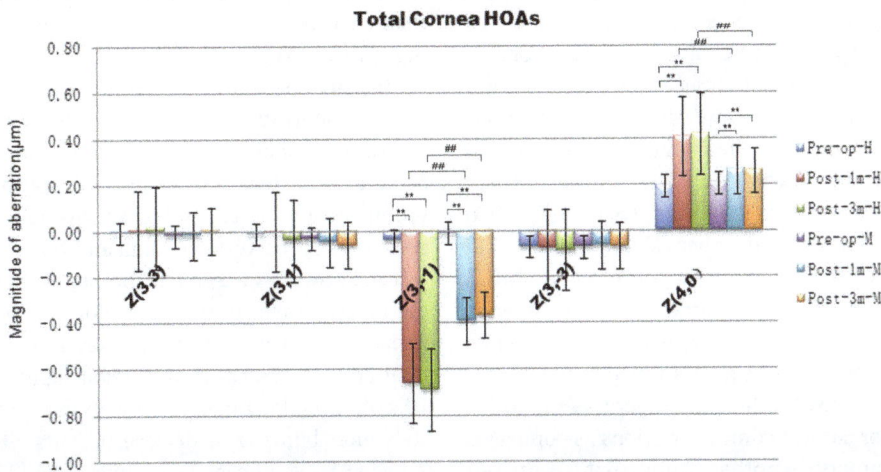

Fig. 4 Higher-order aberrations (HOAs) of the total cornea before and after SMILE surgery in Group H and group M. *p, #$p < 0.0167$ (the modified Bonferroni correction, 0.05/3 tests)

Table 3 Correlations between SE and induced corneal HOAs after SMILE surgery

Cornea aberrations	r	p
RMS HOA (CF)	−0.631	0.000
RMS HOA (CB)	0.011	0.867
RMS HOA (cornea)	−0.648	0.000
Oblique trefoil $Z^{3,3}$ (CF)	0.047	0.516
Horizontal coma $Z^{3,1}$ (CF)	0.028	0.692
Vertical coma $Z^{3,-1}$ (CF)	0.616	0.000
Vertical trefoil $Z^{3,-3}$ (CF)	0.076	0.290
Spherical aberration $Z^{4,0}$ (CF)	−0.582	0.000
Oblique trefoil $Z^{3,3}$ (CB)	−0.046	0.517
Horizontal coma $Z^{3,1}$ (CB)	0.026	0.718
Vertical coma $Z^{3,-1}$ (CB)	−0.323	0.000
Vertical trefoil $Z^{3,-3}$ (CB)	−0.060	0.398
Spherical aberration $Z^{4,0}$ (CB)	0.037	0.601
Oblique trefoil $Z^{3,3}$ (cornea)	0.027	0.702
Horizontal coma $Z^{3,1}$ (cornea)	0.026	0.715
Vertical coma $Z^{3,-1}$ (cornea)	0.613	0.000
Vertical trefoil $Z^{3,-3}$ (cornea)	0.070	0.329
Spherical aberration $Z^{4,0}$ (cornea)	0.561	0.000

RMS-HOA-CF: third-order to eight-order aberrations of anterior corneal surface (cornea front, CF); RMS-HOA-cornea: third-order to eight-order aberrations of total corneal surface; RMS-HOA-CB: third-order to eight-order aberrations of posterior corneal surface (cornea back, CB)

indicating that the posterior corneal surface plays a compensatory role in the balance of corneal aberrations in myopic eyes.

This study also found that spherical aberrations induced by the SMILE procedure increased in the anterior corneal surface and total cornea. The induction of spherical aberrations was significantly greater in the high myopic group than mild to moderate group. However, spherical aberrations of the posterior corneal surface remained almost unchanged in both groups after surgery. SMILE-induced coma aberrations, especially vertical coma aberrations of the anterior surface, posterior surface, and total cornea changed in both groups, with a significantly greater increase in vertical coma aberrations in the high myopic group than mild to moderate group. These results were similar to study of Wu et al. [3] Their study indicated that FS-LASIK, FLEx, and SMILE surgeries induced spherical aberrations and coma of the anterior surface and total cornea. The SMILE surgery induced fewer spherical aberrations of the anterior cornea and total cornea than FLEx procedure, and posterior corneal spherical aberrations significantly increased after FS-LASIK surgery. Thus, the SMILE surgery seems to induce fewer posterior corneal coma aberrations as compared with the FLEx surgery. Another study that compared aberrations induced by FLEx and wavefront-guided LASIK procedures indicated that FLEx induced fewer spherical

aberrations but the same amount of coma aberrations as compared with that observed using wavefront-guided LASIK1 [14]. Gertnere et al. found a reduced incidence of spherical aberrations in a FLEx group but a higher incidence of induced coma aberrations in an FS-LASIK group [15]. Lin et al. compared changes in aberrations induced by FS-LASIK and SMILE surgery and found a significantly lower incidence of spherical aberrations in the SMILE procedure [16]. The aforementioned studies used different LASIK ablation techniques and different microkeratomes for cutting the LASIK flap. The use of different LASIK ablation techniques and diverse methods of flap creation may result in substantial differences in HOAs [13]. The increased number of induced aberrations observed with the FS-LASIK procedure seems to be primarily associated with the ablation of corneal tissue rather than the creation of the flap, as the flap-dependent FLEx procedure does not seem to be different from that used in SMILE [13]. In the present study, there were significantly more surgically induced aberrations in the high myopia group than mild and moderate myopia group, and more central corneal tissue was removed in the high myopia group than mild to moderate myopia group. The correlation study also indicated changes in the induction of aberrations in the two groups were related to the preoperative SE, which was consistent with the findings of the study by Chen et al. [17].

Previous studies indicated that centeration and wound healing might influence the induction of coma aberrations [18, 19]. Li et al. demonstrated that horizontal decentration induced horizontal coma aberrations but that there appeared to be no association between the magnitude of vertical decentration and induction of vertical coma aberrations [20]. In our previous study, we reported that spherical aberrations and horizontal coma aberrations increased significantly after SMILE surgery and that the increase of spherical aberrations was higher in Group H than that in Group M [8]. This result was similar to findings presented by Liang et al. [21]. The difference in these results may be due to different methods used to evaluate corneal aberrations. In our previous study, we used a Hartmann–Shack WASCA aberrometer (Carl Zeiss Meditec AG, Jena, Germany). To optimize postoperative vision quality, more studies are needed to investigate the resources of the vertical coma and horizontal coma.

It is known that tear film problems that might influence the measurement of the aberrations of the anterior corneal surface, especially in dry eyes. Recently, Jung reported that total HOA RMS, coma and trefoil significantly increased at 10 s after blinking compared with those measured immediately after blinking in dry eye patients after LASEK (Laser Assisted Subepithelial Keratomilesusis) [22]. In the study of Elmohamady [23], they evaluated dry eye after LASIK, FS-LASIK, and SMILE. They found the mean ocular surface disease index (OSDI) scores were significantly elevated in all groups postoperatively but were significantly lower in the SMILE group 3 months postoperatively. The mean tear breakup time (TBUT) was significantly decreased in all groups postoperatively but was significantly higher in the SMILE group 6 months postoperatively. This result indicated the influence on dry eye was minimal after SMILE surgery. In our study, there were no significant differences in aberrations in the two groups after SMILE surgery 1 and 3 months postoperatively. This result may be due to the relatively small interference of SMILE on the tear film. Of course, long-term follow-up is still needed.

There were some limitations in this study. First, this study included 197 eyes, the two groups were not of equal size, and available data covered only 3 months. Longer term follow-up visits would have been desirable. Second, for bilaterally treated patients, there may be a correlation between the two eyes of one patient. This is a common mistake in ophthalmology research, for the overall variance of a sample of measurements combined from both eyes is likely to be an underestimate of the true variance resulting in an increased risk of a Type 1 error [24]. Future studies of the association of HOAs and corneal biomechanics with vision quality are needed to shed light on.

In conclusion, third-order to eight-order aberrations, particularly spherical aberrations and vertical coma aberrations of the anterior cornea and total cornea significantly increased after SMILE surgeries. In contrast, posterior corneal surface HOAs remained relatively unchanged. The induction of aberrations postoperatively was related to the preoperative SE. Further and larger studies, with longer-term follow-ups are needed.

Abbreviations
CB: Posterior cornea surface/Cornea Back; CF: Anterior cornea surface/Cornea Front; FLEx: Femtosecond lenticule extraction; FS-LASIK: Femtosecond laser-assisted LASIK; HOAs: High-order aberrations; LASEK: Laser Assisted Subepithelial Keratomilesusis; LASIK: Laser-assisted in situ keratomileusis; OSDI: Ocular surface disease index; PRK: Photo Refractive Keratectomy; RMS: Root mean square; SE: Spherical equivalent; SMILE: Small incision lenticule extraction; TBUT: Tear breakup time

Acknowledgements
None.

Funding
This study was funded by National Natural Science Foundation of China (No. 81500694), Zhejiang Province Key Research and Development Program(No. 2015C03042).

Authors' contributions
HYJ conceived of the study and drafted the manuscript. TW collected the data. YXN performed the statistical analysis. FW collected the data. KY revised the manuscript. All authors read and approved the final manuscript.

Competing interests
The authors declare that they have no competing interests.

References
1. Li L, Cheng GPM, Ng ALK, Chan TCY, Jhanji V, Wang Y. Influence of refractive status on the higher-order aberration pattern after small incision lenticule extraction surgery. Cornea. 2017;36(8):967–72.
2. Maeda N, Nakagawa T, Kosaki R, Koh S, Saika M, Fujikado T, Nishida K. Higher-order aberrations of anterior and posterior corneal surfaces in patients with keratectasia after LASIK. Invest Ophthalmol Vis Sci. 2014;55(6):3905–11.
3. Wu W, Wang Y. Corneal higher-order aberrations of the anterior surface, posterior surface, and total cornea after SMILE, FS-LASIK, and FLEx surgeries. Eye Contact Lens. 2016;42(6):358–65.
4. Shah R, Shah S, Sengupta S. Results of small incision lenticule extraction: all-in-one femtosecond laser refractive surgery. J Cataract Refract Surg. 2011;37(1):127–37.
5. Sekundo W, Kunert KS, Blum M. Small incision corneal refractive surgery using the small incision lenticule extraction (SMILE) procedure for the correction of myopia and myopic astigmatism: results of a 6 month prospective study. Br J Ophthalmol. 2011;95(3):335–9.
6. Kim JR, Hwang HB, Mun SJ, Chung YT, Kim HS. Efficacy, predictability, and safety of small incision lenticule extraction: 6-months prospective cohort study. BMC Ophthalmol. 2014;14:117–23.
7. Reinstein DZ, Carp GI, Archer TJ, Gobbe M. Outcomes of small incision lenticule extraction (SMILE) in low myopia. J Refract Surg. 2014;30(12):812–8.
8. Jin HY, Wan T, Wu F, Yao K. Comparison of visual results and higher-order aberrations after small incision lenticule extraction (SMILE): high myopia vs. mild to moderate myopia. BMC Ophthalmol. 2017;17(1):118–25.
9. Shen Y, Chen Z, Knorz MC, Li M, Zhao J, Zhou X. Comparison of corneal deformation parameters after SMILE, LASEK, and femtosecond laser-assisted LASIK. J Refract Surg. 2014;30(5):310–8.
10. Pedersen IB, Ivarsen A, Hjortdal J. Three-year results of small incision lenticule extraction for high myopia: refractive outcomes and aberrations. J Refract Surg. 2015;31(11):719–24.
11. Tan DK, Tay WT, Chan C, Tan DT, Mehta JS. Postoperative ocular higher-order aberrations and contrast sensitivity: femtosecond lenticule extraction versus pseudo small-incision lenticule extraction. J Cataract Refract Surg. 2015;41(3):623–34.
12. Juhasz E, Kranitz K, Sandor GL, Gyenes A, Toth G, Nagy ZZ. Wavefront properties of the anterior and posterior corneal surface after photorefractive keratectomy. Cornea. 2014;33(2):172–6.
13. Gyldenkerne A, Ivarsen A, Hjortdal JØ. Comparison of corneal shape changes and aberrations induced by FS-LASIK and SMILE for myopia. J Refract Surg. 2015;31(4):223–9.
14. Kamiya K, Shimizu K, Igarashi A, Kobashi H, Komatsu M. Comparison of visual acuity, higher-order aberrations and corneal asphericity after refractive lenticule extraction and wavefront-guided laser-assisted in situ keratomileusis for myopia. Br J Ophthalmol. 2013;97:968–75.
15. Gertnere J, Solomatin I, Sekundo W. Refractive lenticule extraction (ReLEx flex) and wavefront-optimized Femto-LASIK: comparison of contrast sensitivity and high-order aberrations at 1 year. Graefes Arch Clin Exp Ophthalmol. 2013;251(5):1437–42.
16. Lin F, Xu Y, Yang Y. Comparison of the visual results after SMILE and femtosecond laser-assisted LASIK for myopia. J Refract Surg. 2014;30:248–54.
17. Chen X, Wang Y. Comparison of ocular higher-order aberrations after SMILE and wavefront-guided femtosecond LASIK for myopia. J Ophthalmol. 2017;17(1):42.
18. Yu Y, Zhang W, Cheng X, Cai J, Chen H. Impact of Treatment Decentration on Higher-Order Aberrations after SMILE. J Ophthalmol. 2017;2017:9575723.
19. Li X, Wang Y, Dou R. Aberration compensation between anterior and posterior corneal surfaces after small incision lenticule extraction and femtosecond laser-assisted laser in-situ keratomileusis. Ophthalmic Physiol Opt. 2015;35:540–51.
20. Li M, Zhao J, Miao H, Shen Y, Sun L, Tian M, Wadium E, Zhou X. Mild decentration measured by a Scheimpflug camera and its impact on vision quality following SMILE in the early learning curve. Invest Ophthalmol Vis Sci. 2014;55(6):3886–92.
21. Liang G, Zha X, Zhang F. Analysis of higher-order aberrations (HOAs) and related factors after small incision lenticule extraction (SMILE) surgery. Clin J Optom Ophthalmol Vis Sci. 2015;17(11):644–8.

22. Jung HH, YS J, Oh HJ, Yoon KC. Higher order aberrations of the corneal surface after laser subepithelial keratomileusis. Korean J Ophthalmol. 2014;28(4):285–91.
23. Elmohamady MN, Abdelghaffar W, Daifalla A, Salem T. Evaluation of femtosecond laser in flap and cap creation in corneal refractive surgery for myopia: a 3-year follow-up. Clin Ophthalmol. 2018;12:935–42.
24. Armstrong RA. Statistical guidelines for the analysis of data obtained from one or both eyes. Ophthalmic Physiol Opt. 2013;33:7–14.

24

Programme choice for perimetry in neurological conditions (PoPiN): a systematic review of perimetry options and patterns of visual field loss

Lauren R. Hepworth and Fiona J. Rowe[*]

Abstract

Background: Visual field loss occurs frequently in neurological conditions and perimetry is commonly requested for patients with suspected or known conditions. There are currently no guidelines for how visual fields in neurological conditions should be assessed. There is a wide range of visual field programs available and the wrong choice of program can potentially fail to detect visual field loss. We report the results of a systematic review of the existing evidence base for the patterns of visual field loss in four common neurological conditions and the perimetry programs used, to aid the design of future research and clinical practice guidelines.

Methods: A systematic search of the literature was performed. The inclusion criteria required studies testing and/or reporting visual field loss in one or more of the target conditions; idiopathic intracranial hypertension, optic neuropathy, chiasmal compression and stroke. Scholarly online databases and registers were searched. In addition articles were hand searched. MESH terms and alternatives in relation to the four target conditions and visual fields were used. Study selection was performed by two authors independently. Data was extracted by one author and verified by a second.

Results: This review included 330 studies; 51 in relation to idiopathic intracranial hypertension, 144 in relation to optic neuropathy, 105 in relation to chiasmal compression, 21 in relation to stroke and 10 in relation to a mixed neuro-ophthalmology population.

Conclusions: Both the 30–2 and 24–2 program using the Humphrey perimeter were most commonly reported followed by manual kinetic perimetry using the Goldmann perimeter across all four conditions included in this review. A wide variety of other perimeters and programs were reported. The patterns of visual field defects differ much more greatly across the four conditions. Central perimetry is used extensively in neurological conditions but with little supporting evidence for its diagnostic accuracy in these, especially considering the peripheral visual field may be affected first whilst the central visual field may not be impacted until later in the progression. Further research is required to reach a consensus on how best to standardise perimetry for neurological conditions.

Keywords: Perimetry, Visual field loss, Idiopathic intracranial hypertension, Chiasmal compression, Stroke, Optic neuropathy

* Correspondence: rowef@liverpool.ac.uk
Department of Health Services Research, University of Liverpool, Waterhouse Building, Block B, First Floor1-5 Brownlow Street, Liverpool L69 3GL, UK

Background

Perimetry is the systematic measurement of visual field function using different types and intensities of stimuli. Visual fields may be assessed by using moving (kinetic) targets which outline the boundaries of visual field or by using static (stationary on-off) targets which map the sensitivity within the visual field [1]. The visual field is the full area which can be seen by each eye and includes both central and peripheral vision.

Perimetry programs can be chosen to measure the central or peripheral visual field, or both [1]. Typically, the central visual field is assessed as approximately 60% of all retinal nerve fibres originate from the central 30 degrees of the visual field [1]. Therefore, assessment of the central visual field tends to show the majority of visual field loss caused by common ophthalmic disease/conditions. Peripheral visual field assessment is indicated where pathology is known to affect the visual field outside the central 30 degrees.

Visual field assessment is an important clinical tool in the assessment of patients with acute and chronic ocular and/or neurological diseases and is often considered a 'corner-stone' assessment in ophthalmology services. Glaucoma is the most common ocular condition for which visual field assessment is required [2]. Visual field assessment using standard automated perimetry with a central thresholding test is listed as a key priority for implementation in the diagnosis of glaucoma [3]. Specifically the 24–2 program is referred to as the reference standard in assessing visual fields [3].

Given the choice of many perimetry programs across a variety of perimeters on the market, it is important to understand the designs of the programs available and apply them according to the type of visual field loss expected in order to improve diagnostic accuracy. In neuro-ophthalmology, perimetry has three important functions: 1) diagnostic, 2) monitoring and 3) functional assessment [4].

Diagnostic accuracy is important for any condition affecting the visual pathway particularly as a missed diagnosis of visual field loss can delay diagnosis of neurological pathology with serious life consequences. The recommendation for the 24–2 programme in glaucoma has streamlined clinical practice, allowing interchange of results across hospitals and providing a clinical result that clinicians worldwide recognise and accept. Such significant practice must be applied to other commonly occurring conditions to afford the same benefits.

It is not yet known how best to assess the visual field of individuals with neurological conditions. As visual field loss occurs frequently in neurological conditions, perimetry is commonly requested at eye clinics for patients with suspected or known diagnoses. There are currently no guidelines for how visual fields in neurological conditions should be assessed. There is a pressing need to identify reference standard visual field program for neurological conditions.

The aim of this study is to undertake a systematic review of the existing evidence base for perimetry in common neurological conditions. This will aid the design of future research and clinical practice guidelines. The primary objective is to determine the common patterns of visual field defects in chiasmal compression, idiopathic intracranial hypertension (IIH), stroke and optic neuropathy, and the secondary objective is to identify the common perimeters and visual field programmes used to investigate these conditions.

Methods

This review was registered with PROSPERO [Ref: CRD42017080742] [5].

Types of studies

The following types of studies were included in the review: randomised controlled trials, controlled trials, prospective and retrospective cohort studies, observational studies and case controlled studies. Case reports, editorials and letters were excluded. All languages were included and translations were obtained when necessary. Studies of participants reporting visual field loss relating to chiasmal compression, IIH, stroke and optic neuropathy were included. The search was limited to publications after 1990; this date restriction was chosen to coincide with the switch to the use of the Humphrey Field Analyser II-*i* Series which is still currently and commonly used within ophthalmology clinics.

Target conditions

Common neurological conditions of IIH, optic neuropathies, chiasmal compression and stroke were targeted [2].

In IIH, loss of visual function may occur at any stage [6]. Monitoring of visual fields is crucial in this population as visual loss can be insidious and asymptomatic for a considerable amount of time [7]. The frequency of subclinical visual loss underscores the need for thorough ophthalmological examination with perimetry [8].

Two common optic neuropathies include optic neuritis and anterior ischaemic optic neuropathy (AION), however there are many other optic neuropathy aetiologies [7]. Visual field loss in optic neuropathy is an important factor in diagnosis [9]. Within this review the following types of optic neuropathy were included: AION, non-arteritic anterior ischaemic optic neuropathy (NAION), optic neuritis, thyroid/Grave's, toxic and traumatic.

Visual field loss is a common mode of presentation for chiasmal compression. There is clinical significance to the detection of visual field loss in chiasmal compression and capturing peripheral loss is important to early diagnosis, which is essential to allow prompt neurosurgical intervention [10].

The prevalence of visual field loss following stroke has been reported in approximately one third of stroke survivors [11]. UK national guidelines recommend that every patient with stroke be examined for the presence of visual field loss [12]. Repeated perimetry in stroke-related visual field loss is important to track recovery [13].

Information sources and search strategy
A systematic strategy to search key electronic databases, including Cochrane registers and electronic bibliographic databases was used: Cochrane Stroke Group Trials Register, Cochrane Eyes and Vision Group Trials Register, Cochrane Central Register of Controlled Trials (CENTRAL), MEDLINE, EMBASE, CINAHL, AMED, PsycINFO, Dissertations & Theses (PQDT) database, British Nursing Index, PsycBITE (Psychological Database for Brain Impairment Treatment Efficacy), ClinicalTrials.gov, Current Controlled Trials, Trials Central, Health Service Research Projects in Progress, National Eye Institute Clinical Studies Database, Orthoptic Search Facility and Proceedings of Association for Research in Vision and Ophthalmology. Search terms are detailed in Table 1.

Selection process and quality assessment
The titles and abstracts identified from the search were independently screened by the two authors through each phase of the review (screening, eligibility and inclusion) using the pre-stated inclusion criteria. The full papers of any studies considered potentially relevant were considered and the selection criteria applied independently by two reviewers. We resolved disagreements at each step by discussion between the two review authors; all were solved in this manner without the need to seek the opinion of a third reviewer.

The data being extracted from the studies was not related to the study methodology, therefore quality assessment of the individual studies was not required.

Data extraction for included studies
A pre-designed data extraction form was used to gather information on sample size, study design, defect type, severity and location and choice of visual field program. The data was extracted and documented by one researcher (LH) and verified by another (FR).

Table 1 Search terms

OR	OR
AND	
Pituitary	Visual Fields
Pituitary adenoma	Vision Disorders
Craniopharyngioma	Vision
Pseudotumour cerebri	Visual field loss
Idiopathic intracranial hypertension	Visual field defect
Benign intracranial hypertension	Perimetry
Chiasm	Perimeter
Stroke	Visual field assessment
Cerebrovascular disorders	Humphrey™
Brain ischaemia	Octopus™
Intracranial Haemorrhage	
Optic neuropathy	
Anterior ischaemic optic neuropathy	
Multiple sclerosis	
Optic neuritis	
Demyelination	
Neuromyelitis optica	
Devic's disease	
Compressive neuropathy	
Toxic neuropathy	

™ Humphrey (Carl Zeiss AG, Germany), Octopus (Haag Streit International, Switzerland)

Results
The search results are outlined in Fig. 1. Three hundred and thirty studies were included. Fifty-one of the studies reported on IIH, 144 studies reported on optic neuropathy, 105 studies reported on chiasmal compression, 21 studies reported on stroke and 10 studies reported on a mixed neuro-ophthalmology population.

The most commonly used perimeters and programmes for IIH, optic neuropathy, chiasmal compression and stroke are outlined in Table 2.

All the reported patterns of visual field loss for IIH, optic neuropathy, chiasmal compression and stroke are outlined in Fig. 2.

For the purposes of identifying perimetry programs, papers which were clearly associated with the same study i.e. Idiopathic Intracranial Hypertension Treatment Trial (IIHTT)[23–27] and Optic Neuritis Treatment Trial (ONTT)[19, 28–40], the study was counted once as the same protocol applied to all papers.

Idiopathic intracranial hypertension
Perimetry choices
Of the 44 studies reporting visual field testing in IIH, the majority (n = 38) of studies reported using a Humphrey perimeter[8, 23, 41–76]. Of the studies which

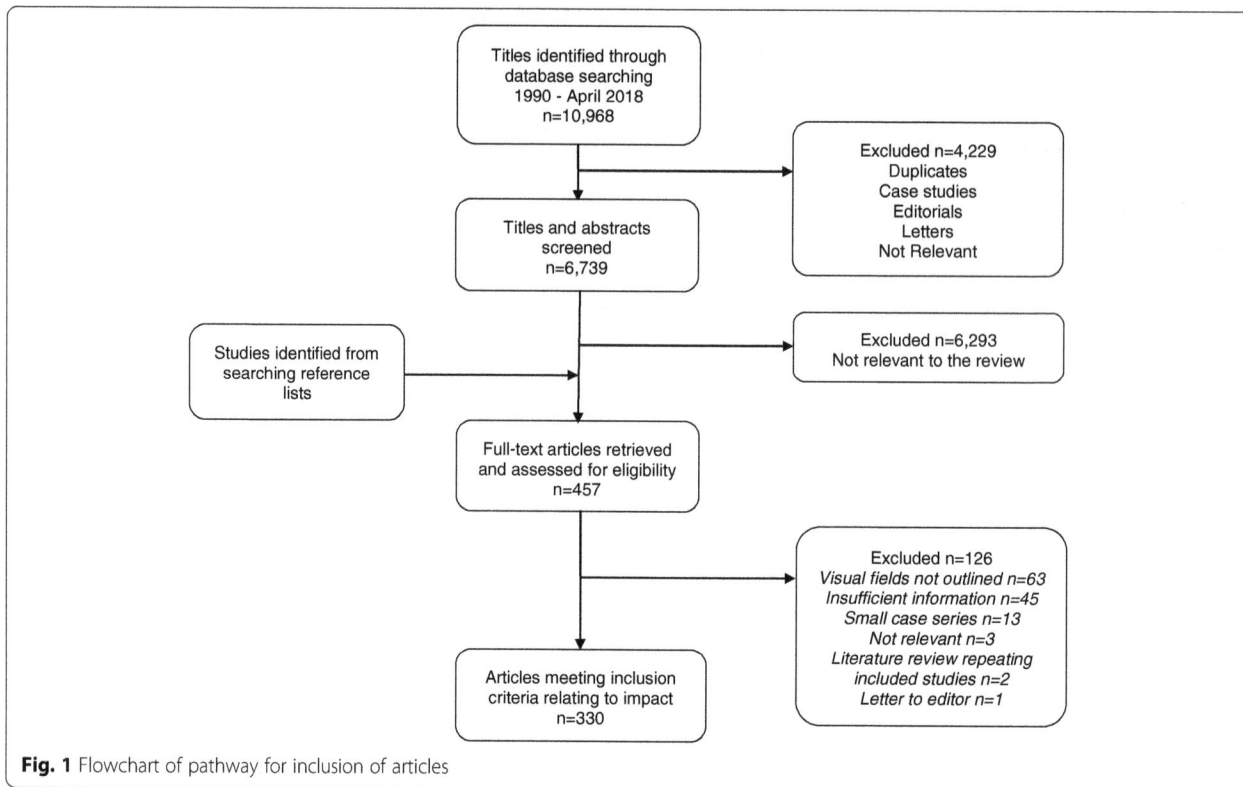

Fig. 1 Flowchart of pathway for inclusion of articles

reported the specific program there was an almost even split between the 30–2 ($n = 16$)[41–43, 47, 52, 60–62, 64–66, 71–73, 75, 76] and 24–2 ($n = 14$)[8, 23, 41, 43–46, 56, 57, 64, 67–69, 73] programs. The stategy used in these two programs was a mixture of full threshold[46], SITA Standard[23, 24, 52, 65–69, 72, 75] and SITA Fast[49, 60–62, 70]. The use of the Goldmann perimeter was reported by 22 studies[8, 43, 45, 46, 48, 50, 51, 53–55, 58, 59, 62, 63, 67, 72, 76–81] and the Octopus perimeter in six studies[59, 70, 76, 78–80]. The variety of specific programs used on the Octopus perimeter

Table 2 Number of most commonly reported perimeters and programmes used for the four neurological conditions of interest, including if more detail on programme was specified or not. ™ Humphrey (Zeiss Meditec, USA), Octopus (Haag Streit International, Switzerland)

n=		Neurological condition			
		Idiopathic intracranial hypertension	Optic Neuropathy	Chiasmal compression	Stroke
Perimeter used	Multiple	26	27	31	5
	Humphrey	38	86	60	11
		10 unspecified 28 specified	5 unspecified 81 specified	7 unspecified 51 specified	3 unspecified 8 specified
	Humphrey 30-2	16	46	20	4
		6 unspecified 10 specified	22 unspecified 24 specified	10 unspecified 10 specified	0 unspecified 4 specified
	Humphrey 24-2	14	39	22	5
		7 unspecified 7 specified	11 unspecified 28 specified	5 unspecified 17 specified	1 unspecified 4 specified
	Goldmann	22	31	41	8
		18 unspecified 4 specified	30 unspecified 1 specified	41 unspecified	7 unspecified 1 specified
	Octopus	6	9	9	1
		6 unspecified	1 unspecified 8 specified	2 unspecified 7 specified	1 unspecified

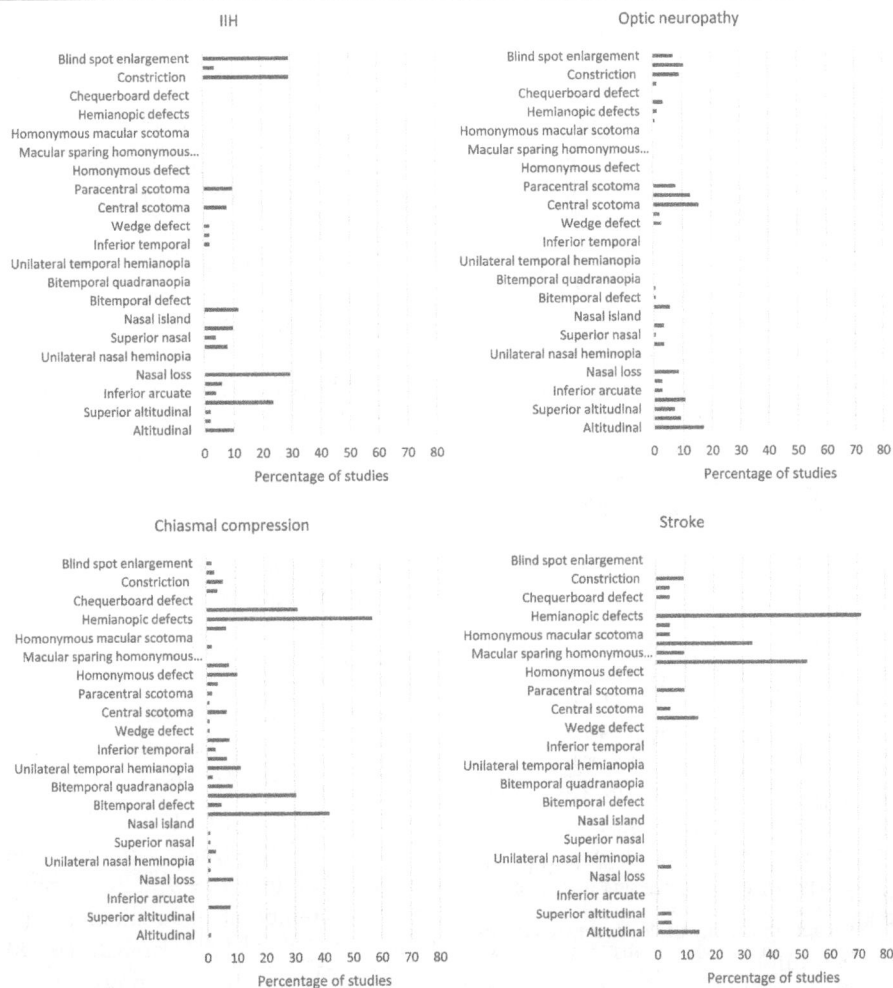

Fig. 2 Percentage of reported patterns of visual field loss in the four neurological conditions of interest

included 32 program[78], 24 program[78], 30 degree static[76], 90 degree static[79] and kinetic[70]. Twenty-six studies reported the use of multiple perimeters and/or programs[8, 41, 43–46, 48–51, 53–55, 58, 59, 62–64, 67, 70, 72, 73, 76, 78–80, 82], with two citing an indication such as poor vision or concentration[62, 72] for using an alternative and a further two changing perimeter or program at a set time point[76, 80].

A variety of other perimeters/perimetry included motion periemtry[41, 44], Tangent screen[43, 49], high pass resolution (Ophthimus)[44], Rarebit perimetry[82] and macro automated MP 30-2 [82].

Patterns of visual field loss

The most common patterns of visual field loss reported by the included studies were blind spot enlargement (n = 15)[41, 42, 47, 48, 53, 54, 58, 64, 77–81, 83, 84], constriction (n = 15)[8, 24, 42, 47–49, 53, 54, 58, 64, 76, 77, 80, 83, 84], nasal loss (n = 15)[8, 41, 42, 47–49, 53, 54, 58, 64, 76, 81, 83–85] and arcuate defects (n = 12)[8, 24, 41, 48,

53, 54, 58, 64, 76, 80, 84, 85]. Other patterns of loss reported included altitudinal (n = 5)[41, 42, 53, 54, 64], nasal step (n = 5)[8, 48, 49, 64, 85], paracentral scotoma (n = 5)[8, 48, 54, 64, 74], temporal loss (n = 5)[42, 53, 64, 81, 83] and central scotoma (n = 4)[41, 54, 64, 74].

Optic neuropathy
Perimetry choices

Of the 129 studies reporting visual field testing in optic neuropathy, the majority (n = 86) of studies used a Humphrey perimeter[32, 86–170]. Of the studies which reported the specific program the majority used the 30–2 program (n = 46)[32, 86–88, 94–97, 106–120, 127–149] compared to the 24–2 program (n = 39)[89–91, 98–102, 111, 117, 119, 121–126, 135, 139, 150–168, 170]. The stategy used in these two programs was a mixture of full threshold[39, 88, 97, 100, 101, 113–115, 121, 136], STATPAC[116], SITA Standard[100, 119, 120, 125, 126, 141–147, 154, 157–168], SITA Fast[148, 149, 169] and short wavelength automated perimetry (SWAP)[97, 128]. The use of the Goldmann perimeter was reported by 31 studies[9, 32, 92, 93, 98, 100, 103–105, 108, 130, 171–190]. The Octopus perimeter was reported in nine studies[178, 179, 191–197], and a variety of specific programs were reported; 32 program[179], 24 program[192], 07 program[191], G program[178, 197], 30°[193, 195], 60°[195], 90°[196] static and kinetic/semi-kinetic[194]. Twenty-eight studies reported the use of multiple perimeters and/or programs[32, 87, 92, 93, 97, 98, 100, 103–105, 108, 111, 117, 119, 128, 130, 135, 139, 175, 177–180, 185, 194, 195, 198]; two cited indications of poor vision[194] or concentration[178] for using an alternative.

A variety of other perimeters/perimetry were reported; motion perimetry, Tangent screen[179], high pass resolution (Ophthimus) [199, 200], 4–28° program [201], frequency doubling perimetry[178] including the C-20[87] and N-30[97] programs, Bjerrum screen[202, 203], Tuebingen perimeter 30° static[194, 204] and manual[194], Metrovision 30° static[205] and Amsler grid[175, 180, 185].

Patterns of visual field loss

The most common patterns of visual field loss reported by the included studies were altitudinal ($n = 24$)[9, 28, 98, 99, 103, 109, 122, 124, 126, 154, 155, 160, 168, 171, 174, 178, 180, 186, 187, 194, 206–209], central scotoma ($n = 22$)[9, 28, 93, 99, 103, 118, 127, 168, 171, 174, 178, 180, 186, 187, 190, 194, 203, 206, 208–211], cecocentral scotoma ($n = 18$)[9, 28, 93, 109, 116, 118, 122, 127, 155, 168, 178, 180, 194, 206, 209, 210], arcuate ($n = 15$)[9, 28, 93, 98, 99, 109, 126, 154, 155, 171, 178, 181, 203, 206, 208] and diffuse depression (n = 15)[28, 99, 109, 118, 122, 154–156, 160, 168, 178, 180, 194, 199, 207]. Other patterns of loss reported included constriction ($n = 13$)[9, 37, 93, 98, 103, 152, 155, 168, 171, 180, 186, 203, 210], blind spot enlargement ($n = 10$)[9, 37, 93, 109, 171, 178, 181, 194, 208], nasal step ($n = 5$)[9, 28, 93, 98, 109], quadrant defect ($n = 5$)[34, 93, 152, 168, 206] and wedge defect ($n = 4$)[9, 109, 194, 203].

Chiasmal compression
Perimetry choices

Of the 105 studies reporting visual field testing in chiasmal compression, the majority ($n = 58$) of studies used a Humphrey perimeter[10, 13, 212–267]. Of the studies which reported the specific program the majority used the 24–2 program ($n = 22$)[213, 214, 216, 217, 221, 224–226, 231–242, 250, 268] compared to the 30–2 program ($n = 20$)[10, 212, 216, 220–223, 229, 230, 245–255]. The strategy used in these two programs was a mixture of full threshold[213, 223, 225, 232–234, 248–252], STATPAC[214], FASTPAC[226], SITA Standard[232, 237, 239–242, 254, 258–267], SITA Fast[255, 268] and SWAP[230]. Another program reported for the Humphrey perimeter was the 10–2 program[224]. The use of the Goldmann perimeter was reported by 41 studies[214, 215, 218–220, 225, 227, 232, 244, 266, 269–299]. The Octopus perimeter was reported in nine studies[10, 244, 247, 269, 288, 294, 295, 300, 301]; a variety of specific programs were

reported including 32 program[300], 24 program[300], 30° static[295, 301] and kinetic/semi-kinetic[10]. Thirty-one studies reported the use of multiple perimeters and/or programs[10, 214–216, 218–221, 224, 225, 227, 230, 232, 238, 244, 247, 250, 253, 266, 269–271, 273, 288, 292, 294, 295, 300, 302–304]; four cited indications of poor vision[304], concentration[273], symptoms[224] or diagnosis[221] for using an alternative.

A variety of other perimeters/perimetry were reported; Bjerrum screen[218], camprimetry[294, 295], frequency doubling perimetry[232], C-20[221, 238] and 20–1[238], high pass resolution 30° (Ophthimus)[214, 303], Metrovision kinetic[305], Metrovision STAT 95 30°[306], motion perimetry, Rarebit perimetry 24°[303], Tangent screen[271], Topcon perimter[273], Tuebingen perimeter 30°[307, 308] and Vision monitor 30°[270].

Patterns of visual field loss

The most common patterns of visual field loss reported by the included studies were bitemporal hemianopia ($n = 32$)[213, 217, 218, 223, 224, 226, 229, 238, 239, 243, 246, 248, 255, 258, 261, 273, 275, 276, 279, 285, 286, 289, 291, 297, 299, 304, 305, 309–313], other temporal loss ($n = 21$)[215, 217, 218, 229, 238, 245, 250, 253, 255, 256, 258, 261, 269, 271, 274, 279, 294, 302, 305, 312, 313] and unilateral temporal hemianopia ($n = 12$)[217, 218, 220, 246, 258, 279, 280, 289, 291, 309–311]. Other patterns of loss reported included nasal loss ($n = 9$)[214, 215, 217, 255, 256, 274, 279, 302, 314], bitemporal quadrantanopia ($n = 9$)[229, 253, 275, 279, 285, 289, 309, 310, 313], arcuate ($n = 8$)[214, 215, 217, 256, 274, 275, 311, 312], homonymous hemianopia (n = 8)[218, 224, 255, 258, 279, 291, 302, 313], central scotoma ($n = 7$)[218, 224, 246, 256, 274, 302, 313], three-quadrant loss ($n = 7$)[223, 254, 258, 273, 285, 293, 311], unilateral temporal quadrantanopia ($n = 7$)[217, 258, 289, 309–312] and constriction ($n = 6$)[214, 215, 218, 274, 296, 302].

Stroke
Perimetry choices

Of the 21 studies reporting visual field testing in stroke, the majority ($n = 11$) of studies reported using a Humphrey perimeter[21, 315–325]. Of the studies which reported the specific program there was an almost even split between the 24–2 program ($n = 5$)[318–321, 323] and the 30–2 program ($n = 4$)[21, 319, 320, 324]. The strategy used in these two programs was a mixture of full threshold[318–320], SITA Standard[319–321] and SITA Fast[319, 320, 324]. Other programs used on the Humphrey perimeter were the 10–2[323], 76 supra-threshold screening[315], full field 120[318] and Esterman[318] programs. Ten studies reported the use of multiple perimeters and/or programs[21, 316–319, 321–323, 325, 326], with two changing perimetry/program at a set time point[319, 320].

The use of the Goldmann perimeter was reported by eight studies[21, 316, 317, 319, 322, 325, 327, 328] and the Octopus perimeter by two studies[325, 329].

A variety of other perimeters/perimetry were reported; Competer 750[330], Humphrey Matrix ZEST[321], ShP-31[331], Peritest semi-automated[326] and Tangent screen[322, 332].

Patterns of visual field loss

The most common patterns of visual field loss reported by the included studies were homonymous hemianopia ($n = 11$)[317–320, 322, 324–327, 333, 334] and homonymous quadrantanopia ($n = 7$)[318, 322, 324–327, 334]. Other patterns of loss were reported including altitudinal[322, 325, 334], temporal crescent[319, 325, 331] ($n = 3$), constriction[325, 331], paracentral scotoma[329, 331] ($n = 2$), binasal heminaopia[325], central scotoma[331], chequerboard loss[325], homonymous macular scotoma[327], unilateral blindness[325], 3-quadrant loss[325] ($n = 1$).

Mixed neuro-ophthalmology population
Perimetry choices

Of the 10 studies reporting visual field testing in mixed neuro-ophthalmology populations, the majority ($n = 9$) of studies reported using a Humphrey perimeter[4, 335–342]. Of the studies which reported the specific program there was an even split between the 30–2 program ($n = 5$)[335–337, 339, 340] and the 24–2 program ($n = 5$)[337–339, 341, 342]. The strategy used these two programs was a mixture of full threshold[337, 339], FASTPAC[337], SITA Standard[339, 340], SITA Fast[4, 339] and SWAP[336]. Other programs used on the Humphrey perimeter were the peripheral 68 and full field 120 programs[335].

The use of the Goldmann perimeter was reported by five studies[4, 335, 337–339], and the Octopus perimeter by three studies[335, 337, 338]. The variety of specific programs used on the Octopus perimeter included 32 program[335, 337], 07 program[335], G program[337] and TOP program[338].

A variety of other perimeters/perimetry were reported; frequency doubling perimetry[4, 337], high pass resolution (Ophthimus)[337] and Humphrey Matrix 30–2[340].

The super-scripted references included in this meta-analysis are listed in full in Additional file 1.

Discussion

Across all four neurological conditions a wide variety of perimeters and perimetry programs are being used. It is clear from these findings that there is no standardisation for assessment of visual fields for the neurological conditions (IIH, optic neuropathy, chiasmal compression and stroke) at the focus of this review.

The majority of studies reported using the Humphrey perimeter. The Humphrey II-i Series mainly performs static perimetry programs, both central and peripheral. Kinetic perimetry was available on the 750i model and was optional on 740i and 745i models [14]. The most commonly used static perimetry programs were the 30–2 and 24–2. Both these programs assess the central portion of the visual field. The 30–2 program assesses a grid of 76 points over the central 30° of the visual field. The 24–2 program has limitations in that its assessment of visual field is restricted on superior, inferior and temporal sides to 24° with an extension to 27° nasally, assessing a total grid of 54 points [1]. As a result, it can miss visual field loss outside these extremities leading to poor diagnostic accuracy in certain conditions [10, 15]. Although static automated perimetry has been shown to be adequate in neuro-ophthalmology practice, kinetic perimetry is useful for patients with severe visual and neurological deficits and patients with peripheral visual field defects [16, 17].

The second most commonly reported perimeter was the Goldmann perimeter, used in 100 of the included studies. The Goldmann perimeter is primarily used to perform manual kinetic perimetry [1]. In addition to the use of the Goldmann perimeter, a number of studies reported using semi-kinetic/kinetic perimetry using the Octopus 900 perimeter. The Octopus 900 perimeter was the replacement for the Goldmann perimeter when Goldmann production ceased in 2007. The Octopus 900 is capable of performing both kinetic and static perimetry programs. Kinetic perimetry programs can be pre-set and run as an automatic program or performed manually in the equivalent way as Goldmann kinetic perimetry. A comparison of kinetic perimetry using Goldmann and Octopus perimeters, found strong agreement in detecting the presence of all visual field defects for type and location of defect between the two instruments [17].

Comparative studies have contrasted different combinations of static and kinetic perimetry in single and mixed neuro-ophthalmic conditions. Szatmáry and colleagues compared the Humphrey SITA Fast 24–2 program to Goldmann manual perimetry in a mixed neuro-ophthalmic population, with similar defects found on both tests in 61.5% [18]. The authors concluded for central defects the SITA Fast program may be useful but the development of program extending further into the peripheral visual field would be more appropriate for neuro-ophthalmology [18]. Rowe and colleagues compared a Humphrey peripheral static screening program (full field 120) to an Octopus peripheral kinetic strategy in a mixed neuro-ophthalmology population [16]. A match for normal or abnormal visual field results was reported for 87% of the cases. The authors concluded that although the full field 120 was useful for detection of visual field defects, Octopus kinetic perimetry was advantageous providing added information of defect depth and size plus a more representative view of the visual field defect [16]. Keltner and colleagues compared central (30–2 program) and peripheral (manual kinetic) perimetry in optic neuritis, they reported a greater number of visual field defects were within the central area (97.1%) compared to the peripheral area (69.9%) at baseline [19]. The authors concluded in the majority of cases optic neuritis could be monitored using a central program, but in more severe cases peripheral perimetry would be required [19]. Rowe et al. compared the Humphrey 30–2 and 24–2 programs and Octopus semi-automated kinetic perimetry in a population with pituitary disease, they reported kinetic perimetry to be the favoured option when available and recommends the 30–2 over the 24–2 program in this population [10]. Wong and colleagues compared the Goldmann perimeter (manual kinetic), Humphrey perimeter (30–2 program) and tangent screen (manual kinetic) for the detection and localisation of occipital lesions [20]. The detection of visual field defects was achieved by all three techniques, however the Humphrey 30–2 program failed to be in agreement in 33% of cases in terms of localisation. This study also reported the 10–2 program detection of macular sparing was in agreement with that of the manual kinetic perimetry. The authors concluded all were suitable for screening, however more information was provided by kinetic perimetry [20]. Pineles and colleagues compared an automated combined static and kinetic program using an Octopus perimeter to standard static (24–2 or 30–2 programs) or Goldmann manual perimetry in a mixed neuro-ophthalmic population, 86% of visual field defects matched [21]. The authors argued that the combination of both static and kinetic perimetry overcome the limitations the individual types of perimetry [21]. These comparative studies have highlighted there are advantages and disadvantages within the range of available perimetry options.

The most commonly reported patterns of visual field defect for IIH included arcuate (predominantly superiorly), constriction and blind-spot enlargement.The patterns of visual field defect most commonly reported in cases of optic neuropathy are the most diverse of the four conditions; these were altitudinal defects, central, cecocentral and paracentral scotomas, diffuse depression, arcuate defects and constriction. The most commonly reported patterns of visual field defect for chiasmal compression included hemianopic and quadrantanopic defects, predominantly to the temporal side. In the case of stroke, the most commonly reported patterns of visual field defect were homonymous hemianopic and quadrantanopic defects.

With the exception of optic neuropathy and IIH, the majority of patterns of visual field defects reported are peripheral defects. The 30–2 program and equivalents detect the presence of central defects however, do not show peripheral defects so cannot display the full extent of the visual field loss and may not detect visual field loss until it is further advanced such that it also affects the central field.

A limitation of this review was the restriction of targeting four common neurological conditions which cause visual field loss. Furthermore the types of optic neuropathy were also limited. It is therefore not inclusive of all neurological conditions.

Conclusion

The common perimeter programs and the common patterns of visual field defect and for IIH, optic neuropathy, chiasmal compression and stroke have been reported. Both the 30–2 and 24–2 program using the Humphrey perimeter are most commonly reported followed by manual kinetic perimetry using the Goldmann perimeter across all four conditions included in this review. The patterns of visual field defects reported differ much more greatly across the four conditions. In IIH, blind spot enlargement, constriction, nasal loss and arcuate defects were most commonly reported. In optic neuropathy, altitudinal defects, arcuate defects, diffuse depression, central and cecocentral scotomas were most commonly reported. In chiasmal compression, the most commonly reported were bitemporal hemianopia, unilateral temporal hemiaopia and other temporal defects. In stroke, homonymous hemianopia and quadrantaopia were the most commonly reported defects.

It is apparent that the 24–2 perimetry strategy is used extensively for visual field assessment in neurological conditions but with little supporting evidence for its diagnostic accuracy in these particularly where visual field loss may affect the peripheral visual field first and may not impact the central visual field until later in the progression, if at all. It is important now to research this topic further in order to reach consensus on how best to standardise perimetry for neurological conditions.

Abbreviations
AION: Anterior ischaemic optic neuropathy; IIH: Idiopathic intercranial hypertension; NAION: Non-arteritic anterior ischaemic optic neuropathy

Acknowledgements
We acknowledge the funding support for this research from the Liverpool Clinical Commissioning Group.

Funding
This systematic review was funded by Liverpool CCG RCF 2017/148093. The funding organisation had no role in the design or conduct of this research.

Authors' contributions
FR was involved in the conception and design of the study. Data collection was carried out by FR and LH. Both authors were involved in analysis and interpretation of the data. Both authors helped to draft the manuscript, and both read and approved the final manuscript.

Competing interests
The authors declare that they have no competing interests.

References
1. Rowe FJ. Visual fields via the visual pathway, 2nd edition edn. Boca Raton: CRC Press; 2016.
2. Johnson CA, Keltner JL. Incidence of visual field loss in 20,000 eyes and its relationship to driving performance. Arch Ophthalmol. 1983;101:371–5.
3. National Institute for for Health and Clinical Excellence. Glaucoma: Diagnosis and management of chronic open angle glaucoma and ocular Hypertension. London: National Collaborating Centre for Acute Care at The Royal College of Surgeons of England; 2009.
4. Kedar S, Ghate D, Corbett JJ. Visual fields in neuro-ophthalmology. Indian J Ophthalmol. 2011;59(2):103–9.
5. Moher D, Liberati A, Tetzlaff J, Altman DG. Preferred reporting items for systematic reviews and meta-analyses: the PRISMA statement. PLoS Med. 2009;6(7). https://doi.org/10.1371/journal.pmed.1000097.
6. Corbett JJ, Savino PJ, Thompson S, Kansu T, Schatz NJ, Orr LS, Hopson D. Visual loss in pseudotumour cerebri. Arch Neurol. 1982;39:461–74.
7. Pane A, Burdon M, Miller NR. The neuro-ophthalmology survival guide. Edinburgh: Mosby Elsevier; 2007.
8. Rowe FJ, Sarkies NJ. Assessment of visual function in idiopathic intracranial hypertension: a prospective study. Eye. 1998;12:111–8.
9. Hayreh SS, Zimmerman B. Visual field abnormalities in nonarteritic anterior ischemic optic neuropathy their pattern and prevalence at initial examination. Arch Ophthalmol. 2005;123:1554–62.
10. Rowe FJ, Chenye CP, Garcia-Fiñana M, Noonan C, Howard C, Smith J, Adeoye J. Detection of visual field loss in pituatary disease: peripheral kinetic versus central static. Neuro-Ophthalmology. 2015;39(3):116–24.
11. Rowe F, Hepworth L, Hanna K, Howard C. Point prevalence of visual impairment following stroke. Int J Stroke. 2016;11(Suppl 4):7.
12. Intercollegiate Stroke Working Party. National clinical guideline for stroke. 5th ed. London: Royal College of Physicians; 2016.
13. Jones SA, Shinton RA. Improving outcome in stroke patients with visual problems. Age Ageing. 2006;35(6):560–5.
14. Humphrey Field Analyzer - HFA II-i Series: Technical data. www.zeiss.com/meditec/int/products/ophthalmology-optometry/glaucoma/diagnostics/perimetry/humphrey-hfa-ii-i.html#technical-data. Accessed 4 Sept 2018.
15. Khoury JM, Donahue SP, Lavin PJM, Tsai JC. Comparison of 24-2 and 30-2 perimetry in glaucomatous and non-glaucomatous optic neuropathies. J Neuroophthalmol. 1999;19(2):100–8.
16. Rowe FJ, Noonan CP, Manuel M. Comparison of Octopus semi-automated kinetic perimetry and Humphrey peripheral static perimetry in neuro-ophthalmic cases. ISRN Ophthalmol. 2013:753202. https://doi.org/10.1155/2013/753202.
17. Rowe FJ, Rowlands A. Comparison of diagnostic accuracy between Octopus 900 and Goldmann kinetic visual fields. Biomed Res Int. 2014:214829. https://doi.org/10.1155/2014/214829.
18. Szatmáry G, Biousse V, Newman NJ. Can Swedish Intractive thresholding algorithm fast perimetry be used as an alternative to Goldmann perimetry in neuro-ophthalmic practice? Arch Ophthalmol. 2002;120(9):1162–73.
19. Keltner JL, Johnson CA, Spurr JO, Beck RW. Comparison of central and peripheral visual field properties in the optic neuritis treatment trial. Am J Ophthalmol. 1999;128(5):543–53.
20. Wong AM, Sharpe JA. A comparison of tangent screen, goldmann, and Humphrey perimetry in the detection and localization of occipital lesions. Ophthalmology. 2000;107(3):527–44.
21. Pineles SL, Volpe NJ, Miller-Ellis E, Galetta SL, Sankar PS, Shindler KS, Maguire MG. Automated combined kinetic and static perimetry: an alternative to standard perimetry in patients with neuro-ophthalmic disease and glaucoma. Arch Ophthalmol. 2006;124:363–9.

25

Outcomes and costs of Ranibizumab and Aflibercept treatment in a health-service research context

Martin K. Schmid[1,2], Oliver Reich[3], Eva Blozik[3], Livia Faes[2], Nicolas S. Bodmer[4], Silvan Locher[2], Michael A. Thiel[1,2], Roland Rapold[3], Maximilian Kuhn[5] and Lucas M. Bachmann[1,4*]

Abstract

Background: To compare anti-VEGF treatments for macular disease in terms of costs and clinical outcomes.

Methods: We identified patients suffering from macular disease and treated either with aflibercept, ranibizumab or both at the largest public eye clinic in Switzerland between January 1st and December 31st 2016 who were insured in one of the two participating health insurance companies. Clinical data were extracted from the electronic health record system. The health insurers provided the health claim costs for the ophthalmologic care and the total health care costs of each patient in the observation period. Using multivariate regression models, we assessed the monthly ophthalmologic and the monthly total costs of patients with no history of switching (ranibizumab vs. aflibercept), patients with a history of switching from ranibizumab to aflibercept, patients switching during the observation period and a miscellaneous group. We examined baseline differences in age, proportion of males, visual acuity (letters), central retinal thickness (CRT) and treatment history before entering the study. We investigated treatment intensity and compared the changes in letters and CRT.

Results: The analysis involved 488 eyes (361 patients), 182 on ranibizumab treatment, and 63 on aflibercept treatment, 160 eyes with a history of switching from ranibizumab to aflibercept, and 45 switchers during follow-up and 38 eyes of the miscellaneous group. Compared to ranibizumab, monthly costs of ophthalmologic treatment were slightly higher for aflibercept treatment + 175.0 CHF (95%CI: 1.5 CHF to 348.3 CHF; $p = 0.048$) as were the total monthly costs + 581.0 CHF (95%CI: 159.5 CHF to 1002.4 CHF; $p = 0.007$). Compared to ranibizumab, the monthly treatment intensity with aflibercept was similar (+ 0.057 injections/month (95%CI -0.023 to 0.137; $p = 0.162$), corresponding to a projected annual number of 5.4 injections for ranibizumab vs. 6.1 injections for aflibercept. During follow-up, visus dropped by 0.7 letters with ranibizumab and increased by 0.6 letters with aflibercept ($p = 0.243$). CRT dropped by − 14.9 μm with ranibizumab and by − 19.5 μm with aflibercept ($p = 0.708$). The monthly costs of all other groups examined were higher.

Conclusion: These real-life data show that aflibercept treatment is equally expensive, and clinical outcomes between the two drugs are similar.

Keywords: Claims data, Health insurance, Cost analysis, Macular degeneration, Aflibercept, Ranibizumab

* Correspondence: bachmann@medignition.ch
[1]University of Zurich, Zurich, Switzerland
[4]Medignition Inc. Research Consultants, Verena Conzett-Strasse 9, P.O. 9628, 8036 Zurich, CH, Switzerland
Full list of author information is available at the end of the article

Background

Two years ago, we published a study comparing the reimbursed treatment costs and clinical outcomes of ranibizumab and aflibercept in the treatment of macular conditions in Switzerland, when adjusting for patients' characteristics and clinical status [1]. We found that the two anti-VEGF medications do not differ in clinical outcomes, injection frequency and costs. Differences in costs could be explained by the underlying clinical condition. Also, patients' characteristics and duration of medication were associated with the variability in cost. The study also showed that aflibercept and ranibizumab were used in a similar fashion in Switzerland when applying the same treatment scheme, which was unexpected in view of the fact that aflibercept was assumed to require less injections. Consequently the total health care expenditures for both these anti-VEGF agents [2] were comparable.

A major drawback of our study was the low number of patients receiving aflibercept overall and de novo. Consequently, the comparison between the two drugs lacked precision and robustness. To verify our initial findings we decided to repeat and expand the analysis by adding the health claims data of a second, large health insurance company. By interconnecting health care data with clinical data, we expected to find a solid depiction of the actual status quo in the real-life treatment of patients. In this study, we compared the reimbursed costs and clinical follow-up of ranibizumab and aflibercept treatment considering differences in patients' characteristics and clinical status in the analysis.

Methods

This study received Ethics approval from the Ethics Commission for North-East and Central Switzerland (EKNZ 2014–110 Amendment) and adhered to the Declaration of Helsinki and the principles of good clinical practice [3].

Clinical visits

All patients followed an optical coherence tomography (OCT) guided pro re nata [4] treatment pattern. Accordingly, patients were seen on a monthly basis at the hospital's retinal service. A fundoscopy, visual acuity (ETDRS) and OCT scanning (Spectralis, Heidelberg Engineering GmbH, 69,121 Heidelberg, Germany) was performed at each visit. The final decision for an injection was based on intra or subretinal fluid found in the OCT and an injection was made on the same day. Patients missing a follow-up visit were approached by the clinic to settle a new visit date. The clinical data were entered into the clinic's electronic health record system (EHRS).

Patient identification and matching

Patients with a Helsana or a CSS health insurance in the year 2016 who received either ranibizumab or aflibercept at the eye clinic were considered. From the electronic health record system, we obtained all available clinical data of these patients, also the data of previous years. On the other hand, Helsana and CSS provided the corresponding health care claims data of these patients for the same observation period. The databases were matched into one analysis file. We checked the quality of matching by comparing the health claims of the hospital's system and the health insurer's database. If the entries were inconsistent, we matched the clinical recordings of a specific visit to the entry date of the corresponding health claim, if the discrepancy between the two dates was less than 30 days. The data management adhered to the current data protection protocols and the requirements of the Ethics committee. Patient information was anonymized and de-identified prior to analysis.

Clinical data

The target condition, gender and age, the visual acuity and retinal thickness (CRT) at study entry, the number of IVI per treatment, the visual outcome and the central retinal thickness (CRT) at the last visit of follow-up was well as vital status were secured. The medical history prior to the observation period in terms of treatment duration, number of injections and treatment changes were also extracted. The data for these parameters were complete. We used the data of both eyes if a patient had a binocular condition. The minimum follow-up period was 1 month.

Outcomes

The outcome parameter total costs comprised the total of health care claims of 2016 in the numerator and number of months of follow-up in the denominator. This outcome was chosen to study global treatment effects within the various clinical groups. Costs for ophthalmologic treatment included all health care claims of the eye clinic that could be directly attributed to the anti-VEGF management in the numerator and duration of follow-up (months) in the denominator.

Statistical analysis

Continuous variates were summarised with means, standard deviations and ranges and dichotomous variates were summarised with percentages. In univariate analyses, the association between clinical parameters and costs were examined. Between groups comparisons of continuous variates were made using the parametric t-test. Dichotomous variates were compared using the non-parametric chi-square test. Cost per month was computed by dividing the sum of costs (total or for eye treatment) with the number of month in the follow-up. These costs parameters were used throughout the analyses.

Statistical modelling was made on the level of eyes rather than patients. Normality of the error distribution was confirmed visually and statistically using the Anderson-Darling test. In separate multivariate linear regression models we compared global costs/month and ophthalmologic costs/month (dependent variables) between different patient-groups using four indicator variables for five therapies (only ranibizumab, only aflibercept, switchers from ranibizumab to aflibercept prior to the observation period, switchers to aflibercept during the observation period and a miscellaneous group) (independent variates). We adjusted for differences in the duration of treatment prior to study entry, patients' age and female gender as well as for visual acuity at study entry and the CRT. We repeated these analyses for the subgroup of patients with diabetic macular edema. Statistical analyses were performed using the Stata 14.2 statistics software package. (StataCorp. 2015. Stata Statistical Software: Release 14. College Station, TX: StataCorp LP.)

Results
Patients' characteristics
The analysis involved 488 eyes (361 patients), 182 eyes on ranibizumab treatment, and 63 eyes on aflibercept treatment, 160 eyes with a history of switching from ranibizumab to aflibercept prior to study entry, 45 switchers during follow-up and 38 eyes of the miscellaneous group including 13 patients with a double switch (ranibizumab, aflibercept, ranibizumab) before entering the study. Median follow-up period was 11 months (Interquartile range 11 to 12 months), mean age was 78.2 years (standard deviation (SD) 9.5), and 61.8% of all patients were female. In the ranibizumab group, 21 eyes (11.5%), and in the aflibercept group 8 eyes (12.7%) had a diabetic macular edema (DME) ($p = 0.806$). Among switchers prior to study entry (15.6%) and during the observation period (17.8%) the proportion of DME was similar. The miscellaneous group had the highest proportion of DME (18.4%).

At study entry, mean visus in letters was 65.3 letters (SD 24.0) and CRT was 318.5 (SD 106.6). Compared to ranibizumab, patients receiving aflibercept were significantly younger (75.1 years vs. 80.0, $p < 0.001$), and were more often male (46.0% vs. 34.6%, $p = 0.107$). They had a slightly better visus (69.4 letters vs. 64.7 letters, $p = 0.159$) and had a higher CRT (361.2 μm vs. 314.3 μm, $p = 0.006$) at study entry. Anti-VEGF treatment was initiated in 60 eyes during the observation period. Of them, 38 eyes (18.4%) started with ranibizumab and 22 eyes (9.3%) started with aflibercept ($p = 0.005$). the salient patient characteristics is shown in Table 1.

Assessment of costs
Compared to ranibizumab ($n = 182$ eyes), monthly costs of ophthalmologic treatment were slightly higher for aflibercept ($n = 63$ eyes) treatment + 175.0 CHF (95%CI: 1.5 CHF to 348.3 CHF; $p = 0.048$) as were the total monthly costs + 581.0 CHF (95%CI: 159.5 CHF to 1002.4 CHF; $p = 0.007$). When excluding patients with DME from this analysis, the monthly costs of ophthalmologic treatment were almost identical (+ 54.6 (95% CI: -118.1 CHF to 227.14 CHF; $p = 0.534$), while the total monthly cost remained slightly higher in the aflibercept ($n = 55$ eyes) group (+ 574.2 CHF (95% CI: 164.6 to 983.8; $p = 0.006$) compared to the ranibizumab group ($n = 161$ eyes). Irrespective of treatment, patients with DME had slightly, albeit not significantly higher, mean monthly costs for ophthalmologic (1284 CHF vs. 1224 CHF; $p = 0.483$) and mean total monthly costs (2412 CHF vs. 2321 CHF; $p = 0.642$). There was no interaction between treatment (ranibizumab or aflibercept) and presence of DME in respect to mean monthly ophthalmologic ($p = 0.576$) and mean monthly total costs ($p = 0.386$).

Frequency of treatment and clinical follow-up
Compared to ranibizumab, the monthly treatment intensity with aflibercept was similar (+ 0.057 injections/month (95%CI -0.023 to 0.137; $p = 0.162$), corresponding to a projected annual number of 5.4 injections for ranibizumab vs. 6.1 injections for aflibercept. When excluding patients with DME the monthly injection frequency was almost identical (+ 0.02 injections/month (95% CI: -0.06 0.10; $p = 0.619$).

During follow-up, visus dropped by 0.7 letters with ranibizumab and increased by 0.6 letters with aflibercept ($p = 0.243$). CRT dropped by – 14.9 μm with ranibizumab and by – 19.5 μm with aflibercept ($p = 0.708$).

Patients switching from ranibizumab to aflibercept
Compared to ranibizumab, ophthalmologic and total monthly costs of those switching from ranibizumab to aflibercept prior to study entry were significantly higher (+ 362.8 CHF (95CI: 204.9 CHF to 520.63 CHF; $p < 0.001$) and 443.2 CHF (95%CI; 70.8 CHF to 815.6 CHF; $p = 0.020$). Similarly, the ophthalmologic costs of those switching from ranibizumab to aflibercept during the observation period were + 269.0 CHF (95%CI: 61.7 CHF to 476.2 CHF; $p = 0.011$), but total monthly costs were slightly albeit not significantly higher (+ 378.8 CHF (95%CI: -110.1 CHF to 867.7; $p = 0.129$). The higher ophthalmologic costs were due to the higher treatment intensity compared to ranibizumab (+ 0.14 injections/month (95% CI: 0.06 to 0.22; $p < 0.001$) and + 0.16 injections/months (95%CI: 0.08 to 0.24; $p < 0.001$), corresponding to a mean of 6.5 injections and 7.4 injections per year, respectively.

Table 1 Shows the distribution of salient clinical characteristics of the different treatment groups at study entry

Therapy	# Eyes (patients)	Age (sd[a])	Male (%)	Visus (sd[a])	CRT (sd[a])	DME (%)	CRVO (%)	Mean # IVI before	Treatment duration prior study [months]
Only ranibizumab	182 (144)	80.0 (8.9)	63 (34.6)	64.7 (23.7)	314.3 (100.3)	21 (11.5)	7 (3.8)	8.7	19.5
Only aflibercept	63 (52)	75.1 (9.4)	29 (46.0)	69.4 (18.8)	361.2 (152.3)	8 (12.7)	6 (9.5)	4.7	7.9
p-values		< 0.001	0.107	0.159	0.006	0.806	0.083	0.002	< 0.001
Switching from ranibizumab to aflibercept prior study	160 (128)	77.4 (10.2)	66 (41.3)	65.8 (25.4)	304.0 (86.7)	25 (15.6)	7 (4.4)	27.4	51.3
Switching from ranibizumab to aflibercept during study	45 (36)	76.8 (8.7)	19 (42.2)	66.7 (23.8)	323.2 (93.9)	8 (17.8)	6 (13.3)	9.9	19.1
Miscellaneous[b]	38 (34)	78.9 (8.5)	10 (26.3)	57.2 (26.7)	302.7 (64.3)	7 (18.4)	2 (5.3)	31.8	63.5

[a]sd = standard deviation
[b]including eyes with various treatment regimens. The largest group consisted of 13 eyes with a double switch from ranibizumab to aflibercept and back to ranibizumab prior to study entry

Miscellaneous group

In terms of treatment history, this was a heterogeneous group. The largest subgroup consisted of 13 eyes with a double switch (ranibizumab – aflibercept – ranibizumab) before entering the study. These patients were older (mean age 81.9 years (Range 75 to 94 years), had a lower visus (mean 57.4 letters (range 14 to 87 letters), had a mean CRT of 291.8 μm (range 214 to 432 μm) had received anti VEGF treatment for over 5 years (mean treatment duration in months 63.2 (range 36 to 93) with a mean of 39.4 injections (21 to 72). The mean monthly and total costs were 1308.9 CHF (range 515.5 to 2146.7 CHF) and 2280.7 CHF (range 661.5 to 3930.6 CHF) respectively. A summary of number of IVI and (unadjusted) monthly costs is shown in Table 2.

Discussion

Main findings

The results of this study show that aflibercept is equally expensive as ranibizumab in a pro re nata treatment scheme, while clinical outcomes between the two drugs are similar, when correcting for possible confounding due to differences in baseline characteristics. The higher total monthly cost in the aflibercept group may be due to the slightly higher number of patients with DME in this group.

Results in context of the existing literature

Both the efficacy [5–7] and cost-effectiveness [8, 9] of ranibizumab and aflibercept has been thoroughly studied. A paper by Johnston and co-workers assessed first-line anti-VEGF management patterns in AMD using claims data [10]. They found no differences between the two drugs for number of injections and healthcare costs. Very recently, two studies assessed the efficacy of ranibizumab and or aflibercept in the clinical routine [11, 12]. One study found a similar effect of aflibercept as reported in the pivotal clinical studies [11] and Rasmussen, via retrospective chart review, found a 15% reduction in treatment frequency among patients receiving aflibercept rather than ranibizumab [12].

The findings presented here mostly corroborate those of our previous study [1]. By including a larger number of patients receiving aflibercept de novo, the study also overcomes a relevant shortcoming our previous report. While the pervious study showed equivalence between the two drugs, this update showed a small, albeit statistically significant higher costs at a similar clinical outcome. Again,

Table 2 Shows the distribution of number of IVI, mean monthly ophthalmologic and total cost of the different treatment groups. Note that these are unadjusted values

Therapy	# Eyes (patients)	Mean # IVI (sd[a])	Ophthalmologic costs per months [CHF] (sd[a])	Total costs per months [CHF] (sd[a])
Only ranibizumab	182 (144)	4.3 (2.3)	1063.9 (549.3)	2060.5 (1274.4)
Only aflibercept	63 (52)	5.1 (2.5)	1238.8 (735.6)	2641.5 (1912.3)
Switching from ranibizumab to aflibercept prior study	160 (128)	5.9 (2.7)	1336.1 (742.2)	2486.8 (1702.0)
Switching from ranibizumab to aflibercept during study	45 (36)	6.9 (2.4)	1337.1 (443.1)	2408.5 (1133.6)
Miscellaneous[b]	38 (34)	6.6 (3.0)	1470.8 (770.5)	2404.5 (1141.9)

[a]sd = standard deviation
[b]including eyes with various treatment regimens. The largest group consisted of 13 eyes with a double switch from ranibizumab to aflibercept and back to ranibizumab prior to study entry

patients receiving aflibercept were younger and had a slightly better vision at study entry. Why selection occurs, remains unclear. The use of either ranibizumab or aflibercept was fully at the discretion of the treating physician. Also, total costs for patients with DME was not as high as in the previous study, which may be due to the mean shorter observation period of 11 vs. 33 months. Patients with a history of switching or switching during the observation period were clinically different to those staying on either ranibizumab or aflibercept. Also, treatment costs were higher in the switching groups.

Strength and limitations

By matching health claims with clinical data we were able to study cost consequences of treatment in a real life setting in a straightforward fashion. This dataset allows studying and contextualising the variability of costs as seen in the health claims with help of the clinical information that is available. The findings of this study are also useful to improve the understanding of healthcare delivery in the whole country and help improving the interpretation of health claim data of the health insurer. By identifying patients who had switched treatment prior the study entry or during the observation period, we were able to assess three different treatment groups: the non-switched ranibizumab and aflibercept groups and the (heterogeneous) group of treatment switchers. This excluded an important possible source of bias. However, this study also has its limitations. Data collected in the daily routine are inferior to those from clinical studies adhering to strict protocols. While missing data were uncommon, findings from repeated fundus fluorescein angiography examinations and also the rationale to switch treatment were unavailable, as they are not performed and recorded in a systematic fashion in clinical routine. Second, matching of the two datasets was problematic sometimes, because the entries were inconsistent. Although we carefully validated thousands of records by hand, we cannot fully exclude that the analysis file contained small errors. Nevertheless, we believe that this does not jeopardize our results. Although we included patients with DME and CRVO we were unable to perform meaningful statistical comparisons against AMD due to the limited number of participants in these two groups. By treating patients with a pro re nata scheme irrespective of drug they received, we may have equalized the number of intravitreal injections. Finally, as only one clinic was involved in this study, generalisations of the findings may be limited.

Implications for research

Health service research is urgently needed to understand and improve clinical care [13]. These studies allow validating the expectations that were met when approving a new drug based on the results of clinical studies. Previous research has clearly highlighted the gap between the trial world and clinical reality of treatment delivery after the approval [14]. Second, the collaboration between all involved stakeholders should be intensified to tackle the challenges of a healthcare system. Real-world studies like ours contribute to the transparency within the healthcare system which ultimately serves to the advantage of the patients.

Implications for practice

The clinical equality of the two treatment substances in AMD patients, supporting our previous results and also the findings of Johnston et al. [10] are the most interesting finding of this study The higher costs of aflibercept treatment, remains incompletely understood.

Conclusions

Both currently licensed anti-VEGF medications showed similar clinical outcomes, and were equally expensive. These findings contradict previous studies and also the findings of those trials that were used to negotiate reimbursement in Switzerland. By linking health care claims to clinical data, this study succeeded to examine and interpret routine clinical care.

Abbreviations

AMD: Age-related macular degeneration; Anti-VEGF: Anti-vascular endothelial growth factor; CHF: Swiss Francs; CRVO: Central vein occlusions; DME: Diabetic macular edema; IVI: Intravitreal Injection; OCT: Optical coherence tomography; PRN: Pro re nata

Acknowledgements

Not applicable

Funding

An unrestricted educational grant was awarded to Oliver Reich (OR), Roland Rapold (RR) and Eva Blozik (EB) by Novartis Pharma Schweiz AG, Switzerland. The funder had no role in study design; collection, analysis, and interpretation of data; writing of the paper; or in the decision to submit the paper for publication.

Authors' contributions

All authors were involved in the study design. MKS, LMB, MAT and OR conceived and designed the experiments. LMB analysed the data. LMB, LF and NSB drafted the manuscript. OR, RR, MKS, SL, MAT, EB and MK revised the manuscript. All authors participated in the interpretation of data, critically reviewed for important intellectual contents and gave the final approval of the version to be published.

Competing interests

Financial support for this study was provided by Novartis Pharma, Switzerland. The sponsor had no role in collection, analysis, and interpretation of data; writing of the paper; or in the decision to submit the paper for publication.

Lucas Bachmann (LB), Livia Faes and Nicolas Bodmer are employees of medignition Inc. EB, RR and OR are employees of the Helsana Health Insurance Company, and Maximilian Kuhn is an employee of CSS Group. These funders provided support in the form of salaries but did not have any additional role in the study design, data collection and analysis, decision to publish, or preparation of the manuscript.

Author details
¹University of Zurich, Zurich, Switzerland. ²Eye Clinic, Cantonal Hospital of Lucerne, Lucerne, Switzerland. ³Department of Health Sciences, Helsana Group, Zurich, Switzerland. ⁴Medignition Inc. Research Consultants, Verena Conzett-Strasse 9, P.O. 9628, 8036 Zurich, CH, Switzerland. ⁵CSS Group, Luzern, Switzerland.

References
1. Schmid MK, Reich O, Faes L, Boehni SC, Bittner M, Howell JP, Thiel MA, Signorell A, Bachmann LM. Comparison of outcomes and costs of Ranibizumab and Aflibercept treatment in real-life. PLoS One. 2015;10(8):e0135050.
2. Reich O, Bachmann LM, Faes L, Bohni SC, Bittner M, Howell JP, Thiel MA, Rapold R, Schmid MK. Anti-VEGF treatment patterns and associated health care costs in Switzerland: findings using real-world claims data. Risk Manag Healthc Policy. 2015;8:55–62.
3. General Assembly of the World Medical A. World medical association declaration of Helsinki: ethical principles for medical research involving human subjects. J Am Coll Dent. 2014;81(3):14–8.
4. Holz FG, Amoaku W, Donate J, Guymer RH, Kellner U, Schlingemann RO, Weichselberger A, Staurenghi G. Safety and efficacy of a flexible dosing regimen of ranibizumab in neovascular age-related macular degeneration: the SUSTAIN study. Ophthalmology. 2011;118(4):663–71.
5. Mitchell P. A systematic review of the efficacy and safety outcomes of anti-VEGF agents used for treating neovascular age-related macular degeneration: comparison of ranibizumab and bevacizumab. Curr Med Res Opin. 27(7):1465–75.
6. Schmid MK, Bachmann LM, Fas L, Kessels AG, Job OM, Thiel MA. Efficacy and adverse events of aflibercept, ranibizumab and bevacizumab in age-related macular degeneration: a trade-off analysis. Br J Ophthalmol.
7. Vedula SS, Krzystolik MG. Antiangiogenic therapy with anti-vascular endothelial growth factor modalities for neovascular age-related macular degeneration. Cochrane Database Syst Rev. 2008;2:CD005139.
8. Raftery J, Clegg A, Jones J, Tan SC, Lotery A. Ranibizumab (Lucentis) versus bevacizumab (Avastin): modelling cost effectiveness. Br J Ophthalmol. 2007; 91(9):1244–6.
9. Aflibercept solution for injection for treating wet age-related macular degeneration. NICE technology appraisal guidance 294, guidanceniceorguk/ta294 2013, ISBN 978-1-4731-0234-7.
10. Johnston SS, Wilson K, Huang A, Smith D, Varker H, Turpcu A. Retrospective analysis of first-line anti-vascular endothelial growth factor treatment patterns in wet age-related macular degeneration. Adv Ther. 30(12):1111–27.
11. Duval MV, Rougier MB, Delyfer MN, Combillet F, Korobelnik JF. Real life visual and anatomic outcomes of aflibercept treatment for treatment-naive patients with exudative age-related macular degeneration. J Fr Ophtalmol. 2017;40(4):270–8.
12. Rasmussen A, Sander B, Larsen M, Brandi S, Fuchs J, Hansen LH, Lund-Andersen H. Neovascular age-related macular degeneration treated with ranibizumab or aflibercept in the same large clinical setting: visual outcome and number of injections. Acta Ophthalmol. 2017;95(2):128–32.
13. Committee on Quality of Health Care in America. Crossing the quality chasm: a new health system for the 21st century Institute of Medicine. 2001.
14. Black N. Why we need observational studies to evaluate the effectiveness of health care. BMJ. 1996;312(7040):1215–8.

Permissions

The contributors of this book come from diverse backgrounds, making this book a truly international effort. This book will bring forth new frontiers with its revolutionizing research information and detailed analysis of the nascent developments around the world.

We would like to thank all the contributing authors for lending their expertise to make the book truly unique. They have played a crucial role in the development of this book. Without their invaluable contributions this book wouldn't have been possible. They have made vital efforts to compile up to date information on the varied aspects of this subject to make this book a valuable addition to the collection of many professionals and students.

This book was conceptualized with the vision of imparting up-to-date information and advanced data in this field. To ensure the same, a matchless editorial board was set up. Every individual on the board went through rigorous rounds of assessment to prove their worth. After which they invested a large part of their time researching and compiling the most relevant data for our readers.

The editorial board has been involved in producing this book since its inception. They have spent rigorous hours researching and exploring the diverse topics which have resulted in the successful publishing of this book. They have passed on their knowledge of decades through this book. To expedite this challenging task, the publisher supported the team at every step. A small team of assistant editors was also appointed to further simplify the editing procedure and attain best results for the readers.

Apart from the editorial board, the designing team has also invested a significant amount of their time in understanding the subject and creating the most relevant covers. They scrutinized every image to scout for the most suitable representation of the subject and create an appropriate cover for the book.

The publishing team has been an ardent support to the editorial, designing and production team. Their endless efforts to recruit the best for this project, has resulted in the accomplishment of this book. They are a veteran in the field of academics and their pool of knowledge is as vast as their experience in printing. Their expertise and guidance has proved useful at every step. Their uncompromising quality standards have made this book an exceptional effort. Their encouragement from time to time has been an inspiration for everyone.

The publisher and the editorial board hope that this book will prove to be a valuable piece of knowledge for researchers, students, practitioners and scholars across the globe.

List of Contributors

Yingyan Ma, Senlin Lin, Jianfeng Zhu, Xun Xu, Lina Lu, Xiangui He and Haidong Zou
Department of Preventative Ophthalmology, Shanghai Eye Disease Prevention and Treatment Center, Shanghai Eye Hospital, No. 380 Kangding Road, Shanghai, China

Department of Ophthalmology, Shanghai General Hospital, Shanghai Jiao Tong University, No.100, Haining Road, Shanghai, China

Senlin Lin and Zhiyuan Hou
School of Public Health, National Key Laboratory of Health Technology Assessment (National Health and Family Planning Commission), Fudan University, Shanghai, China

Rong Zhao
Shanghai Shen Kang Hospital Development Center, No.2 Kangding Road, Shanghai, China

Huijuan Zhao and Qiangqiang Li
Baoshan Center for Disease Prevention and Control, No. 158 Yueming Road, Shanghai, China

Nasser J. Gili, Sven Crafoord and Anders Bäckman
Department of Ophthalmology, Örebro University Hospital, SE-701 85 Örebro, Sweden

Torbjörn Noren and Anders Bäckman
Faculty of Medicine and Health, Örebro University, Örebro, Sweden

Torbjörn Noren and Eva Törnquist
Department of Laboratory Medicine, Örebro University Hospital, Örebro, Sweden

Anders Bäckman
Department of Clinical Research Laboratory, Örebro University Hospital, Örebro, Sweden

Nathalie J. S. Patty, Marc Koopmanschap and Kim Holtzer-Goor
Erasmus School of Health Policy & Management, Erasmus University, 3000, DR, Rotterdam, The Netherlands

Yuan He, Shi-Ming Li, Meng-Tian Kang, Shi-Fei Wei, An-Ran Ran and Ningli Wang
Beijing Tongren Eye Center, Beijing Tongren Hospital, Beijing Ophthalmology & Visual Science Key Lab, Beijing Institute of Ophthalmology, Capital Medical University, Beijing, China

Luo-Ru Liu and He Li
Anyang Eye Hospital, Anyang, Henan, China

Jing Wang, Jiangyue Zhao, Jun Xu and Jinsong Zhang
Department of Ophthalmology, the Fourth Affiliated Hospital of China Medical University, Eye Hospital of China Medical University, The Key Lenticular Laboratory of Liaoning Province, Shenyang 110005, China

Ziqian Zhu, Hongmin Zhang, Juan Yue, Susu Liu and Liya Wang
People's Hospital of Zhengzhou University and Henan Provincial People's Hospital, Henan Eye Institute, Henan Eye Hospital, Zhengzhou 450003, China

Zhijie Li
Department of Pediatrics, Baylor College of Medicine, Houston, TX, USA

Zelalem Tilahun and Teferi Gedif Fenta
Social and Adminstrative Pharmacy Working Group, Departement of Pharmaceutics and Social Pharmacy, College of Health Sciences, Addis Ababa University, Addis Ababa, Ethiopia

Shiva Pirhadi
Department of Biomedical Engineering, Tehran Science and Research Branch, Islamic Azad University, Tehran, Iran

Neda Mohammadi
Department of Epidemiology and Biostatistics, School of Public Health, Tehran University of Medical Sciences, Tehran, Iran

Seyed Aliasghar Mosavi and Hossein Aghamollaei
Vision Health Research Center, Semnan University of Medical Sciences, Semnan, Iran

Hashem Daryabari and Khosrow Jadidi
Department of Ophthalmology, Baqiyatallah
University of Medical Sciences, Tehran, Iran

**Eugene Appenteng Osae, Reynolds Kwame
Ablorddepey and David Ben Kumah**
Department of Optometry and Visual Science,
Kwame Nkrumah University of Science and
Technology, PMB, Kumasi, Ghana

**Eugene Appenteng Osae, Jens Horstmann and
Philipp Steven**
Department of Ophthalmology, Faculty of Medicine,
University of Cologne, Cologne, Germany

Jens Horstmann and Philipp Steven
Cellular Stress Response in Aging – associated
Diseases (CECAD), University of Cologne, Cologne,
Germany

Yousef Shanti
Department of Ophthalmology, An-Najah National
University Hospital, 44839 Nablus, Palestine, Palestine

**Yousef Shanti, Ahlam Abu-Samra, Areen Abu-
Qamar, Reem Barakat and Reham Shehada**
Department of Medicine, College of Medicine and
Health Sciences, An-Najah National University,
44839 Nablus, Palestine, Palestine

Ithar Beshtawi
Department of Optometry, College of Medicine and
Health Sciences, An-Najah National University,
44839 Nablus, Palestine, Palestine

Sáed H. Zyoud
Department of Clinical and Community Pharmacy,
College of Medicine and Health Sciences, An-
Najah National University, 44839 Nablus, Palestine,
Palestine

**William Fusi-Rubiano, Chandoshi Mukherjee,
Mark Lane, Marie D. Tsaloumas, Nicholas Glover,
Andrej Kidess, Alastair K. Denniston, Helen E.
Palmer, Avinash Manna and Rupal Morjaria**
Ophthalmology Department, Queen Elizabeth
Hospital Birmingham, University Hospitals
Birmingham NHSFT, Mindelsohn Way, Birmingham
B15 2TH, United Kingdom

**William Fusi-Rubiano, Chandoshi Mukherjee,
Mark Lane and Rupal Morjaria**
Sandwell & West Birmingham NHS Trust, Dudley
Road, Birmingham B18 7QH, United Kingdom

Alastair K. Denniston
Academic Unit of Ophthalmology, Institute of
Inflammation & Ageing, University of Birmin-
gham, Edgbaston, Birmingham B15 2TT, United
Kingdom

**Shintaro Shirahama, Toshikatsu Kaburaki, Hisae
Nakahara, Rie Tanaka and Makoto Aihara**
Department of Ophthalmology, University of
Tokyo Graduate School of Medicine, 7-3-1 Hongo,
Bunkyo-ku, Tokyo 113-8655, Japan

Mitsuko Takamoto
Department of Ophthalmology, Saitama Red Cross
Hospital, 1-5 Shintoshin, Chuo-ku, Saitama-shi,
Saitama 330-8553, Japan

Yujiro Fujino
Department of Ophthalmology, Tokyo Shinjuku
Medical Center, 5-1 Tsukudo-cho, Shinjuku-ku,
Tokyo 162-8543, Japan

Hidetoshi Kawashima
Department of Ophthalmology, Jichi Medical
University, 3311-1 Yakushiji, Shimotsuke-City,
Tochigi, Japan

**Song Wang, Chenjun Guo, Xiaona Ning and
Hong Yan**
Department of Ophthalmology, Tangdu Hospital,
Fourth Military Medical University, 1 Xinsi Road,
Xi'an, Shaanxi 710038, People's Republic of China

Mengsi Yu
Department of Dermatology, Xijing Hospital, Fourth
Military Medical University, 169 West Changle
Road, Xi'an, Shaanxi 710032, People's Republic of
China

Bo Yan, Jing Zhao and Angang Yang
The State Key Laboratory of Cancer Biology,
Department of Biochemistry and Molecular
Biology, Fourth Military Medical University, 169
West Changle Road, Xi'an, Shaanxi 710032, People's
Republic of China

Hong Yan
Chongqing Key Laboratory of Ophthalmology
and Chongqing Eye Institute, The First Affiliated
Hospital of Chongqing Medical University, 1 Youyi
Road, Chongqing 400016, People's Republic of
China

Milad Azami
Student Research Committee, Ilam University of Medical Sciences, Ilam, Iran

Zahra Jaafari and Shoboo Rahmati
Student Research Committee, Ilam University of Medical Sciences, Ilam, Iran

Afsar Dastjani Farahani
Iranian National ROP Committee, Tehran, Iran

Gholamreza Badfar
Department of Pediatrics, Behbahan Faculty of Medical Sciences, Behbahan, Iran

Min Chen, Lina Zhang, Wei Wang, Xinyi Chen, Xiaoning Yu and Kaijun Wang
Eye Center, the 2nd Affiliated Hospital, Medical College of Zhejiang University, Hangzhou, China

Min Chen, Wei Wang, Xinyi Chen and Xiaoning Yu
Zhejiang Provincial Key Lab of Ophthalmology, Hangzhou, China

Aimin Wu
Department of Ophthalmology, Fenghua People's Hospital, Fenghua, Zhejiang, China

Lina Zhang
Department of Ophthalmology, Lishui People's Hospital, Lishui, Zhejiang, China

Yueqin Chen, Qian Cao, Chunyan Xue and Zhenping Huang
Department of Ophthalmology, Jinling Hospital, School of Medicine, Nanjing University, 305 East Zhongshan Road, Nanjing, People's Republic of China

Mohammad T. Akkawi
Department of Special Surgeries, Faculty of Medicine and Health Sciences, An-Najah National University Hospital, An-Najah National University, Nablus, Palestine

Jamal A. S. Qaddumi, Hala R. M. Issa and Liana J. K. Yaseen
An-Najah National University, Nablus, Palestine

Debora Goetz Goldberg and Riddhi Shah
Department of Health Administration and Policy, George Mason University Peterson Family Health Sciences Hall, 4400 University Drive, Virginia 22030, USA

Michael H. Goldberg, Jane N. Meagher and Haresh Ailani
Eye Consultants of Northern Virginia, 8134 Old Keene Mill Rd., Ste. 300, Springfield, VA 22152, USA

Huina Zhang, Tiepei Zhu and Juan Ye
Department of Ophthalmology, the Second Affiliated Hospital, Zhejiang University School of Medicine, Hangzhou, Zhejiang, China

Hongjie Zhou
Hangzhou Hospital for the Prevention and Treatment of Occupational Diseases, Hangzhou, Zhejiang, China

Yongseok Mun and Joo Youn Oh
Department of Ophthalmology, Seoul National University Hospital, 101, Daehak-ro, Jongno-gu, Seoul 03080, South Korea

Ji-Won Kwon
Department of ophthalmology, Hanyang University College of Medicine Myongji Hospital, 14 Bungil 55, Hwasu-Ro, Deokyang-Gu, Goyang-si, Gyeonggi-do 14075, South Korea

Joo Youn Oh
Laboratory of Ocular Regenerative Medicine and Immunology, Biomedical Research Institute, Seoul National University Hospital, 101 Daehak-ro, Jongno-gu, Seoul 03080, South Korea

Zhen Li, Zhike Xu, Yaqin Wang, Qiang Liu and Bin Chen
Department of Ophthalmology, The People's Hospital of Leshan, 635 Wanghaoer Street, Leshan, Sichuan Province 614000, People's Republic of China

Syunsuke Araki, Atsushi Miki, Katsutoshi Goto, Tsutomu Yamashita, Go Takizawa, Kazuko Haruishi, Tsuyoshi Yoneda, Yoshiaki Ieki and Junichi Kiryu
Department of Ophthalmology, Kawasaki Medical School, 577 Matsushima, Kurashiki, Okayama 701-0192, Japan

Atsushi Miki, Tsutomu Yamashita and Tsuyoshi Yoneda
Department of Sensory Science, Faculty of Health Science and Technology, Kawasaki University of Medical Welfare, 288 Matsushima, Kurashiki, Okayama 701-0193, Japan

Goro Maehara
Department of Human Sciences, Kanagawa University,
3-27-1 Rokkakubashi, Yokohama, Kanagawa 221-
8686, Japan

Kiyoshi Yaoeda
Yaoeda Eye Clinic, 2-1649-1 Naga-Chou, Nagaoka,
Niigata 940-0053, Japan

**Hong-Ying Jin, Ting Wan, Xiao-Ning Yu, Fang
Wu and Ke Yao**
Eye Center, 2nd Affiliated Hospital, School of
Medicine, Zhejiang University, Hangzhou 310009,
China

Lauren R. Hepworth and Fiona J. Rowe
Department of Health Services Research, University
of Liverpool, Waterhouse Building, Block B, First
Floor1-5 Brownlow Street, Liverpool L69 3GL, UK

**Martin K. Schmid, Michael A. Thiel and Lucas
M. Bachmann**
University of Zurich, Zurich, Switzerland

**Martin K. Schmid, Livia Faes, Silvan Locher and
Michael A. Thiel**
Eye Clinic, Cantonal Hospital of Lucerne, Lucerne,
Switzerland

Roland Rapold, Oliver Reich and Eva Blozik
Department of Health Sciences, Helsana Group,
Zurich, Switzerland

Nicolas S. Bodmer and Lucas M. Bachmann
Medignition Inc. Research Consultants, Verena
Conzett-Strasse 9, 8036 Zurich, CH, Switzerland

Maximilian Kuhn
CSS Group, Luzern, Switzerland

Index

Nuclear Cataract, 102, 107-111
Nuclear Opacity, 102-103, 106-107

O
Ocular Surface, 11-13, 73-80, 160, 164, 166-167, 183, 189
Ophthalmic Viscosurgical Device, 137-138, 140-143
Ophthalmology, 1, 8-11, 14-15, 26, 36-39, 45, 54, 65, 71-73, 79-82, 84-87, 94, 100, 102, 111, 122, 125, 127-128, 135, 137-138, 142-143, 148, 154, 161-163, 170, 177, 181, 183, 189, 193, 197, 205
Optic Neuropathy, 191-195, 197-199
Optical Coherence Tomography, 39, 45, 66, 71-72, 87-88, 151, 154, 176-178, 180-181, 201, 204
Oxidative Stress, 102-106, 108-110, 124

P
Pediatricians, 144-148
Pentacam, 72, 81-82, 85, 155-159, 161, 170, 183, 187
Perimetry, 191-193, 195-199
Phakic Intraocular Lens, 169, 175
Pocketmaker Microkeratome, 65-66, 69
Posterior Cornea, 170, 182, 184, 186-187, 189
Preeclampsia, 114, 122, 124
Prematurity, 113-114, 117-118, 120-121 123-126, 144-148
Primary Iris, 169-175
Progression, 1-9, 48, 81, 84-85, 99, 102, 110-111, 124, 157, 159-161, 191, 198

R
Ranibizumab, 88-89, 91, 93, 200-205
Retinal Arteriolar Diameter, 26, 31-32
Retinal Venular Diameter, 26, 28-29, 31, 33, 36
Retinopathy, 27, 36-37, 39, 87-88, 93, 96-98, 100-101, 113-114, 117-118, 120-121, 123-126, 138, 144-148

S
Small-gauge Vitrectomy, 10-11, 14
Spherical Equivalent Refraction, 1, 3, 5-6, 8, 28-29, 128, 135
Stroke, 27, 31, 36-37, 48-49, 54, 89, 191-194, 196-199

T
Tear Film, 73-74, 76-80, 159, 163-168, 183, 188-189
Tear Syndrome, 74
Toric Intraocular Lens, 39, 45, 137, 143
Trachoma Elimination, 56, 58, 63, 80

U
Ultrasound Biomicroscope, 169
Uveitis, 39, 88, 94-101

V
Visually Impaired, 16-17, 19, 22, 24-25
Vitrectomy, 10-12, 14-15, 89, 93, 95, 99, 108, 111, 143